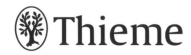

Orthopedic Manual Therapy

Assessment and Management

Jochen Schomacher, PhD, PT-OMT, DPT, MCMK

Physical Therapist
Küsnacht, Switzerland

534 illustrations

Thieme
Stuttgart • New York • Delhi • Rio

Library of Congress Cataloging-in-Publication Data is available from the publisher.

This book is an authorized translation of the 5th German edition published and copyrighted 2011 by Georg Thieme Verlag, Stuttgart. Title of the German edition: Manuelle Therapie. Bewegen und Spüren lernen

Translator: Stephanie Kramer, Berlin, Germany

Illustrators: Friedrich Hartmann, Nagold, Germany; Helmut Holtermann, Dannenberg, Germany

1st Italian edition 2001

© 2014 Georg Thieme Verlag KG
Thieme Publishers Stuttgart
Rüdigerstrasse 14, 70469 Stuttgart, Germany,
+49 [0]711 8931 421
customerservice@thieme.de

Thieme Publishers New York
333 Seventh Avenue, New York, NY 10001, USA,
1-800-782-3488
customerservice@thieme.com

Thieme Publishers Delhi
A-12, second floor, Sector-2, NOIDA-201301, Uttar Pradesh, India, +91 120 45 566 00
customerservice@thieme.in

Thieme Publishers Rio
Thieme Publicações Ltda.
Argentina Building, 16th floor, Ala A, 228 Praia do Botafogo, Rio de Janeiro 22250-040 Brazil, +55 21 3736-3631

Cover design: Thieme Publishing Group
Typesetting by STM Media, Köthen (Anhalt), Germany
Printed in China by Everbest Printing Co. Ltd.

ISBN 978-3-13-171451-0

Also available as an e-book:
eISBN 978-3-13-171461-9

Foreword by Ola Grimsby

Scientific evidence has increased tremendously in physical therapy during the last two decades, so far however without resulting in a single, evidence-based approach for patients with musculoskeletal dysfunction. Consequently clinicians must complement their evidence-based knowledge with clinical expertise—that is, via thorough individual examination of each patient—in order to achieve competent clinical decision-making. This is the focus presented in this book, which offers a systematic approach based on manual examination and treatment of the locomotor system. The thoroughness and insight into the biomechanics of extremity and spinal joints makes a valuable contribution to the reference works of orthopedic manual therapy worldwide. With well-structured and logical sequences of assessments and interventions, clear illustrations, and graphics this book assists the clinical special-

ist in teaching clinical competence; it also constitutes a useful resource for any student or therapist interested in expanding their physical/manual therapy skills. The emphasis on traction as an essential, low-risk technique for pain and joint stiffness is justified for one simple reason: it works and has survived for thousands of years.

Dr. Jochen Schomacher has received an extensive education from internationally recognized programs. This updated English translation of the fifth German language edition of *Orthopedic Manual Therapy* is a valuable asset to any medical library and is warmly recommended to colleagues interested in orthopedic manual therapy as a means to optimal treatment outcome for patients with musculoskeletal complaints.

Ola Grimsby, PT, DMT, FAAOMPT

Foreword by Freddy Kaltenborn

Physical therapy with postgraduate training in Manual Therapy and Orthopedic Manual Therapy (OMT) has developed steadily over the past 50 years into an independent discipline around the world.

OMT is embedded in a biopsychosocial model of disease and gives physiotherapists the skills they need to examine and treat postural and movement dysfunction. This is important in all areas of the physical therapy profession and often helps to avoid surgery. Thus physical therapists around the world view Manual Therapy as an important foundation for examining and treating the locomotor system. This is reflected by the numerous international journals and professional associations for Manual Therapy.

The road to such developments is paved by a solid education, which provides the necessary current medical knowledge. Yet the most important thing for the physical therapist is—and will continue to be—the practical skills needed to identify, evaluate, and positively influence the patient's dysfunction.

For the past 14 years, this book has opened the door to this area for many physical therapists and has enabled them to use movement and feeling to examine and treat dysfunction of the locomotor system. The first English edition contains important new information and also presents tried and tested material in an even better way. Thus it remains an excellent companion for physical therapists on the road to Manual Therapy and Orthopedic Manual Therapy.

I wish this book continued success, and I also hope that readers make the effort to carefully study the information contained in it. More important, they should apply what they learn to physical therapy practice in order to gain an understanding of how vital the skills of moving and feeling are in the physical therapy profession.

Professor Freddy Kaltenborn, ATC, PT, OMT

Preface

In this latest and first English edition of the book, the chapters continue to emphasize the guiding and sensing of movements, as well as the documentation of logical processes, which is the basis for well-thought-out treatment in manual therapy. Specific technical aspects are illustrated with full color images.

This edition has been updated with information detailing thought and decision-making processes (clinical reasoning) encompassing aspects drawn from pain physiology, biomechanics, neurodynamics, and the biopsychosocial model of disease, which together form the foundation for manual therapy. Actual practice is now more clearly structured and described in greater detail using key questions and classification systems pertaining to the physical examination of the patient as well as six categories of treatment. Numerous bibliographic references also enable the interested reader to broaden his or her background knowledge.

The English edition contains links to the Thieme Media-Center, where the reader can download the document templates in chapter 19 and find videos accompanying the treatments presented in the book. The model shown in the videos is not a physical therapist, nor were the filmed sequences practised in advance. These are intended to represent an actual examination situation with a real patient.

Thus certain maneuvers which are shown there do not necessarily work perfectly the first time around.

I am pleased to see that the information contained in this book down the years has proved its usefulness in teaching, in continuing education courses, and in the treatment of patients. Since the first edition of this book was published, my own experiences have continually convinced me of the value of the procedures described here. When teachers and students work closely together, a high level of agreement on the results of physical examination is quickly achievable, especially for rotational movement tests. The treatments derived from the summary (physical therapy diagnosis) work surprisingly well with the techniques described here if they are performed at optimal dosages and for suitable indications. Often, the use of complicated techniques is not actually necessary. More information on the necessary supplementary measures such as active exercises and self-treatments is available from continuing education programs. A description of these here, however, would be beyond the scope of the book.

I hope that the English edition will help many colleagues on the road toward responsible and successful physical therapy practice. Comments and constructive criticism are welcome.

Jochen Schomacher

Contents

Practice

Appendix

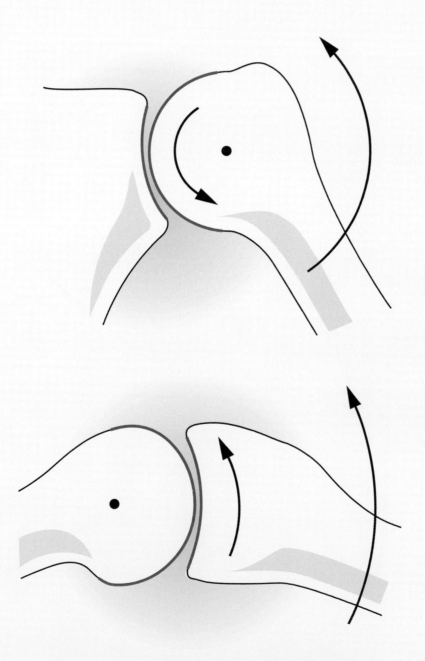

1 The History and Definition of Orthopedic Manual Therapy

*"All thinking is repetition,
but with increasing consolidation."*
(Egon Friedell)

1.1 What Is Manual Therapy?

The term orthopedic manual therapy (OMT) refers to treatment or healing (from the Greek word for "therapy") using the hands (from the Latin word "manus"), which allows for a range of interpretations. In a more literal sense, the term *manual* underscores the importance of the *hands* as tools in the concept of OMT. When Freddy Kaltenborn introduced the term in the 1950s, he was emphasizing the complementary role that manual therapy brought to physical therapy (PT), which at that time mainly consisted of giving instructions for performing certain exercises and behavioral changes. This was particularly true in Germany where massage, as a classic manual treatment, was largely the domain of the masseur profession that was steeped in tradition. Yet even now, in an age of high-tech medicine and unwavering belief in scientific data, the emphasis on the hands has not lost any of its significance.

Treatment with the hands includes the manual therapy *examination* as a necessary precondition of any therapeutic measure. Although the results of the manual assessment of core criteria are not always scientifically quantifiable in precise terms, they can often lead to specific *manual therapy*, which offers the patient more than could mere movements.

Still, doctors and physical therapists often use their hands as a part of patient care without it being manual therapy. What, then, is behind the term manual therapy? In order to answer this question, we must first take a brief look at history to see how the current branch of manual therapy namely OMT arose from the various manual forms of therapy.

1.2 History

The **history of medicine** shows that the separation of joint partners was long referred to as *traction* and is found in many pre-Christian medical texts. Traction is one of the main features of OMT. In what is probably the oldest surviving image of traction therapy, from India, Lord Krishna is shown stretching the deformed back of the faithful Kubja by standing on her feet and pulling her up by her chin (ca. 3500–1800 BC) (Kumar 1996). Hippocrates (ca. 460–377 BC) too emphasized the importance of spinal treatments for various problems. He used axial traction, for instance, by binding patients by their legs upside-down to a ladder, which he then carefully dropped to the ground from a low height, presumably causing a sudden traction force. The Greek notion of medicine was later consolidated by Claudius Galen (ca. 129–199 AD) in Rome. Galen's views continued to influence medicine in Europe for more than 1,000 years. There are numerous depictions, dating back to Galen, of treating spinal deformities using the hands and feet along with simultaneous axial traction. Ibn Sina (980–1037 AD, whose name was Latinized as Avicenna) brought the Greek view of medicine to the Orient and described various manual corrective techniques. Many of these were performed on the spine by using traction while assistants applied traction caudally and cranially to the treated region. Many of these treatment forms, which were largely based on Hippocrates and later revised by his followers, have been handed down to us through works from the Middle Ages (**Figs. 1.1** and **1.2**). During the Renaissance, physicians in Europe continued to be concerned with the treatment of joint problems, especially those affecting the spine. The use of traction is an often-mentioned method.

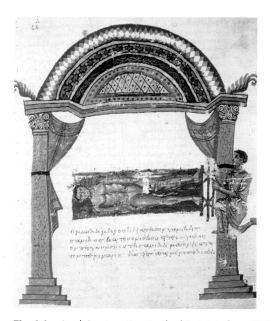

Fig. 1.1 Applying traction to the hip joint, from "Hippocratis Chirurgica" (Florence, The Biblioteca Medicea Laurenziana, ms. Plut. 74,7. With kind permission of the Ministry for Goods and Cultural Activities. Any further reproduction by any means is prohibited).

Since the Black Death in 1348, to which nearly two-thirds of the European population succumbed, medical doctors avoided direct contact with patients for fear of infection (Greenman 1998). Many manual treatment techniques survived among folk medicine practitioners, like bonesetters. In the late 19th century, two highly influential schools of manual therapy arose in America. One was osteopathy, which was established in 1874 by the physician Andrew Taylor Still (1828–1917). Osteopathy primarily views dysfunction as a result of a malfunction in a part of the body ("osteopathic lesion") which may be treated with soft-tissue techniques, mobilization, and manipulation. The other was chiropractic, which was founded in 1895 by Daniel David Palmer (1845–1913). With the aid of radiographic diagnosis, joint malalignment (especially subluxation or "displacement") is viewed as a common cause of pain symptoms and is corrected often using manipulations. Both Still and Palmer originally treated not only musculoskeletal complaints with manipulation, but numerous diseases as well.

From historical sources of academic medicine, folk medicine as well as osteopathic medicine and chiropractic and—with the help of some uncommonly talented laypersons—manual therapy by physicians developed in Europe during the 20th century; today it is known as manual medicine (Cramer et al 1990). Recent research in history, however, has shown that in 19th-century Europe, physical therapy essentially fashioned manual treatment in Manual Medicine and Orthopedic Medicine (Ottosson 2010 a and b). It also suggests

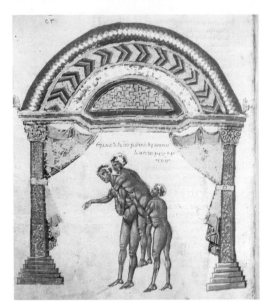

Fig. 1.2 Applying traction to the back after placing it in a flexed position, from "Hippocratis Chirurgica" (Florence, The Biblioteca Medicea Laurenziana, ms. Plut. 74,7. With kind permission of the Ministry for Goods and Cultural Activities. Any further reproduction by any means is prohibited).

a possible European influence with regard to the North American traditions of manual therapy (Ottosson 2011).

1.3   The History of Physiotherapeutic Manual Therapy

In Europe the physical therapy profession arose in 1813 with the foundation of the Royal Central Institute of Gymnastics (RCIG) in Stockholm (Sweden) by Pehr Henrik Ling (1776–1839). His followers—Jonas Henrik Kellgren (1837–1916) and his son-in-law Dr. Edgar Ferdinand Cyriax (1874–1955), father of Dr. James Cyriax (1904–1985), amongst others—disseminated the treatment methods developed at the RCIG all over Europe, where also medical doctors learned and practised them (Ottosson 2010). Only in a round-about way—mainly via Dr. James Mennell and Dr. James Cyriax with his Orthopedic Medicine—did many of these techniques finally find their way back into physical therapy (Ottosson 2011).

From 1916 to 1954, the London physician **James Mennell** instructed physical therapists in the "Art and Science of Joint Manipulation" (Mennell 1945, 1949, 1952). His successor was **James Cyriax** (Cyriax 1971, 1982) who continued this tradition (Lamb et al 2003). As teachers, both these physicians had a significant influence on Kaltenborn, who worked together with Cyriax for several decades.

Around 1950, two physical therapists each began to develop a separate concept of OMT that emphasized the use of manual interventions in physical therapy, which at that time largely consisted of active exercises. They were **Geoffrey Maitland** and **Freddy Kaltenborn**.

Maitland trained under Cyriax and others in Europe during his travels around the world, which largely shaped his development. Interested readers are referred to the literature for more information about his remarkable journey through life (e.g., Bucher-Dollenz and Wiesner 2008). As an illustrative historical example, the following presents a summary of how Kaltenborn developed his approach to manual therapy on which the techniques presented in this book are based.

During his education as a sports/gymnastics teacher, Kaltenborn discovered his desire to help the sick, which later led him to continue his studies in physical therapy in Norway. An important experience in his development was related to the test of forearm pronation/supination. This had been taught to him using a handshake-greeting grip. Yet Kaltenborn questioned whether the limited movement came from the forearm joints (and, if so, which ones?) or from the wrist. This gave him the idea to perform the most specific test possible and to treat movements of a single joint or vertebral segment.

During the 1950s and 1960s, immobilization was a widely used form of orthopedic treatment, much as it is today (Ushida and Willis 2001). The two major pathological joint changes that arise from immobilization are joint capsule stiffness and cartilage degeneration (Trudel et al 2001). These used to be more common, given the more widespread use of cast immobilization at that time compared with osteosynthesis procedures which are more common today and which enable early functional treatment. At the time, the prevailing mobilization technique consisted of exerting extra pressure in the direction of the limitation at the end of the movement. Kaltenborn wondered why in some patients this did not function well or was even painful. If, instead of using classic rotatory mobilization, he used gliding mobilizations and (especially) traction mobilizations, the pain disappeared and the range of motion increased more rapidly (Kaltenborn 2002). It was above all his teacher, Mennell, who had pointed out such traction and gliding techniques to him.

Kaltenborn found the explanation he was looking for in arthrokinematics, or the study of how joint surfaces move with respect to each other (Mac Conaill and Basmajian 1977; Williams et al 1989). In the view of arthrokinematics, in a dysfunctional joint there is insufficient gliding of articular surfaces along with excessive rolling, leading to impingement on one side of the joint and gaping on the other. Signs of presumed cartilage damage due to impinging joint surfaces are visible, for instance, in impingement syndrome of the ankle joint (Schomacher 2010).

Together with a group of his colleagues, Kaltenborn continued to develop his techniques of mobilization and manipulation in Norway. In London, he trained under Cyriax, whose clinical examinations greatly impressed him. There Kaltenborn also visited lectures by Alan Stoddard on osteopathic treatment of the locomotor system. In Germany he became a member of the physician's society of manual medicine (known then as the German Research Foundation for Arthrology and Chirotherapy [Forschungsgemeinschaft für Arthrologie und Chirotherapie, FAC], now the German Society of Manual Medicine [Deutsche Gesellschaft für Manuelle Medizin, DGMM]). There he taught physicians from 1958 to 1982 (Cramer et al 1990; Kaltenborn 2005).

In the 1950s and 1960s Kaltenborn selected from these areas the procedures that he felt were most suitable for physical therapy. Thus he created MT ad modum Kaltenborn, which became a core element of the Nordic system, which he and his colleagues developed, starting in 1962. Oddvar Holten, a member of this group, further developed the training into Medical Exercise Therapy (MET) which he integrated into the Nordic system. It includes not only actual "strengthening" of the muscles, but the entire locomotor system along with the cardiovascular and respiratory systems. A further focus is on exercises that the patients may perform on their own for joint mobilization, muscle relaxation and stretching, and for stabilization and movement control of the joints. Individual practice is vital to the concept which Kaltenborn expanded with his colleague Evjenth in 1973 into the OMT Kaltenborn–Evjenth concept, which he presented in 1974 at a congress of the World Confederation for Physical Therapy (WCPT) with a video of self-mobilization exercises. From 1968 onward, Kaltenborn worked closely together with his colleague **Olaf Evjenth**. Kaltenborn was strongly interested in joint mechanics and straight-lined translatoric motion. This was at the heart of "manual therapy according to Kaltenborn." The collaboration with Evjenth resulted in additional emphasis on the muscles in regard to stretching and training and specific symptom localization, especially by using tests for relief of symptoms. Kaltenborn and Evjenth also integrated various developments from medicine and physical therapy, such as the examination and treatment of the neural system, into their concept, which is geared toward the evidence-based medicine/practice (EBM/EBP) and undergoes continuous development.

Cyriax (1971) recommended following Kaltenborn's concept in all physical therapy schools worldwide as an example of a comprehensive approach. In 1973 the first exams in Orthopedic Manual Therapy (OMT) were held. The doctors James Cyriax, Alan Stoddard, Harald Brodin, and Walter Hinsen examined Kaltenborn, Evjenth and several colleagues on Gran Canaria. Successful completion of the exam was considered the mark of expert knowledge and proficiency in OMT. Together with the physicians Cyriax, Stoddard, and Hinsen, in 1973 Kaltenborn and Evjenth founded an association for the further development and spread of OMT (Kaltenborn 2005).

The influence of Kaltenborn was far-reaching, and in many countries OMT would not have become such a well-established part of physical therapy without his efforts (Hüter-Becker 1998). This is certainly true for Germany, where in 1981 he initiated the founding of the "working group on manual therapy," which is part of the Central Association of Physical Therapists. Today there are a number of training establishments and books in German-speaking regions and many other countries for manual therapy based on Kaltenborn's principles.

1.4 Orthopedic Manual Therapy around the World

Around the same time as the development of the OMT Kaltenborn–Evjenth concept, there was also a kind of merging of various OMT concepts across the world. In 1967 Kaltenborn and Maitland met for the first time in London. Along with several of their colleagues, they worked toward a forum for cooperation that resulted in the formation in 1974 of the IFOMPT (International Federation of Orthopedic Manipulative Physical Therapists) (Lamb et al 2003). The founders were Kaltenborn, Maitland, Gregory Grieve, and Stanley Paris (Kaltenborn 2008). Members of IFOMPT are manual therapists from around the globe who aim for and support a high level of standardized training. Kaltenborn was closely involved in the formulation of the preliminary guidelines for training (Lamb et al 2003), which have been further developed and are central to learning OMT (see www.ifompt.com). In addition, more physical therapy further education programs in manual therapy are being offered by universities as master's degree courses in Europe and elsewhere, underscoring the significance that this physical therapy specialization has achieved.

1.5　Definition of Orthopedic Manual Therapy

Manual therapy is a specialty within the field of physical therapy that focuses on the examination and treatment of symptoms and functional disorders of the locomotor system. The concept of orthopedic manual therapy is clearly defined internationally and is continually evolving:

> **Note**
>
> **Definition of Orthopedic Manual Therapy according to the IFOMPT (2008)**
>
> Orthopedic Manual Therapy is a specialized area of physiotherapy / physical therapy for the management of neuromusculoskeletal conditions, based on clinical reasoning, using highly specific treatment approaches including manual techniques and therapeutic exercises.
>
> Orthopedic Manual Therapy also encompasses, and is driven by, the available scientific and clinical evidence and the biopsychosocial framework of each individual patient (IFOMPT 2008).

As with any development, that of manual therapy did not occur in a vacuum, but happened alongside changes in other medical/technical areas. The initial emphasis on joint techniques in the 1950s and 1960s pertained at a time when cast immobilization was still more common in orthopedics/traumatology. The increasing use of osteosynthesis procedures, starting at the end of the 1960s and continuing in the 1970s, allowed for early postoperative mobilization of the joints. Joint stiffness was reduced thanks to improved surgical techniques. Nowadays, there seems to be a relationship between our high-tech, more sedentary lifestyle and an apparent increase in hypermobility due to muscular de-conditioning, although scientific evidence on this hypothetical cause of hypermobility is lacking and would be difficult to gather. The proportion of active exercises and self-exercises in OMT has increased greatly over the past three decades.

There have also been advancements in joint techniques. In the early years, for example, manipulations were also performed with rotatory movements. Yet, given related risks, Kaltenborn eliminated their use on the extremities in his own concept in 1979 and on the spine in 1991. Since then, all manipulations are taught and applied only in a straight line with translatoric movements (Kaltenborn 2008). Further developments in regard to the physical therapy examination and treatment of the neural system, and especially neurodynamics, were and are being integrated into the concept. Similarly, the results of the enormous advances in pain research since 1965 (Melzack and Wall 1965) have also been integrated in the concept. This is merely to illustrate that manual therapy is a specialization within physical therapy. Thus, manual therapy develops in conjunction with physical therapy, bringing greater depth to new knowledge and skills from research and development related to the locomotor system. The same is true for medicine of which OMT is also an integral part. The manual therapist seeks to cooperate with doctors as each side has a clearly defined area of expertise and the two are complementary. To enhance communication, OMT thus uses the same terminology generally used in PT and medicine. Only a few terms have distinct definitions, for example, the "treatment plane."

As this brief historical overview illustrates, treatment forms that were originally limited to OMT—such as specific muscle stretching or MET—have been incorporated into general physical therapy. As a result of the passing down of manual therapy knowledge, Kaltenborn's goal of an overall improvement in PT is gradually being realized. The differences between OMT and PT continue to diminish. This also applies to differences among other concepts within PT, which are adopting more principles from each other and thus becoming increasingly similar—despite perhaps wanting to see themselves as unique.

Of the four special features of manual therapy in the OMT–Kaltenborn–Evjenth concept (Kaltenborn 2005), three have already been integrated into PT: the **trial treatment** (see p. 27), the **combined use of several techniques**, and the **use of ergonomic principles** (see p. 63).

The attention to joint mechanics may still be considered a unique feature which hopefully will soon also become a "normal" part of physical therapy (see p. 10 and 48). This includes terms such as straight-lined translatoric movements in relation to the treatment plane and the convex-concave rule, which are often associated with OMT.

A further characteristic of OMT as presented in this book is its **systematic, step-by-step approach to the clinical reasoning process** for examination and treatment in contrast to the hypothetic–deductive approach that is also used in OMT (see p. 21). All the different approaches (and concepts) existing within OMT should merge in the future and refrain from the defending their unique selling positions. In order to achieve this, physical therapists should clearly define what they do and why they do it and open their minds to discussion. A useful aid to the study of OMT is the training guidelines which are set forth by the IFOMPT (2012; see "Standards" at www.ifompt.com). The contents of this book form a solid basis for specialization in OMT as well as for proficiency in PT.

The primary indication for orthopedic manual therapy (OMT) is symptoms which correlate with movement, or —more exactly—which may be influenced by posture or movement. Manual therapy is therefore not limited to areas such as orthopedic medicine, rheumatology, traumatology, and sports medicine. Rather, it is also indicated for disorders in areas such as neurology, internal medicine (e.g., respiratory mechanics), pediatrics, and whenever movement and/or posture are related to the patient's symptoms (Kaltenborn 2005). Manual therapy uses a **biopsychosocial model** for understanding the patient and his or her problem. To understand this model, the physical therapist must first understand how it describes the original causes of the pain and how the pain can be influenced by OMT. Then, the principles of joint mechanics and the use of a systematic procedure—a special feature of the technique based on the OMT Kaltenborn–Evjenth Concept—may be integrated into the approach.

2.1   The Biopsychosocial Model as a Basis for OMT

In "traditional" medicine and physical therapy (PT), the biomedical and biopsychosocial views are the predominant models. The biomedical model is based on the assumption of a specific cause, a predictable course of disease, and one single adequate therapy. This concept is still valid today in certain areas such as traumatology and infectious diseases. Yet in other areas, such as chronic diseases, it is inadequate. Structural changes such as osteoarthritis or herniated disks often fail to sufficiently explain the pain. Indeed, such changes may occur without any pain, or, alternatively, there may be pain without any (persistent) underlying structural cause. During the 1970s, the biopsychosocial model was introduced as an expansion of the biomedical model (Engels 1977). The biopsychosocial model views nociception (= signaling of [impending] damage) as a phenomenon which may be influenced by various factors. These include the patient's attitude, his or her management of psychosocial problems such as stress, learned behaviors in response to illness, and social environment (Waddell 1998). The biomedical and biopsychosocial models are reflected in two systems used by the World Health Organization (WHO) for the classification of diseases in society: the ICD and the ICF. The 10th **International Statistical Classification of Diseases and Related Health Problems** (ICD) describes disease from a biomedical standpoint, that is, on structural and functional levels. The WHO classification is used for coding of diseases. Every diagnosis is given a code number which enables collection of statistics. This is the system primarily used by physicians. The **International Classification of Functioning, Disability and Health** (ICF) complements the ICD with the addition of the biopsychosocial perspective. The ICF is a phenomenological description of the patient's situation in which, in particular, the consequences of disease and the interactions with personal and environmental factors are itemized. The ICF therefore does not describe related causal factors, nor does it enable causative treatment. The ICF allocates code numbers to the observed health problem manifestations. These are intended to facilitate the collection of statistics in order to better describe the consequences of disease. This makes the ICF an ideal physical therapy instrument for the description of the patient and his or her problem (Huber and Cieza 2007; Schomacher 1999). This classification system of the consequences of disease has so far found little use in statistical analyses. The introduction of ICF intervention categories, ICF model pages, and core sets is intended to facilitate its use (Allet et al 2007; Kirschneck et al 2007a, b). The psychosocial aspects in the biopsychosocial model of disease of the ICF are widely discussed in physical therapy (Gifford 2002a, b; Klemme et al 2007). Cultural and economic factors have also been added. The view of OMT does not diverge from the overall PT view in this regard. In a holistic view of the patient, the **ICF activities and participation domains** play an important role in examination and treatment. In terms of the ICF, the characteristic features of OMT are physical functioning and structures, that is, they are within the realm of biomedicine.

2.2   The Biomedical Model

According to the definition of the World Confederation of Physical Therapy (WCPT), movement is the core element of physical therapy. PT **diagnoses are based on movement and posture** for targeted therapy. Individual psychosocial factors are also viewed in their relation to movement and posture, as well as to symptom (pain) management. Central to OMT diagnosis is a description of potentially abnormal movement and postural function(s) and tissue alterations which correlate with the patient's symptoms. **Core questions** are used to identify the problem (Schomacher 2001 , 2004a) and the responses given by the patient, and the examination, form the basis for diagnosis. Various core questions are described in more detail in the section concerning systematic examination structure (see p. 24).

2.2.1   The Pathomechanical Model

In the mechanical model, the central factor in symptoms related to movement is tissue tension (Cyriax 1982). Tissue tension may increase or decrease with movement. The resulting changes in the input in the pain-modulating and autonomic nervous system can alter symptoms. The goal of the examination is therefore to search for a **correlation between tissue tension and symptoms**. Tissue tension may be caused by either pressure or elongation of tissue (Panjabi 1992). OMT consequently searches for the movement and/or posture that produce changes in tissue tension, which are related to symptoms such as pain. Changes may be quantitative alterations in range of motion and/or qualitative changes like uniformity or speed of the movement. In postural causes, a search is made for any deviations from ideal posture. Static posture ideally distributes weight on all structures evenly according to their physiological function (bones under pressure and ligaments under tension, etc.). Dynamic posture should ensure an optimal balance between loading and unloading for stimulation of growth and maintenance and relief for recovery and regenerative processes. Deviations from physiological motion and ideal posture can result in lasting changes to the structures of the locomotor system. The stabilizing connective tissue of the joints can loosen and the stabilizing muscles can become insufficient. This can lead to hypermobility. Alternatively, lack of movement can result in atrophy with shortening of muscles and shrinkage of joint capsules. Loss of tissue function and restricted mobility might result. Such structural changes can also cause increased tissue tension. Tissue tension in turn stimulates—potentially sensitized—peripheral receptors like nociceptors. Under certain conditions, their afferent impulses may be interpreted by the central nervous system (CNS) as chronic or acute pain. The associations between pain **physiology** and **biomechanics** are fundamental to understanding OMT. Pain physiology describes the development, transmission, and processing of nociceptive information which leads one to experience pain. Biomechanics refers to the reactions of living tissue in the movement apparatus to mechanical (internal and external) forces (Debrunner 1995; Niethard and Pfeil 2003). It explains how shortening and lengthening of tissue occur and how tissue reacts to loading and movement in physiological and unphysiological ways.

2.2.2   Pain Physiology

Pain can be classified by the length of its duration. Acute pain is usually defined as lasting up to six weeks, or sometimes less. Pain is generally considered chronic if it lasts more than 12 weeks. Pain that falls in between acute and chronic is referred to as subacute. The key to understanding pain physiology in terms of duration is the physiological differences between acute and chronic pain.

> **Note**
> **Physiological differences between acute and chronic pain**
> - In **acute pain**, the extent of unphysiological tissue tension, or lesion, is proportional to the intensity of perceived pain: the greater the tissue tension or lesion size, the greater the pain.
> - In **chronic pain**, there is no proportionality between tissue tension and pain: even slight increases in tissue tension without any external stimulus, or minimal lesions, can trigger intense pain.

Pain physiology further distinguishes between peripheral and CNS pain mechanisms as well as between receptor pain and neurogenic pain (Schomacher 2001a, b).

Peripheral Pain Mechanisms

In **receptor pain** (also known as "nociceptive pain"), external and internal forces act on the tissue as stress, causing strain by pressure-tension and/or elongation-tension (Niethard and Pfeil 2003). The resulting increased tissue tension stimulates the mechanoreceptors. If the intensity of the stimulus increases, the nociceptors are stimulated as well, a protective mechanism that is necessary for survival (Melzack and Wall 1996).

- **"Fast" nociceptors** with myelinated A-delta nerve fibers trigger a withdrawal reflex which is intended to avoid or reduce damage. A classic example is walking onto a nail. The pain in the foot causes a flexion reflex in the painful leg and a crossed extension reflex in the leg on the other side (Bruggencate 1996).

- **"Slow" nociceptors** with minimally myelinated or unmyelinated C nerve fibers cause protection of the affected site to allow physiological wound healing to proceed undisturbed.

In order to enhance protection and disuse of the affected site, there is increased sensitivity of the peripheral nervous system (= peripheral sensitization). Pain is perceived as greater than normal (= **peripheral hyperalgesia**). **Peripheral neurogenic pain** does not occur due to stimulation of nociceptors, but rather through axonal damage in the peripheral nerve. During wound healing of such an axonal lesion the nerve sometimes forms more ion channels at the injury site. With sufficient numbers, these can spontaneously trigger an action potential even without any external stimuli. The lesion site thus is transformed into an **ectopic pacemaker**, that is, a nonphysiological site for development of action potentials. The patient perceives pain in the area supplied by the nerve. An example is phantom pain experienced after a nerve is severed during amputation.

Central Pain Mechanisms

Acute pain is designed to activate protection and disuse of the affected site. Similar to the peripheral nervous system, the central nervous system (CNS) also increases its sensitivity to enhance protection and physiological healing. If sensitization of the CNS lasts longer than physiological wound healing, protection and disuse of the area loses its sense. Sensitization of the nervous system can generate **central neurogenic pain**, which can become a disease in itself if it becomes chronic (Cervero and Laird 1991). Sensitization of the CNS can occur at the synapses in the spinal cord, brain stem, or thalamus, or in various regions of the brain which are associated with perception. Complex mechanisms lead to permanent changes in the nervous system. This is known as neuroplasticity, and is one explanation for pain memory as well as pain that occurs in the absence of a physical stimulus. The increased pain perception in **CNS sensitization** is referred to as **central hyperalgesia**. In **allodynia**, even normal afferent impulses from mechanoreceptors, thermoreceptors, and chemorecep-

tors may be perceived as pain. In **hyperpathia**, the pain can last longer than the triggering stimulus. An **ectopic pacemaker** can also arise in the CNS if, for example, there is axonal membrane damage due to hemorrhage.

Disease-Induced Hyperalgesia and Biopsychosocial Aspects

Nociceptors react not only to mechanical stress, but also to thermal and chemical stimuli. For example, chemical substances are released during inflammation or with generalized disease. These may reduce the threshold for activation of nociceptors and directly stimulate them (Weiss and Schaible 2003a: 4). The pain in **disease-induced hyperalgesia** is caused by activation of the immune system following inflammation, tissue damage, or illness (Logiudice 2003). A common example is general joint pain that occurs with a fever or the flu, which is not due to dysfunction of the locomotor system but rather to "hypersensitization of the system."

The fact that stress can also alter the immune system and facilitate pain (Logiudice 2003) shows why therapists must analyze patients not only in terms of biomedical aspects, but also must use the biopsychosocial model. Stress-reducing measures may be integrated into treatment as needed.

Pain Mechanisms and Consequences for Treatment

Receptor pain and neurogenic pain, peripheral and central pain mechanisms commonly occur together. Often only a broad distinction is possible. Yet these help with clinical reasoning and decision-making. **Clinical reasoning** refers to the thinking and decision-making processes of the therapist during examination and treatment measures (Jones 1997; Higgs and Jones 2000).

The differentiation between acute and chronic pain has therapeutic consequences.

- In receptor pain, which is **acute pain**, treatment of the dysfunction and the related tissue lesion is paramount, taking into consideration physiological wound healing. The therapist must respect guarding mechanisms and disuse of the affected body part which are associated with the acute pain.

- In **chronic pain**, which is largely neurogenic pain, the symptomatic dysfunction in the periphery is often very small (Giamberardino 2003). The therapist must use extremely precise examination and treatment methods. In addition, nervous system **desensitization** must be done using systematic and progressive adaptation to movement. This treatment probably need not be specific.

Painful stimuli may threaten to sustain chronic pain or even exacerbate it. The therapist must therefore avoid causing any pain during treatment. In certain situations, such as desensitization of the nervous system and counter irritation, pain may be an acceptable part of treatment, as long as one quickly returns to the former level and keeps the pain under control. Counter irritation involves painful stimulation of a nonpainful area, diminishing the original pain (Melzack and Wall 1996).

■ The Relationship between Pain and Dysfunction

Asking the patient about his or her pain is of limited value. While superficial pain occurring near or at the level of the skin may provide precise information about the origin, extent, and type of pain, it is more difficult to locate deeper pain, which is often reported by patients undergoing physical therapy. The descriptions of articular, neuro-genic, muscular, and visceral pain are frequently similar and thus are virtually an open invitation to misinterpretation (Zusman 2003).

Thus it is more important to locate and treat the dysfunction related to the pain. The preliminary interview about the pain, assuming there are no warning signs alerting the therapist to serious disease or dysfunction—such clinical flags are discussed later (see p. 56)—is typically brief so that the functional examination can proceed. The purpose of functional tests is to search for malfunctions in terms of postural/movement and/or tissue changes which are related to the pain. The relationship between deviations from correct physiological posture/movement and tissue changes is discussed in the following from a biomechanical standpoint.

2.2.3   Biomechanics—Stress and Strain

The tissues of the locomotor system are created for **stress** and **strain**. Stress describes the force acting from outside on a structure, while strain is the mechanical effect of this force within a structure (Panjabi and White 2001).

External stresses may be influenced by the rules governing behavioral ergonomics (see p. 63). The ability of the tissues to withstand mechanical stress—along with genetics and other factors—depends on its use.

All living tissues follow the **biological principle of adaptation** (Arndt-Schulz rule; Pschyrembel 2007). This rule states that:

- minimal stimuli diminish life functions,
- habitual stimuli maintain them,
- moderate stimuli (exceeding the threshold) encourage them (= training),
- strong stimuli inhibit life functions, and
- extremely strong stimuli suspend them.

■ Consequences of Inadequate Activity

If one applies the biological principle of adaptation, then regular movement should sustain the functioning of the tissue. This illustrates the dependence of all connective and supporting tissues (Akeson et al 1992) and the other tissues (Schomacher 2005a) on stress.

Insufficient activity carries a risk of:

- Loss of strength (muscle atrophy)
- Poorer coordination (neuromuscular insufficiency)
- Decreased bone density (osteoporosis)
- Diminished ability of cartilage to withstand stress (osteoarthritis)
- Loss of connective tissue stability (risk of micro- or macrorupture)

Insufficient activity or immobilization can lead to **joint contractures** with **stiffness of the capsule** and **degeneration of the cartilage** as the two most important pathological joint changes (Trudel et al 2001; Trudel and Uhthoff 2000). This explains the importance of (early) mobilization and progressive training during physical rehabilitation in order to increase the ability of the tissue to withstand stress.

■ Consequences of Overload

Overloading the locomotor system can also result in weakening of tissue functions or even partial destruction of structures. In **"overtraining,"** intense training sessions can lead to a loss of strength and coordination and may damage the noncontractile structures of the locomotor system.

Similarly, persistent **poor posture** or **repeated end-range movements** may, over time, elongate the structures which are intended to limit movement. Patients should participate in training to increase the tissue's ability to withstand stress as well as train motor control to limit the range of motion (see p. 46).

The tissue responses to the influence of stress are not only mechanical in nature. Various other aspects such as histological, biochemical, neurological, and endocrine factors should also be considered (Schomacher 2005b). The complexity of the process explains why not all patients respond in the same manner to outside force—for example, during mobilization or training—and why these reactions cannot be fully anticipated. For more detailed information, the reader is referred to the literature (e.g., Schomacher 2005b; van den Berg 2010).

In manual therapy, the **attention to joint mechanics** means applying functional anatomy to the patient. Along with other basic medical sciences such as biomechanics, pain physiology, and neurophysiology, it helps form the theoretical basis of clinical reasoning in Orthopedic Manual Therapy (OMT).

To understand joint mechanics, this chapter first discusses kinematics in order to derive consequences for treatment. Afterward, joint positions are described that are relevant for OMT.

Kinematics, the study of motion, examines and describes movement without consideration of the forces that cause them. Kinematics is an essential part of OMT given that assessment of range of motion and quality of movement are central to the concept.

Depending on how many bones or joints are involved in a movement, a distinction may be made between general and specific movements:

- *General movements*: several bones or extremity joints (e.g., shoulder girdle) or several vertebral segments (e.g., lumbar spine) move actively or are moved passively.

- *Specific movements*: only a single bone or extremity joint (e.g., ankle joint) or one vertebral segment (e.g., C3–C4) is moved. Specific movements of the spine can only occur passively, although recent evidence is questioning this and specificity might be limited to movement of some segments of a spinal region (Schomacher and Learman 2010).

Joint kinematics may be divided into *osteokinematics* and *arthrokinematics*.

3.1   Osteokinematics

Osteokinematics examines and describes the manner in which bones move in space. Bones may move with *rotation* or *translation*.

3.1.1   Rotation

Rotation is the spinning of a body around a mechanical axis. If a bone rotates in a joint around multiple instantaneous axes of rotation, a changing angle is formed between it and its bony counterpart. One thus speaks of *angular motion*. Human beings perform such movements passively and actively.

A total of six movements may be defined. These rotate around three rotatory axes in three anatomical planes, in two directions each:

- two in the sagittal plane around a frontal axis: flexion/extension (ventral flexion and dorsal flexion);

- two in the frontal plane around a sagittal axis: abduction/adduction (right and left lateral flexion); and

- two in the horizontal plane around a vertical axis: external/internal rotation (right and left rotation).

Pronation and supination, as well as eversion and inversion, are movements around independent axes. Rotation may be divided into **anatomical** and **functional** movements.

■ Simple Anatomical Movements

Anatomical movements occur in one anatomical plane as rotation around an axis or around multiple instantaneous axes of rotation (e.g., around the flexion/extension axes). These are referred to as *simple* or *uniaxial movements* and they correspond to the above-mentioned rotatory movements.

If a person were to move strictly within the anatomical planes, the movement would take on a robotic quality. Such movements are rarely performed in everyday life. Rather, they are used primarily for the neutral zero method of joint measurement.

Functional, Combined Movements

If one observes a person in motion, one notices that the movement always goes beyond the basic anatomical planes, creating a curved arc of motion. These *functional movements* occur in several anatomical planes around numerous axes or groups of instantaneous axes of rotation. These are referred to as *combined* or *multiaxial movements*, may be performed as coupled or uncoupled movements and they are used in various treatment methods such as proprioceptive neuromuscular facilitation (PNF).

Coupled Movements

If one carefully observes a person in motion, one notices that he or she performs certain movement combinations repeatedly and automatically, without thinking. The knee, for instance, is always extended with external rotation. Hip joint flexion occurs with abduction/external rotation. The shoulder is abducted with external rotation, flexed with internal rotation, and the kyphotic thoracic spine bends sideways with rotation in the same direction. Such combined movements are known as *coupled movements* and are a result of the joint structure. Lateral flexion of the spine is always coupled with a certain degree of rotation, the direction of which depends on whether the spine is in the neutral-null position or whether there is ventral flexion or dorsiflexion. The following are examples of coupled movement patterns:

C0–C2:	in ventral and dorsal flexion:	lateral flexion with rotation in the opposite direction
C2–C7 (–T3):	in ventral and dorsal flexion:	lateral flexion with rotation in the same direction
Thoracic spine:	in ventral flexion and neutral position:	lateral flexion with rotation in the same direction
	in (nearly max.) dorsal flexion:	lateral flexion with rotation in the opposite direction
Lumbar spine:	in (nearly max.) ventral flexion:	lateral flexion with rotation in the same direction
	in dorsal flexion and neutral position:	lateral flexion with rotation in the opposite direction

Uncoupled Movements

Movement combinations that do not occur automatically at the extremity and vertebral joints, whose range of motion tends to be smaller and their end-feel rather more firm or even hard, are known as *uncoupled movements*.

> **!** Given that movement combinations depend on joint structure, and that this varies greatly from one person to the next, combinations other than those mentioned above are possible. For the physical therapist, it is important to evaluate the criteria of coupled movement:
>
> - Spontaneous, automatic, active movement
> - Greater range than the opposite movement combination
> - End-feel is less firm than the opposite movement combination

---

3.1.2   Translation

Translation is the movement of the bone in space without rotation. Translation occurs physiologically with a small range of motion in passive movements. Translatoric movements may describe straight or curved lines.

In OMT, translation is described as rectilinear movements in relation to the treatment plane:

- At a right angle away from the treatment plane → **rectilinear translatoric traction**
  Separation of the joint partners

- At a right angle to the treatment plane → **rectilinear translatoric compression**
  Approximation of the joint partners

- Parallel to the treatment plane → **rectilinear translatoric gliding**
  Displacement of the joint partners anteriorly/posteriorly, medially/laterally, etc.

In everyday practice, OMT views rectilinear translatoric movements as so commonplace that they are simplified as traction, compression, and gliding.

3.1.3   Overview of oteokinematics

Osteokinematics (= the study of the movement of bones in space)			
general (several bones) and specific (single bone) movements			
Rotation is the turning of a bone around an axis = curved motion. It occurs actively and passively.		**Translation** is movement of a bone in space without rotation. It occurs passively (Exception: protraction in the temporo-mandibular joint).	
Anatomical movements <ul><li>*Simple*, single-axis movements such as movements in the zero position method</li></ul>	**Functional movements** <ul><li>*Combined*, multiaxial movements such as everyday movements, PNF movements, etc.</li></ul>	**Rectilinear translatoric movements** *At a right angle* to the treatment plane <ul><li>away from the treatment plane (= traction)</li><li>toward the treatment plane (= compression)</li></ul>	**Rectilinear translatoric movements** *Parallel* to the treatment plane <ul><li>gliding anteriorly/posteriorly, medially/laterally, right, left, etc.</li><li>Note: Curved translations like protraction in the temporomandibular joint are not described here.</li></ul>
Flexion/extension Abduction/adduction (lateral flexion right and left) Inward rotation/outward rotation (rotation right and left)	Coupled movements	Uncoupled movements		

3.2   Arthrokinematics

While most physical therapy concepts are concerned with osteokinematics, clinical reasoning in manual therapy, at the biomedical level, is focused on arthrokinematics (Grimsby and Rivard 2008). In addition to rotatory movements, Kaltenborn also uses translatoric motions occurring in joint play: these are traction, compression, and gliding.

In order for the bones to move through space, the joint surfaces must change their position relative to one another. An analysis of the movements of the joint surfaces with respect to each other is the domain of arthrokinematics. Arthrokinematics plays a central role in OMT. Patients usually perceive their movement dysfunction from the standpoint of osteokinematics as a change in the movement of the bones in space. Typically, patients complain of restricted movement—or too much movement and thus a feeling of instability. The physical therapist can measure the changed range of motion with a goniometer.

Note

According to the basic hypothesis of Kaltenborn (2005), from an arthrokinematic standpoint, limited mobility and hypermobility are caused by impaired gliding of articular surfaces against one another, which alters the osteokinematic range of motion. Restricted gliding may be compensated by rolling in the joint. Increased rolling stresses the connective tissue that stabilizes the joint, however. The gaping and impingement of articulating surfaces occurring at the end of the movement may produce increased tissue tension and thus symptoms such as pain.

When there is a change in range of motion, other possibilities must also be considered such as increase in synovial fluid viscosity, insufficiency of the muscles stabilizing the joints, altered neurodynamics, and increased friction between degenerated joint surfaces. The different causes require different examination and treatment measures. Olaf Evjenth and Jern Hamberg set a technical standard for the examination of muscle length and for muscle stretching (Evjenth and Hamberg 1984a, b). In regard to neurodynamics, OMT is mainly oriented toward the procedures developed by Robert Elvey and David Butler (Butler 1995; Hall et al 1998), which are based on neuroanatomy and have been developed since (Shacklock 2007).

If the hypo- or hypermobility is not due to muscle insufficiency or altered neurodynamics, but rather is caused by the actual joint, the source is restricted physiological movement of the joint surfaces against each other, which must be treated. The proper treatment requires knowledge of arthrokinematics. Arthrokinematics is the study of joint surface movements which may be described as roll-gliding and joint play. When a bone actively or passively moves in space, there is roll-gliding in the joint. If a rectilinear translatoric motion occurs, there is joint play (traction, compression, and gliding).

3.2.1   Roll-gliding

If one observes the movements of the joint partners or joint surfaces in the joint space during their active and passive rotatory movements, one will see the roll-gliding movement. This is a combined movement of rolling and gliding, each of which is present to various degrees.

■ Rolling and Direction of Rolling

During rolling there is a *new* point of contact on the joint surface which touches new points on its counterpart. For this to occur, the joint surfaces must be incongruent, as is the case in human beings. One joint surface rolls along the opposite joint surface.

Rolling action predominates in joints that have low congruence and a small roof over the articulating joint surfaces, such as the femorotibial and distal radioulnar joints. Limited gliding in such joints may be compensated by rolling. Hence patients often do not feel the beginning of limited joint mobility.

The joint surface always rolls in the same direction as that in which the bone moves in space, regardless of whether it is convex or concave (**Fig. 3.1 a, b**).

■ Gliding and Direction of Glide

During gliding, *the same* point of contact of one joint surface is in continuous contact with new points on the other joint surface. Gliding may occur between incongruent or congruent joint surfaces. Completely congruent joint surfaces allow only for gliding, without any rolling, as can be seen, for example, in the joint of a total endoprosthesis of the hip.

In joints with a high level of congruence and a large roof over the articulating joint, surface rolling is virtually impossible as, for example, in the coxofemoral and humeroulnar joints where the concave joint surface is even deeper than is required for a precise congruous fit with the convex joint surface (Bullough et al 1973; von Eisenhart-Rothe et al 1997, 1999). Restricted gliding in this case rapidly results in the patient's sensation of osteokinematically limited movement.

Totally flat surfaces, which are not found in human joints, exhibit straight-lined translatoric gliding (**Fig. 3.2 a**).

In humans, one joint surface glides along the opposing joint surface, describing a curved line. This form of gliding between the joint surfaces is known as *curved gliding* (**Fig. 3.2 b**).

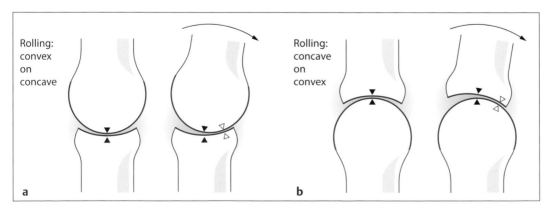

Rolling:
convex
on
concave

Rolling:
concave
on
convex

a   b

Fig. 3.1 a, b
Rolling and direction of rolling.

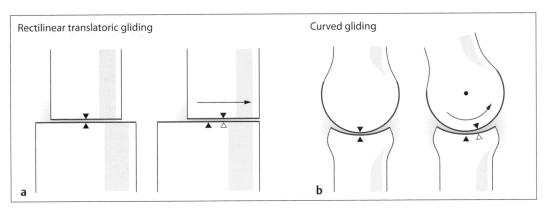

Fig. 3.2 a, b
Gliding and direction of glide.
a Rectilinear translatoric gliding,
b curved gliding pathway.

To improve gliding of the joint surfaces against one another, the therapist must know the direction in which the moved joint surface should actually glide. This indicates the limitation on the gliding action, which must be improved. Experienced therapists can feel this direction of gliding during certain movements. This is the *direct examination method*.

For patients with highly painful or extremely "stiff" joints and amphiarthroses, as well as in situations where palpation is difficult, or if the therapist simply lacks experience in movement palpation, Kaltenborn formulated the convex–concave rule as the *indirect examination method*.

The **Kaltenborn convex–concave rule** for movement of the joints:

- When moving the convex joint partner, the joint surface glides in the opposite direction in relation to the movement of the bone in space (**Fig. 3.3 a**). Because the shaft of the convex bone is on the one side of the

rotatory axis and its joint surface is on the other, this creates a two-armed lever whose arms move in opposite directions (Schomacher 2009a).

- When moving the concave joint partner, there is gliding of the joint surface in the same direction in relation to the movement of the bone in space (**Fig. 3.3 b**). Because the shaft of the concave bone and its joint surface are on the same side of the rotatory axis, there is a single-arm lever whose arms move in the same direction.

The rotatory axis is always located on the more convex joint partner.

Note

Kaltenborn convex–concave rule:
convex = opposite direction
concave = same direction

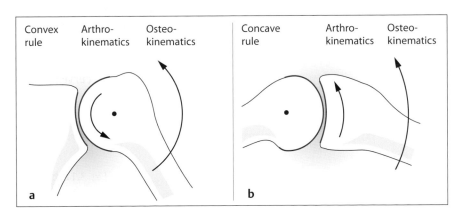

Fig. 3.3 a, b Kaltenborn convex–concave rule.

3.2.2 Joint Play

To examine arthrokinematic movements, the joint surfaces are moved in relation to one another in a straight-lined translatoric motion. This is done in the form of traction, compression, or gliding, which together are known as *joint play* (**Fig. 3.4**).

- **Traction**: One joint surface is moved away from the opposite joint surface at a right angle to the treatment plane.

- **Compression**: One joint surface is briefly pressed against the opposite joint surface. Pressure is exerted at a right angle to the treatment plane.

■ **Gliding**: One joint surface is gliding a small distance parallel to the treatment plane in relation to the other joint surface. Due to the curvature of the joint surfaces, gliding will not occur in a totally straight line. This is not clinically perceptible, however. The therapist moves the mobilizing hand in a straight line and with a translatoric motion.

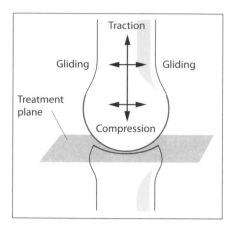

Fig. 3.4
Joint play, which consists of traction, compression and gliding.

Note

■ Traction and compression occur at a right angle to the treatment plane.
■ Gliding occurs parallel to the treatment plane.

3.2.3   Overview of Arthrokinematics

Arthrokinematics (= the study of movements of joint surfaces in relation to one another)		
Roll-gliding Occurs with active and passive rotation of a bone. In normal joint function, rolling and gliding are present = roll-gliding.		**Joint play** Occurs with passive rectilinear translation of a bone with its joint surface in relation to the tratment plane.
Rolling Curved movement in the same direction as the movement of the bone, along the joint surface. The lower the congruence and the smaller the roof over the joint surfaces, the more rolling occurs.	**Gliding** Curved movement in the same (concave) or opposite (convex) direction to the movement of the bone, along the joint surface. The greater the congruence and the larger the roof over the joint surfaces, the more gliding occurs.	**1. Straight-lined translatoric traction** Separation of the joint surfaces at a right angle to the treatment plane **2. Straight-lined translatoric compression** Approximation of the joint surfaces at a right angle to the treatment plane **3. Straight-lined translatoric gliding** Displacement of the joint surfaces parallel to the treatment plane

3.3   Joint Anatomy

"Gray, my friend, is every theory, but green is the golden tree of life."
(Goethe, J. W. v., Faust I)

From a mechanical standpoint, joints are movable connections between bones. At the other extreme are the immobile bony and cartilaginous connections between bones. Examples are the bony connections between the ilium, pubis, and ischium as well as, during growth, the cartilaginous connection between the epiphysis and diaphysis of the tubular bones formed by the epiphyseal plate. Certain cartilaginous joints, such as between the first rib and the sternum, allow for movement owing to their elasticity.

Syndesmoses (e.g., tibiofibular joint) and symphyses (e.g., pubic symphysis, intervertebral joints) connect two bones with ligaments and fibrous/hyaline cartilage.

True joints (= synovial joints, articulatio synovialis, diarthrosis) are characterized by hyaline cartilage-covered joint surfaces, a synovial fluid-producing joint capsule, and a joint space. In an intact joint, the joint space consists of the small gap between the articulating joint surfaces. These are pressed against each other as a result of intraarticular negative air pressure, adhesion forces, and muscular tension. Adhesion is the sticking together of two substances or bodies to one another (e.g., chalk to a chalkboard).

For a more detailed description of the joints and their classification, the reader is referred to the literature. Given that the primary aim of this book is to facilitate an understanding of movement, only a brief explanation is provided here and describes:

- how the shape of the articular surfaces in different joint types determines the motion around an axis,

- the orientations of movements (around axes and planes),
- which joint positions are important for examination and treatment, and
- which structures restrict movement of the joints.

3.3.1 Joint Surface Shape, Joint Types, and Movement Axes

The shape of the joint surfaces (**Fig. 3.5**) determines the movement potential of the joint. This may be compared to a shallow cup, that is, with completely congruent joint surfaces. Thus the movements of the joint partners are clearly defined.

A ball can move in all directions in a socket. For simplicity's sake, three axes are defined which are at a right angle to each other and around which movements can occur (Mac Conaill and Basmajian 1977). Elliptical and saddle shapes move in the socket around two axes while the cylinder can rotate in its hollow cylinder around only one axis.

Using this simplified description, the true joints of classical anatomy may be subdivided into triaxial, biaxial, and uniaxial joints:

- *triaxial*: ball-and-socket joint (spheroidal joint, e.g., glenohumeral joint), cotyloid joint (enarthrodial joint, e.g., coxal joint), and plane joint (e.g., acromioclavicular joint). Plane joints are also often considered as a special type.
- *biaxial*: ovoid joint (ellipsoidal joint, e.g., radiocarpal joint) and saddle joint (sellar joint, e.g., carpometacarpal joint).

- *uniaxial*: hinge joint (ginglymus, e.g., proximal interphalangeal joint) and pivot joint (trochoidal joint, e.g., proximal radioulnar joint, distal radioulnar joint).

Yet upon closer inspection, all joint surfaces exhibit variations in curvature and are therefore incongruent (Mac Conaill and Basmajian 1977; Spalteholz and Spanner 1989; Gray 1989). This means that the human joint does not move around fixed axes, but around instantaneous axes of rotation which change position during movement. This is what produces the varied and harmonious movements of human joints as opposed to the rigid type of motion of a machine. MacConaill reduced this type of variously curved joint surfaces to two basic forms: the ovoid and the sellar joints (**Fig. 3.6**) (MacConaill and Basmajian 1977).

Unaltered, ovoid joint surfaces have three axes of movement. This seemingly flat joint may be imagined as a cutout portion of a giant eggshell. If the egg shape is changed to an elliptical form, the joint becomes a biaxial joint.

If the saddle shape remains unaltered, it corresponds to the classic biaxial saddle joint. If the raised sides are cut off, the result is a cylinder, which represents the classic uniaxial hinge joint.

The condylar joints, which are better called bicondylar joints, are a special type of saddle joint, in which two distinct joint surfaces articulate with one another. An example is the connection between the femoral condyles and

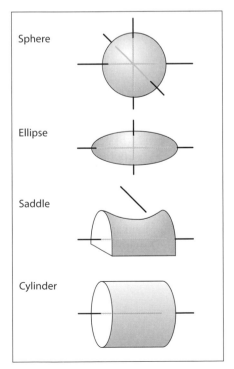

Sphere

Ellipse

Saddle

Cylinder

Fig. 3.5
Shapes of joint surfaces: spheroidal, ellipsoid, saddle-shaped, and cylindrical.

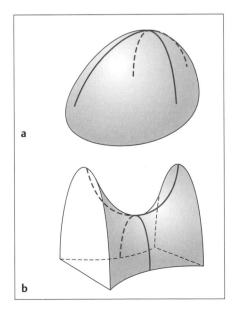

a

b

Fig. 3.6
Basic shapes of the variously curved joint surfaces.
a Ovoid,
b Sellar

the tibia. Such joints allow movements around two axes, for example, at the knee around the flexion/extension axis as well as around the internal/external rotation axis (MacConaill and Basmajian 1977).

An amphiarthrosis is a partially movable joint that allows less than 10° of movement.

> **Note**
>
> ### Classification of joints
>
> | Classic joint type | Ball-and-socket joint | Ovoid joint | Sellar joint | Hinge and pivot joints | |
> |---|---|---|---|---|---|
> | Joint types after MacConaill | Egg-shaped | | Saddle-shaped | | Special type |
> | | ↙ | ↘ | ↙ | ↘ | ↓ |
> | | Unaltered ovoid | Altered ovoid | Unaltered sellar | Altered sellar | Bicondylar joint, e.g., knee |
> | Simplified number of axes of movement | three | two | two | one | two |

3.3.2   Axes and Orientation Planes of Joint Movements

Rotation around an axis is one type of movement. The motion follows a curved path of motion, which in physics is described as rotatory movement. Yet movement can also occur along a linear axis or relative to a plane without any rotation. In physics, this is referred to as translatoric motion.

How the shape of the articulating surfaces determines the number of movement axes has already been discussed. The orientation of the movement axes at a right angle to each other is based on agreement. This is a mechanically adequate concept given that in a plane all momentary axes of movement (e.g., a–a′) may be defined by two (e.g., X–X′ and Y–Y′) of the three basic axes (MacConaill and Basmajian 1977) (**Fig. 3.7**).

The three basic axes are found at the point of intersection of two anatomical planes (frontal, sagittal, and horizontal planes).

Translatoric movements may be performed in relation to any number of planes. In order to define a standard reference point in manual therapy, Kaltenborn introduced the notion of the treatment plane in 1954 (Kaltenborn 2005). This term is somewhat misleading given that it applies to translatoric movements occurring during therapy as well as examination. Yet it has established itself over time, and hence it will also be used in the following.

The treatment plane is an imaginary plane that is located between the articular surfaces and is at a right angle to a line extending from the axis of rotation to the deepest aspect of the articulating concave surface (**Fig. 3.8**).

In clinical practice, the treatment plane is imagined to be on the concave joint partner.

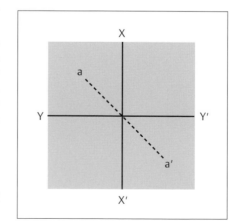

Fig. 3.7
Basic axes of movement. Two basic axes may be used to define any other axis in the same plane.

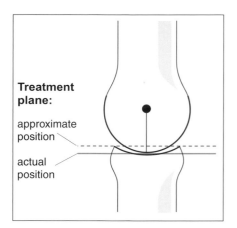

Treatment plane:

approximate position

actual position

Fig. 3.8
The treatment plane.

Note

Joint movements in manual therapy

Occur as rotatory movements curving around **axes**.	Occur as linear translatoric motion in a straight line in relation to the **treatment plane**.
The basic axes of movement are at a right angle to one another and are located at the intersections between two anatomical planes.	This is an imaginary plane between the articular surfaces which is at a right angle to a line passing from the axis of rotation to the deepest aspect of the articulating concave surface.
Due to the curvature of the joint surfaces, movements actually occur around a number of instantaneous axes of rotation.	In clinical practice, the treatment plane is imagined to be on the concave joint partner.

3.3.3 Joint Positions

To document the examination and treatment, as well as for communication with colleagues and physicians, it is important to be aware of standard joint positions.

The Zero Position

The zero position is the reference position from which rotatory, angular movements are measured according to the neutral zero method (Ryf and Weymann 1999). In the zero position, the patient is standing upright with the gaze focused forward, the arms hanging at the sides alongside the trunk with the palms facing forward, and the thumbs in a relaxed neutral position. The feet are placed hip-width apart, pointing forward, and the legs are upright. Measurement of forearm movements is from a slightly different zero position in which the elbows are in 90 degree flexion and the thumbs point vertically upward.

In manual therapy, rotatory movements are tested from the zero position.

Note

The zero position is the reference position from which the measurement of joint motion is made based on the neutral zero method. Testing of rotatory movement is performed from this position.

Resting Position

As already described, the curvatures of the opposing joint surfaces are not congruent. Thus there are many joint positions in which there is only little congruence and one position in which it is greatest. In the position of least contact between the articular surfaces, the capsule/ligament complex is also the most relaxed. Here, in the resting position, the joint surfaces may be most easily moved away from one another at a right angle or moved parallel to the treatment plane. These movements, along with compression, are referred to as joint play. Thus, this is the position used by manual therapists to examine translatoric movements. Pain-alleviating traction—or in some joints gliding, such as in the radioulnar and sacroiliac joints—is also performed in the resting position, as it allows the greatest translatoric movement of the joint capsule which stimulates the mechanoreceptors.

The resting position is defined by the joint anatomy. It is also referred to as "status perlaxus" and the "maximally loose-packed position" (Mac Conaill and Basmajian 1977).

Note

The position of the joint partners relative to one another in which

- the joint capsule/ligament complex is most lax,
- the joint surfaces have the least amount of contact with one another, and
- the joint play is the greatest

is known as the *resting position*.

This is the position in which translatoric motions are tested at the beginning, and pain-reducing traction or gliding may be performed as a form of therapy.

The presence of pathology may change the tension of the joint capsule, and thus the position in which it is loosest. The position in which the therapist feels the greatest joint play is the **actual resting position**. The feeling registered by the therapist at the end of a translatoric movement—the end-feel—is pathologically changed in this position.

According to Kaltenborn, **intra-articular problems** are likely when separation of the articular surfaces is hardly possible. If, when attempting traction, the end-feel is also manipulatable (i.e., firm, less elastic and earlier in the movement pathway than with physiological mobility), this is a classic indication for **straight-lined translatoric traction manipulation** (Kaltenborn 2008).

Extra-articular problems, such as shortening of connective tissues surrounding the joint (e.g., capsular shrinkage), are another common source of diminished traction and gliding. If there is a pathologically firm and less elastic end-feel which occurs earlier than expected, and if a traction manipulation trial treatment failed to produce a positive result, extra-articular problems are likely. Treatment consists of **static mobilization** (grade **III**) to stretch the periarticular structures like the joint capsule.

Distinguishing between intra- and extra-articular problems can be a challenge. Established criteria are still lacking.

Note

The changed resting position due to intra-articular or extra-articular pathologies is called the actual resting position. There is also a pathological end-feel. The actual *resting position* may also be used for the examination of translatoric movements and pain-alleviating traction measures.

In congenital joint deformities, the actual resting position often differs as well from the anatomical norm, but there is a physiological end-feel (Kaltenborn 2004).

■ Close Packed Position

In the close packed position, where contact between joint surfaces is the greatest, the capsule/ligament complex is under maximum tension. Only minimal translatoric movements are possible in this position. In OMT this position is used to place joints in a stable position and reduce their being moved along with the targeted joint during treatment. It is also referred to as "status rigidus" (Mac Conaill and Basmajian 1977).

Note

The position of the joint partners relative to one another

- in which the joint capsule/ligament complex is the tightest,
- in which the articulating surfaces have the greatest contact with one another, and
- in which there is the least amount of joint play,

is referred to as the *close packed position*.

This position serves to stabilize the joints in order to reduce their moving with the treated joint.

3.3.4 Limitations of Joint Movements

When a joint moves, or is passively moved, to the end of its range of motion, certain structures stop the movement. Some are actual joint structures, such as the capsule/ligament complex or bony processes like the olecranon process. Other limiting structures include surrounding soft tissues such as muscles, skin, and nerves. It is important for the physical therapist to recognize whether it is the articular structures or the surrounding soft tissues that are limiting the movement, given that treatment of the limitation requires different structure-specific measures. In OMT, a distinction is made between the actual joint and the complex movement unit which includes all the surrounding soft tissues.

Note

Joint:	**Complex movement unit:**
Bony joint partners along with capsule/ligament complex and intra-articular structures	The joint and surrounding soft tissues as well as blood supply and innervation

Along with a focus on joint mechanics, another cornerstone of Orthopedic Manual Therapy (OMT) is the use of a systematic procedure for examination and treatment.

The use of a system enables methodical follow-up: shortly after undergoing treatment, a change must already be either apparent to the patient (e.g., reduced pain) or measurable by the therapist (e.g., increased range of motion). This constitutes clinical evidence. If relevant studies are available, scientific evidence is used by the therapist for making treatment decisions. Both clinical and scientific evidence enable the best-possible performance of OMT according to the principles of evidence-based medicine (EBM) (Sackett and Rosenberg 1995).

> **Note**
>
> Every manual therapy examination and treatment is tailored individually to the patient and is further adapted each day to his or her response to therapy (Kaltenborn 2005). The aim of the examination is to find a way, through treatment, to help the patient to be able to lead a symptom-free, independent, and more satisfying life. The primary goal of OMT is to relieve pain and improve the functional abilities of the patient (IFOMPT 2008).

Manual therapy uses **systematic procedures** based on the answers to orienting **questions** for examination and treatment. This is best understood against the backdrop of various possible procedures.

There are three main types of procedure: **hypothetical/ deductive examination, pattern recognition**, and a **systematic step-by-step procedure using orienting questions**. In current practice, these methods may overlap, and often they are mixed together. Undoubtedly, spontaneous thoughts about possible hypotheses explaining the patient's problem or pattern detection also occur. This is clearly unavoidable, even with the use of a systematic procedure. The three procedures described here for examination are explained further as follows.

> **Note**
>
> The distinction between a hypothetical/deductive examination, pattern recognition, and a systematic procedure using key questions, is primarily a didactic one and should be understood as enhancing consciousness of the clinical reasoning process. Characteristic for OMT is the use of a systematic step-by-step procedure and the use of orienting questions.

4.1 Hypothetical/Deductive Procedure

In this method, the examiner derives (= deduces) certain conclusions that may be tested (= hypotheses) based on initial information about the patient. These hypotheses are then tested and ruled out one by one until only one remains which is the diagnosis (Jones 1997; Hengeveld 1998).

An example is a patient who has shoulder pain when he raises his arm. Based on the initial symptom, the doctor may form various hypotheses: rheumatoid arthritis, rotator cuff tear, periarthritis humeroscapularis, radiating pain from cervical spine syndrome, etc. Each of these presumptions is checked by the doctor using appropriate examination methods. One by one, the possible hypotheses are ruled out until only one remains which is then the diagnosis.

The **hypothetical/deductive method** is also known as the **"guess and test model"** (Scott 2002) and is widely used in medicine and physical therapy (Cutler 1998). Using the example of shoulder pain, a physical therapist would consider such causes as shrinkage of the joint capsule, inflammation of the supraspinatus tendon, hypermobility, and bursitis. The hypotheses may also be divided into categories. For

instance, using the ICF model (International Classification of Functioning, Disability and Health, see p. 7), categories would be physical functions/structures or activities and participation (Cutler 1998; Jones and Rivett 2004). Using the appropriate methods, the physical therapist then tests his presumptions and, by the process of elimination, arrives at a diagnosis.

One drawback of this procedure is that the number and probability of hypotheses depends on the knowledge of the therapist. Those with less knowledge and experience can hardly come up with further hypotheses and thus may overlook other possible causes. Those with extensive knowledge must organize the many possibilities well, so as not to lose themselves in the possibilities. Furthermore, testing all possible diagnoses can take a significant amount of time.

The advantage is that the experienced therapist can quickly make a diagnosis using the hypothetical/deductive method and can save time and also have a guideline for difficult cases (Cutler 1998).

4.2   Pattern Recognition

Pattern recognition allows for a "**diagnosis at a glance**" (Cutler 1998). It is viewing the patient on a holistic level and assessing similarities between the current and former patient (Newble et al 2002). For instance, seeing an older patient with bent posture and shuffling steps, shaking hands, and a frozen expression on his face would suggest Parkinson disease to the therapist (Cutler 1998).

A significant advantage of pattern recognition is the speed with which a diagnosis can be made. Yet quickly settling on a subjective hypothesis can lead to overlooking clinically important findings. Pattern recognition is also dependent on the knowledge and clinical experience of the therapist.

Pattern recognition should be distinguished from recognition of clinical patterns during the examination. This refers to a comparison of current facts with known clinical presentations. The sum of various symptoms and clinical signs indicates a specific disease.

The following symptoms are an example of the clinical pattern of subacromial impingement: gradual development of pain associated with working with the arms raised overhead, lateral to the acromion at about 160° abduction/elevation without cervical spine involvement. There is pain upon palpation near the tendon insertion site of the supraspinatus muscle as well as a positive resistance test upon abduction (triggering pain and weakness), etc.

4.3   Systematic Examination Structure with Orienting Questions

4.3.1   Systematic Examination Structure

In the systematic step-by-step method, a given series of examination steps is always followed in the same manner. This is a traditional component of manual therapy (Mennell 1949; Cyriax 1982; Frisch 2001; Kaltenborn 2003). Adhering to a strict sequence of steps is intended to avoid missing something in daily routine (Lamb 1994) and to maintain a clear head for interpreting individual signs (Debrunner 1995). A **programmed and systematic examination structure** is also recommended in medicine (Cutler 1998). The procedure may be depicted in algorithmic decision trees (Waddell 1998).

Kaltenborn initially divided the examination structure based on the techniques used. The first step was the patient interview, with five sub-points: current symptoms, course up until present, social history, health development, family history. Next, a functional examination was performed with five main points which were subdivided into five more points (Kaltenborn 1992a, b; Frisch 2001) (**Table 4.1**).

This examination procedure was further developed by Kaltenborn during the 1990s (Kaltenborn and Evjenth 1999). Instead of performing all techniques in a series, Kaltenborn emphasized the significance of each step creating a logical sequence of examination steps. In the clinical reasoning process, he emphasized the well thought-out solution, which must be decided individually—and should nevertheless follow a clear scheme. As Kaltenborn said: "We need thinking therapists!"

The first step in the examination is to define the patient's problem using a precise description (Schomacher 2001a). The often numerous symptoms must then be condensed into a manageable number. Kaltenborn referred to this as a screening **examination** which provides a preliminary orientation (Kaltenborn 2011 and 2012). This primarily means identifying the joint associated with the symptoms. The **specific examination** then analyzes the individual joint features. The results are interpreted as the physical therapy (PT) diagnosis and form the basis for treatment.

Table 4.1 Former structure of the functional examination

I **Inspection**	Everyday movements Posture Form Skin Aids
II **Movement tests**	Active rotatory movements Passive rotational movements Translatoric movements with traction/compression Translatoric movement with gliding Resistance tests
III **Palpation**	Skin and hypoderm Muscles and tendons Tendon sheaths and bursae Joints Nerves and vessels
IV **Neurological tests**	Segment-indicating muscle and reflexes Sensitivity Motor function with strength and reflexes Coordination Cranial nerve examination
V **Additional tests**	Imaging studies Laboratory tests Puncture and excision Electrodiagnosis Organ examination

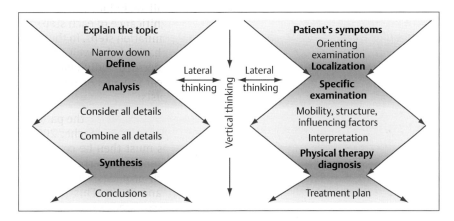

Fig. 4.1 Schematic depiction of dialogue structure based on Plato's "The Phaedrus" (left), and the corresponding steps in the systematic step-by-step examination.

The OMT examination procedure clearly shows similarities to the structure of a dialogue with a definition, analysis, and synthesis of a topic as was already described by Plato in the dialogue between Socrates and Phaedrus (Schomacher 2001a) (**Fig. 4.1**). In this procedure, a distinction may be made between vertically converging and horizontally divergent thinking (Jones and Rivett 2004; Klemme and Siegmann 2006).

4.3.2   Orienting Questions for Patient Classification

Not every examination step is performed on every patient — but every step is considered, as suggested by Kaltenborn's statement about "thinking therapists." The decision to skip a step is also made as part of a deliberate clinical reasoning process. This decision may be facilitated by the use of specific orienting questions. These lead one through the examination and help to classify the patient and his or her symptoms and clinical signs (see **Fig. 4.2**). Once the answer to an orienting question has been found, one may proceed with the next step in the examination without additional testing. Taken together, the answers provide the PT diagnosis.

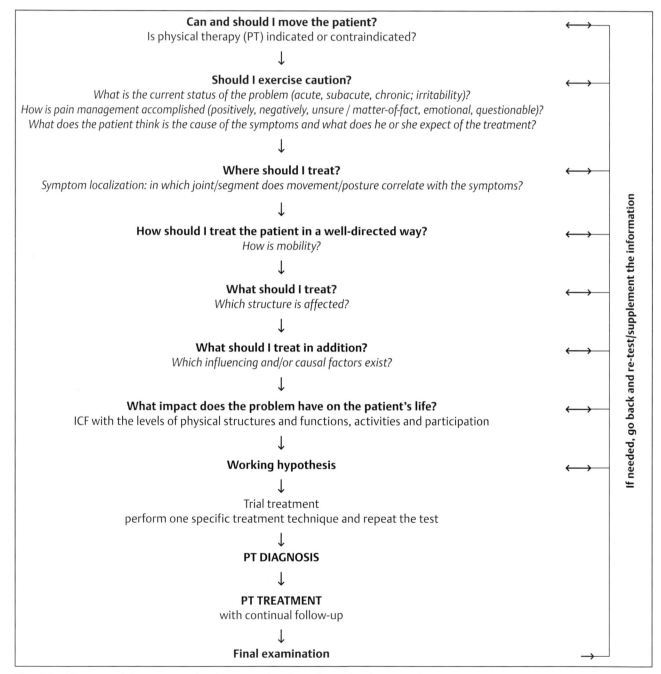

Fig. 4.2   The manual therapy examination procedure based on orienting questions.

Orthopedic manual therapy (OMT) may be divided into

- the examination,
- treatment, and
- research (IFOMPT 2008).

The OMT examination is characterized by a focus on joint mechanics as well as the use of a systemic step-by-step procedure containing orienting questions. This aspect was discussed in Chapters 3 and 4.

Before and during the examination using movement tests, the physical therapist must continually confirm that there are no contraindications to OMT or to a specific movement. Although the prescribing physician has already ruled out the presence of any contraindications, there is always the possibility of a new one arising during the time between the physician consultation and the visit to the physical therapist. With colleagues as well, one must check whether movement is contraindicated. Given the importance of indications and contraindications, these are discussed in a separate chapter (see p. 55).

The aim of the examination is to identify the somatic dysfunction (= physical malfunction) that is correlated with the patient's symptoms. This includes symptoms and functional disorders and consists of:

- Symptoms such as a feeling of physical discomfort, pain, etc.
- Altered mobility such as hypomobility (= restricted movement) or hypermobility (= greater and/or more poorly controlled movement)
- Tissue changes such as edema, atrophy, etc.

The examination and subsequent treatment may alleviate the problem, but those factors should be identified which are causing the problem and which potentially have a negative effect. This is the question posed by the physical therapist in the analysis of additional dysfunction affecting the locomotor system. The therapist should also check the patient's own knowledge of the pathology, self-management measures, and causal or exacerbating factors.

In summary, the OMT examination has the following objectives:

In regard to *symptoms*, the therapist must determine

- whether there are any contraindications to OMT or to a given movement,
- where the symptoms are located, and
- what type of somatic dysfunction is present.

Additional *functional disorders* are analyzed for

- possible causes of the somatic dysfunction, and
- influencing factors.

The *knowledge of the patient* is checked for awareness of

- the causes of the pathology and influencing factors as well as
- self-management measures.

In clinical practice, the techniques are often applied in the following order. Yet it is the treatment goal that is important, and this is determined by the responses to the key examination questions. To answer these, the physical therapist should select the appropriate techniques at every step of the examination.

> **Note**
> The principle of the OMT examination may be stated as follows (Schomacher 2001): **Examine as little as possible**, to avoid worsening the condition with excessive testing, and as **much as necessary** in order to choose targeted and currently appropriate treatment measures.

In actual practice, the examination consists of the following steps.

5.1   Orienting Examination

The orienting examination has the goal of

- determining the acuteness of the problem,
- identifying any contraindications to OMT or a specific movement, and
- locating the responsible area or joint/segment (= symptom localization/localization of region).

Depending on what is needed, the examination may be performed using various techniques: eliciting the patient history, physical inspection, movement tests, palpation, and neurological and vascular tests. In the present book, movement testing consists of the examination of movement around and along the axes, viz. rotatory and translatoric movements.

To collect the patient history, the therapist asks about the history of the problem and current symptoms. This process may be facilitated by using specific questionnaires (Schomacher 2001a). Scales such as the visual analogue scale (VAS) may also help make it easier to describe certain information such as pain intensity (Schomacher 2008a). At the beginning, the therapist should narrow down the questions to focusing on the symptoms (**Table 5.1**).

The patient's medical history may later be expanded during the functional examination, especially after the dysfunction that is correlated to the symptoms has been identified.

During the orienting examination, the physical therapist should select and apply only those techniques which will lead to a preliminary result. These may be:

- symptom alleviation measures (if the symptoms are so severe that they prevent further functional testing that day and the examination must be postponed),
- causal treatment if the problem is readily identifiable,

Table 5.1   The five main symptom questions for the orienting examination

Short question	Note
Where are the symptoms/ where does it hurt?	Where?
How long have you had the symptoms and what happened at the time of their onset?	Since when?
Could you describe the symptoms/pain?	How?
When do symptoms occur during the day and which movements/situations trigger them or make them worse?	When do the symptoms occur and what provokes them?
What are the symptoms related to, e.g., symptoms elsewhere in the body?	What is the complaint related to?

- a certain procedure due to contraindications (e.g., referring the patient back to the physician) and
- with more complex problems, moving on to the specific examination.

The use of an orienting examination is intended to avoid subjecting the patient to a lengthy specific examination, possibly worsening his or her condition given the specific, often end-range movements. This is an essential part of the application of OMT measures.

5.2   Specific Examination

Once the therapist has determined the acuteness of the problem during the orienting examination, ascertained that there are no major contraindications for movement that day, and identified which region or joint or spinal segment is involved, then a thorough, targeted examination may be performed. The results of this examination should clearly identify the somatic dysfunction (symptoms and functional disorder with tissue changes), the causal and influencing factors, as well as the patient's level of knowledge of the problem. The steps in the OMT examination are commonly performed in the following order:

1. Thorough patient history
2. Inspection in resting positions and movement testing (including superficial palpation = "seeing with the fingers")
3. Movement tests
   a) Rotatory movement testing = active and passive movements with end-feel and stability tests
   b) Translatoric movement testing = joint play with end-feel
   c) (Primarily) muscle tests = resistance tests and additional tests (muscle length…)
4. Structure-specific palpation
5. Neurological and vascular tests

5.3 Additional Physician Examinations

Only after the physiotherapeutic functional examination are the physician's findings reviewed or the doctor contacted for further assistance. This avoids searching during the examination for what one has read on paper. The physical therapist's own unbiased examination is complemented by the physician's report and checked against it. An exception, of course, is post-traumatic and postoperative physical therapy for which the therapist collects all relevant information before the examination about previous medical measures.

a. Imaging studies, laboratory tests, puncture aspiration, excision
b. Electrodiagnostic tests (EEG, EMG, etc.)
c. Organ examination by a specialist
d. Medical treatment (medication, sick leave, etc.)

5.4 Summary Evaluation

The summary of the examination results forms a hypothesis upon which to base further action. The most structure-specific treatment possible for the presumed functional disorder should be chosen as a trial treatment (Kaltenborn 2005). This will either lead to improvement, supporting the working hypothesis, or it will worsen or fail to change the symptoms, which means that the examination must be re-evaluated. One should bear in mind the systematic procedure based on orienting questions for the examination (see p. 24).

It should be mentioned that a physical therapy diagnosis of posture and movement is by no means a permanent diagnosis. For instance, after successful treatment of a movement limitation due to shortened muscles, capsular shrinkage may then be identified as a further factor limiting movement. The diagnosis must therefore be checked before and after each treatment session and adjusted as needed according to the new results (Kaltenborn 2005).

> **Note**
> Working hypothesis → Trial treatment → Current diagnosis

The response of the patient to the trial treatment, along with an evaluation of the nature of the problem, allows for an initial prognosis on the possible development of the disorder. This is important for the patient who often wants at least an idea of what may be expected. By presenting the patient with a realistic and positively formulated prognosis, the therapist can encourage his or her cooperation in treatment.

The therapist should also avoid "overexamining" the patient during the specific examination. The number of movements and tests should not make the patient feel worse than before the examination. The art of examination is to choose only those techniques which are considered necessary without overlooking anything. The suggested order is merely meant to serve as a checklist to avoid forgetting something; certain points may be skipped if they do not appear to be necessary for an individual patient.

> **Note**
> **Goal of the examination:**
> Determine
> the *indications and contraindications* to OMT or to a given movement; the *somatic dysfunction:*
> - symptoms (incl. acuteness),
> - mobility: hypomobility, hypermobility, or physiological mobility,
> - tissue change,
> additional *factors* with
> - causal, and
> - influencing effects,
> the *knowledge of the patient* of:
> - the cause,
> - influencing factors, and
> - self-management measures.
>
> **Procedure:**
> **Following the orienting questions**
> *I Orienting Examination*
> *II Specific Examination*
> 1. Comprehensive patient history
> 2. Inspection in resting positions and during movement (including superficial palpation)
> 3. Movement tests
> - Rotatory movement testing = active and passive movements with end-feel and stability tests
> - Translatoric movement testing = joint play and end-feel
> - (Primarily) muscle tests = resistance tests and additional tests (muscle length …)
> 4. Structure-specific palpation
> 5. Neurological and vascular tests
>
> *III Additional Testing by a Physician*
>
> *IV Summary Evaluation*
>
> Working hypothesis → Trial treatment → Current diagnosis

*"If you don't know where you are going,
you risk taking a long time to get there."*
(Tuareg proverb)

The examination implies a search for a problem. Thus it is important for the physical therapist to know what he or she is searching for when testing the patient's movement.

As previously explained, the main goal of the examination is to analyze the symptoms, dysfunction, and level of knowledge of the patient and to understand the relationships between symptoms and dysfunctions as well as the patient's beliefs and attitudes. In this context, the examination of movement is related primarily to the following aspects:

- Quantity of movement
- Quality of movement with end-feel
- Symptoms during movement.

In manual therapy, movement testing uses rotatory and translatoric motions. The point of this approach is briefly outlined in the following before the above-named aspects are further discussed.

6.1   Why Rotatory and Translatoric movement tests?

General rotatory movement tests provide information on the movement direction causing the symptoms, and help to roughly locate which segment of the locomotor system is involved. Specific rotatory and sometimes also translatoric movement tests determine which of the joints or vertebral segments involved produce a change in symptoms (symptom localization tests). The rest of the examination should show whether it is the actual joint/segment that is responsible for the symptoms or whether the surrounding soft tissues are the cause.

In order to find out which joint/segment most strongly correlates with the symptoms, the physical therapist first observes and analyzes which joints/segments are involved in motions that produce pain. Next, each of these joints/segments is tested individually. If there is considerable pain, the therapist may do this with specific movements from the zero position moving toward the painful direction. Alternatively, and often easier with milder symptoms, the therapist may ask the patient to move to the limit of his or her pain threshold and to hold that position. From there the physical therapist moves each of the joints individually further in the symptom-producing direction, asking the patient whether there is a change in symptoms (**Fig. 6.1**). If the patient answers affirmatively, then the joint/segment correlates with the symptoms (Schomacher 2001a, 2006). Depending on the symptoms present and how well they may be controlled, this procedure can be repeated in different variations.

The following four aspects should be taken into account for symptom localization:

1. The tests are performed with the patient and the joints in the position and in the direction which most easily produces the symptoms with the least risk.

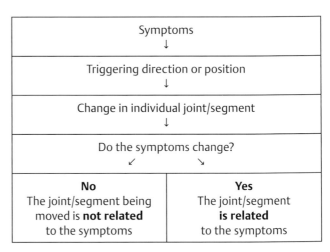

Fig. 6.1   Procedure for symptom localization.

2. The patient should perform the test actively first, if possible. If this does not supply enough information, the therapist should assist with active movement. If the results are still insufficient, passive movements should be performed until the therapist has the required information. Following this procedure helps to avoid any unnecessary risks—especially when testing the spine.
3. The precision of symptom localization may vary from a single region to an individual joint or vertebral segment. The therapist stops searching once sufficient information for determining treatment has been obtained, or once he or she believes that further tests may exacerbate the symptoms.

4. If the symptoms are provoked, they must be controllable by the patient and quickly relieved after provocation. Otherwise, the therapist should use movements for pain-relief or avoid movement testing that day for symptom localization. The examination should never worsen the patient's symptoms.

If a joint is moved around its axes, all of the structures involved undergo a change in stress:

- The articular surfaces and underlying bone are under stress at various sites.
- The intra-articular structures such as menisci are displaced.
- The joint capsule/ligament complex is elongated on one side and relaxed on the other side.
- The surrounding soft tissues are also lengthened on one side and relaxed on the other.

If this produces symptoms or malfunction, a number of structures may be responsible. An evaluation of movement quality gives the therapist the possibility to collect information about the symptom-altering or dysfunctional structure. Rarely is a single test result sufficient for evaluation, however. After testing rotatory movement, the individual structures should be tested specifically. The joint itself is checked with translatoric movement tests and the surrounding soft tissues are evaluated by muscle tests as well as neurological and vascular tests.

Translatoric movement tests specifically

- use traction to relieve the joint surfaces and underlying bones of the pressure on the joint (especially interesting when there is pain at rest), and to test the joint capsule/ligament complex which is placed under tension;
- use compression to increase articular pressure on the joint surfaces and underlying bones;
- use gliding tests to test the gliding ability of the joint surfaces as well as the joint capsule/ligament complex under increased tension.

When testing joint play (= translatoric movement testing), one joint partner is fixated and the other is moved in a straight line and in a translatoric way in relation to the treatment plane.

The amount of translatoric movement is so minimal, especially in the resting position, that there is no significant tension in the surrounding soft tissues like muscels. Thus translatoric movement testing enables one to obtain targeted information on the structures of the actual joint.

The translatoric examination movements are first performed in the resting position because here the range of motion is the greatest and thus assessment is easiest. If palpation is good, the therapist may proceed with tests that are not in the resting position (see p. 19).

6.2 Quantity of Movement

The range of motion shows whether joint movement is limited (= hypomobile), excessive (= hypermobile), or whether there is physiological mobility. For rotatory values, the following guidelines are used for evaluation (normal, comparison of sides, and comparison with overall constitution).

Standardized Normal or Average Values

For each joint, average ranges of motion have been derived from the average population. One should keep statistical variation in mind and that certain patients may have slightly higher or lower physiological mobility. Variation is a statistical measure of deviation of the characteristics of the whole group from the mean.

Comparison of Sides

The joints on either side of the body usually have roughly the same degree of mobility. Slight differences are also possible in physiological mobility. In the spine, the mobility of a single spinal segment/region is compared

(e.g., lower lumbar spine) with the adjacent regions (such as hip joints and middle and upper lumbar spine as well as thoracic spine).

Comparison with the Remainder of the Joints

This enables one to evaluate whether the patient is very flexible or rather more "stiff" in general. Thus one may expect more or less movement than average for a given joint.

To standardize the measurement of angles, these rotatory movements are performed as simple movements around an anatomical axis and in an anatomic plane. Everyday functional movements occur simultaneously, however, as combined movements around several anatomical axes and outside of the anatomic planes (Kaltenborn 2005). As described in the section on osteokinematics (see p. 11), these may be divided into coupled and uncoupled movements. Coupled movements occur automatically, have a larger range of motion and less of a hard or firm end-feel than uncoupled movements. These characteristics should be recalled when testing movement.

The range of rotatory movement is usually given in degrees. In joints in which the range of motion is too small to be measured with a goniometer or in which the placement of a goniometer is difficult, and especially for translatoric movements in which the joint partners do not change their angle to one another, the range of motion must be estimated. A scale of 0 to 6 is commonly used (**Table 6.1**) (Kaltenborn 2004). When examining the quantity of movement, the rotatory movements should be performed slowly. The range of translation until there is an initial, easily palpable barrier may be tested using slower or gentle, quicker movements.

Rotatory movement testing may reveal limitations in various directions. The extent of limitation may also occur in a certain pattern. For instance, at the glenohumeral joint, if external rotation is more limited than abduction, which in turn is more restricted than internal rotation, this suggests capsular shrinkage given the arrangement

of connective tissue fibers. The pathology affects the entire capsule/ligament complex. Similarly, if the direction of movement is painful in a joint-specific order, involvement of the entire capsule/ligament complex may be presumed.

Cyriax called this joint-specific order of limitations and/or painful directions of movement a capsular pattern or capsular sign. When evaluating the capsular pattern, the end-feel is also crucial (Schomacher 2004b). This may be "physiological" or "pathological" and will be discussed later in a separate section on the quality of movement (see p. 31).

> **Note**
>
> A capsular pattern refers to the joint-specific characteristic sequence of limited and/or painful movements in shrinkage or pain affecting the entire joint capsule.

If a contracture or injury affects only a portion of the capsule—for example, following trauma—then the limitation or pain only occurs with those movements that cause tension in that part of the capsule.

Table 6.1 Classification of range of motion

Level		Description
0	Ankylosis	No mobility
1	Restricted mobility	Very limited mobility
2		slightly limited mobility
3	Physiologically mobile	Physiological mobility
4	Hypermobility	Slightly hypermobile
5		very hypermobile
6	Completely unstable	No longer controllable hypermobility

> **Note**
>
> **Quantity of movement**
> describes the extent of movement in comparison
>
> - with standardized average values,
> - with joints on the unaffected side of the body or—in the spine—with adjacent vertebral segments/regions, and
> - with overall individual constitution.
>
> Quantity can be measured by degrees during rotatory movements, or alternatively, rotation and translation may be estimated on a scale of 0 to 6.

6.3   Quality of Movement with the End-Feel

The characteristics of motion are already evaluated while the patient actively performs the movement: whether it is done with trepidation or not, whether the movement is performed smoothly or in a jerky fashion, and whether it can be performed correctly. Passive movement, in particular, provides the therapist with a wealth of information. Every joint in which there is impairment of physiological movement function has an altered quality during passive movement. Restricted joint mobility always begins with restricting gliding of the joint surfaces (Kaltenborn 2004) which the experienced examiner can feel as the altered quality of movement even before any significantly changed range of motion is noticeable. In hypermobility as well, if the capsule/ligament complex becomes looser, the quality of movement changes.

Attention is paid to movement quality during passive rotatory and translatoric movements. The feeling of the

movement from the start to the first more or less easily palpable barrier may reveal more or less resistance than expected. Also, crunching or friction, as well as "jumping," may be felt. Beyond this first barrier, the resistance increases in a characteristic way for each joint until the final barrier for that joint is reached. This criterion is known as the "end-feel" and it provides information about the structures that limit the range of motion. The end-feel begins with the first barrier and continues until the last, which cannot be reached in every patient, depending on whether it produces symptoms (which should be avoided). The range of motion of the end-feel is also a clue to the condition of the structures limiting movement. When palpating the end-feel, additional resistance may sometimes be felt as a second or even third barrier (see examples below) (**Fig. 6.2**).

Note
Quality of movement
describes

- the character of the movement from the start to the first barrier, and
- the end-feel, which represents the quality of movement between the first and last barriers.

The end-feel is basically described as one of two types: physiological or pathological.

The **types of physiological end-feel** are:

- *soft and elastic end-feel:* muscle mass or muscle tension stops the movement, for example, in knee flexion (muscle approximation) or—often—dorsal flexion of the ankle joint with an extended knee joint (muscle lengthening);
- *firm and elastic end-feel:* the capsule and ligaments stop the movement, for example, during external and internal rotation of the femur and humerus;
- *hard and elastic end-feel:* the bony structures stop the movement, for example, as in elbow extension. The elasticity of the end-feel is the result of tension on the capsule/ligament complex when the contact between the bones on one side of the joint causes gaping on the other. During elbow extension, for instance, the olecranon process fits into the olecranon fossa and there is gaping on the anterior joint aspect which is restricted by the capsule/ligament complex.

A hard and nonelastic end-feel occurs physiologically with straight-lined translatoric compression and when closing the mouth.

The **types of pathological end-feel** are:

- an end-feel which occurs at *another place* in the movement pathway and/or has a *different quality* (may also be pain) than typically seen in that joint;
- an empty end-feel, that is, *pain* prevents feeling the actual barrier. This type of end-feel is "void of information" (Cyriax 1982).

It should be noted that not every painful end-feel is empty. The braking tissue may react painfully to increased tension during testing of the end-feel. This results in a soft-elastic, firm-elastic, or hard-elastic and simultaneously painful end-feel.

One example is physiological external rotation of the glenohumeral joint. The therapist begins the passive movement and feels the weight of the arm being moved without any resistance to friction. Then the therapist feels the first barrier, which suggests the start of tightening of the capsule/ligament complex. Continuing the movement, the therapist may evaluate the end-feel, which is firm and elastic up to the last barrier which is caused by the capsule/ligament complex.

If there is slightly painful hypomobility at the glenohumeral joint during external rotation, the therapist may sense increased resistance to movement immediately after beginning the movement. The first barrier is felt earlier than in physiological mobility and may also be unusually soft, suggesting tension in the internal rotators which are beginning to halt the movement. When detecting the end-feel, soon there is a second barrier which is now more clearly felt, and this indicates tightening of the capsule/ligament complex. With continued movement, there is increasingly "firm" resistance up to the last barrier, which causes the pain reported by the patient and occurs earlier than physiologically normal in the movement pathway.

These findings suggest that given the increased resistance to movement upon starting the movement, gliding is restricted, there is defensive musculature tension, and the capsule/ligament complex has shrunk and is rather painful.

During examination of a glenohumeral joint that is hypermobile during external rotation, after beginning movement there may be less resistance than would be expected under physiologically normal conditions. The first barrier is felt late in the movement pathway. There is an increasingly resistant end-feel, which is not soft and elastic, but also not particularly firm and elastic; it feels like pulling on an old rubber band. The last barrier is felt la-

Fig. 6.2 Quality of movement.

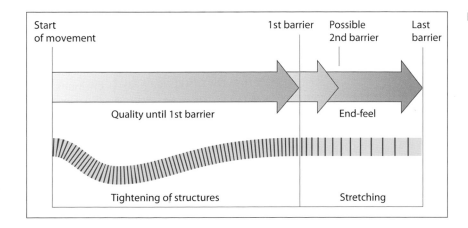

Start of movement   1st barrier   Possible 2nd barrier   Last barrier

Quality until 1st barrier   End-feel

Tightening of structures   Stretching

ter than would be expected under physiologically normal conditions.

It is somewhat difficult to describe the various types of end-feel with words. Perhaps they are better illustrated by an image comparing them with laundry. As every house-wife or house-husband knows, clothes are easier to iron if they have been laid flat and stretched out after washing to eliminate wrinkles when hung up to dry. If one separates the individual items, each one has a different "end-feel."

If new clothes are washed for the first time according to the instructions, the end-feel should stay the same, or "physiologically" normal: a woolen sweater would have a soft and elastic feel, a tightly woven T-shirt would be firm and elastic, and jeans would feel very firm with barely any elasticity. A hard end-feel would not occur unless a pair of overalls had been dropped into concrete mix and came out "rock hard."

If the water is too hot the second time around, the clothes will shrink and have a "pathologically" changed end-feel. With the woolen sweater, the first barrier would be felt earlier, with increased resistance to movement; the end-feel is not as soft and elastic as before. For the T-shirt and jeans as well, the first barrier occurs earlier, the resistance to movement is greater, and the end-feel is more firm than before. The changes suggest "restricted mobility."

Hypermobility may be illustrated using a hand-made cotton shirt with an end-feel that is soft and elastic before the first washing and with each subsequent washing is increasingly softer. The shirt becomes "worn out" and the end-feel becomes softer than "physiologically" normal.

With a little practice, without looking—only by testing the "end-feel"—one can sense which material is being tested. The same is true of human joints. We cannot see how the movement-restricting structures have changed; by sensing the end-feel the therapist can determine which changes of the movement-limiting structures are probably involved.

Note

The evaluation of rotatory and translatoric end-feel is one of the most important aspects of the OMT examination.

Physiological end-feel
may be

- soft and elastic
- firm and elastic, or
- hard and elastic

(during compression of the joint surfaces and when closing the mouth, the end-feel is hard and not elastic)

Pathological end-feel

- occurs at another site in the movement pathway,
- has another quality than typically seen in that joint, and/or
- has an empty end-feel because pain prevents the palpation of the movement-limiting structures.

6.4   Symptoms

Any symptoms such as pain or instability during movement should be noted. This allows the therapist to estimate the irritability of symptoms and also to identify the joint or spinal segment from which the symptoms can best be influenced. In OMT, symptom localization tests are used which consist of specific movements to provoke the symptoms and/or to alleviate them (Kaltenborn 2005). Assuming one has knowledge of anatomy, it is possible to determine which structures are under tension during specific movements. The tests apply mechanical stress to individual structures, selectively placing them under tension. Any symptoms related to this movement should be produced by the structure or structures under tension and alleviated by the opposite movement. The principle of selective tension, developed by Cyriax, is an important foundation for examination (Cyriax 1982).

Movement is thus analyzed from the perspective of functional anatomy. In addition, the symptoms are placed in relation to the examiner's knowledge of pathology. Certain patterns of symptoms and signs of disease suggest the presence of a disorder. Yet in manual therapy, the feeling of movement is paramount. This provides specific information on the quantity and quality of the functions and structures that are involved and possibly changing the symptoms as explained in the foregoing.

Any form of stress can, given a certain degree of intensity, exceed the limits of the joint and damage the structures involved. This also applies to stress due to movement, which is why any test movement should be performed slowly and under control of the patient. If symptoms occur, the movement may be immediately adjusted or interrupted in order to avoid irritation or even injury.

Immediate symptoms may occur with larger lesions or if structures get significant tension. Often they do not occur, however, until some hours after performing the movement. Symptoms can range from mild, uncomfortable tension to debilitating pain. This often indicates that the structures are overstressed in a usually hypermobile capsule/ligament complex.

When learning manual therapy, in the beginning it is not always possible to avoid "overdosing" movement. It is therefore essential that the teacher allows each student to feel the "right" dosage of movement several times. A small overdose of movement usually leads to minimal inflammation of the joint, similar to mild traumatic arthritis, which should generally resolve in 1 to 3 days after initial immobilization and disuse followed by pain-free movements.

The examination of the joints should be performed with extreme care and attention. To return to the example of washing clothing, one should imagine that rather than stretching out an old pair of jeans, one has to stretch out a 500-dollar woolen sweater.

Note

Aspects of movement testing

Aspect	Contents
Quantity	▪ Range of rotatory and trans-latoric movement
Quality with end-feel	▪ Way in which movement is actively performed ▪ Quality of movement from start until the first barrier ▪ Quality and quantity of end-feel (from the first to last barrier)
Symptoms	▪ Irritability of symptoms ▪ Localization of symptoms

As stated earlier, the biopsychosocial model of the manual therapy examination, which is based on pain physiology and biomechanics, is used to describe the relationship between pain and dysfunction. Similarly, the manual therapy treatment model distinguishes between the treatment of symptoms such as pain and the often-related dysfunction.

7.1 Treatment of Pain as a Symptom

Pain, which is probably the most common symptom, may be considered in various ways. Just as one might distinguish between peripheral and central nervous system (CNS) processes in the origin of pain, for didactic purposes it is helpful to consider treatment options at the various levels of the nervous system.

7.1.1 Pain Treatment in the Periphery

At the **peripheral level,** one must reduce the noxious afferents, diminish receptor excitability, allow physiological wound healing to proceed undisturbed, and increase the ability of the tissue to withstand stress. There are various possibilities for pain relief on a peripheral level. The therapist must decide on an individual basis, based on the examination and the response of the patient, which of these is optimal.

Especially in patients with **acute pain**, it is important to **reduce noxious afferents**. The cause of the damage should be eliminated, if possible. Keeping mechanical aspects of the origin of pain in mind, the physical therapist should aim to reduce the increased tissue tension. If mobility is limited, the shortened structures may be lengthened to decrease the tension during end-range movements. If there is hypermobility, the patient must learn to control his or her movements to avoid the maximum range of motion.

Generalized pain relief may be achieved by decreasing receptor stimulation. This may be done in various ways (Schomacher 2001a, b). **Increasing circulation** can wash out the inflammatory mediators which stimulate the nociceptors of the tissue. Application of **cold** can inhibit biochemical pain mediators such as factor P, desensitize peripheral receptors, and close the gateways in the spinal cord to nociceptive afferents (Zusman and Moog-Egan 2003). Given the vasoconstrictive effects of cold, it is a classic first aid measure for treating sports injuries to prevent an excessive inflammatory response. Longer exposure, however, lowers the tissue temperature which reduces the metabolic rate and thus does not aid the wound healing process (Wolf 2005).

Warmth, electrotherapy, vibration, and **oscillation** all have similar effects on reducing receptor stimulation. The nociceptive afferents are also influenced by sympathetic efferents (Jänig 2003). It is uncertain whether sympathetic hyperactivity or altered sensitivity of the sensory and nociceptive system to adrenaline and noradrenaline is the determining factor (Thaker and Gifford 2002). Some physical therapy approaches, such as connective tissue massage, aim at regulation of the sympathetic nervous system (SNS) when treating diseases influenced by the SNS such as complex regional pain syndrome (CRPS). The manual therapist searches for possible dysfunctions, especially in the region of the thoracic spine, which could disrupt the sympathetic system.

7.1.2 Pain Therapy and Wound Healing

In acute trauma, **undisturbed wound healing** is paramount. The physical therapist must provide the patient with the necessary information and prescribe the movement options and dosage instructions that are appropriate to each phase of healing (**Table 7.1**).

Table 7.1 Phases in wound healing with tissue reactions and movement instructions

Duration	Phases	Tissue reaction	Movement instruction
Up to about day 5	**1. Inflammatory phases** I. Vascular phase II. Cellular phase	▪ Generation of new vessels ▪ Infiltration of leukocytes ▪ Migration of cells such as fibroblasts	No tension on the lesion
Day 5–21	**2. Proliferation phase**	▪ Cells and fiber proliferation – Matrix production (fibroblast activity ↑)	Begin careful movement without tension
Day 21–60	**3. Consolidation phase**	– Production of ground substance ↑ – Increasing thickness of collagen fibers – Remodeling of collagen from type III to type I	Begin increasing tension at the end of movement
Day 60–360	**4. Remodeling phase**	– Reduction in fibroblasts – Further remodeling of collagen from type III to type I – Direction of fibers ↑	Increasing end-range movements and stress (tissue tension ↑)
Source: After van den Berg (2010) , de Morree (2001), and Schomacher (2005b). Phases 3 and 4 are often combined in the **organization phase** as they are difficult to distinguish clinically.			

After the wound has healed—especially in patients with chronic pain as well as for prevention—the patient must increase the ability of the tissue to withstand stress through systematic training (see p. 46). This builds the resistance of the tissue and makes it less vulnerable to being overstressed by microtrauma or macrotrauma.

7.1.3 Pain Treatment in the Central Nervous System

At the **central level** it is important to **avoid sensitization of the nervous system**, which is an essential factor in chronic pain development. Treatment should thus not only reduce or avoid nociception and improve the ability of the tissue to withstand stress, but it must also activate pain-inhibiting mechanisms in the CNS. The therapist may influence nociception at the spinal cord level through the **gate control system**, in the brain stem through the **descending inhibitory mechanisms**, and in higher centers with **pain management strategies**. The basic rule of therapy still holds: treatment—with certain exceptions such as counter irritation—should never be painful.

Gate Control System

The gate control system is active (**Fig. 7.1**) at the spinal cord level. Thickly myelinated excitatory A-beta fibers (e.g., from mechanoreceptors), supported by central control, act via the Rolando gelatinous substance to inhibit impulse transmission of thin excitatory A-delta and C fibers (nociceptors) to the T cells (transmission cells) in the posterior horn (Melzack and Wall 1965, 1996).

Of special importance are the excitatory and inhibitory functions in the Rolando gelatinous substance. If the inhibiting interneurons are stimulated by mechanical A-beta afferents, inhibition of the T cell occurs. If instead the excitatory interneurons are stimulated by nociceptive or mechanical afferents, the facilitation of the T cell results. The spatial separation between excitatory and inhibitory interneurons explains the difference between the effects of A-beta afferents: A-beta afferents in the center of the receptive field stimulate the T cell, while A-beta afferents surrounding the receptive field inhibit the T cell (Melzack and Wall 1996). This explains why mechanical stimuli may either alleviate or exacerbate pain.

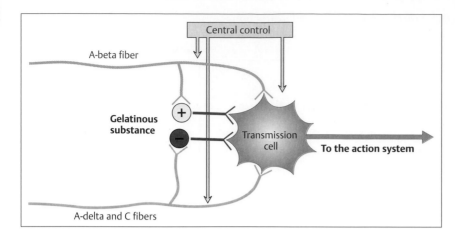

Fig. 7.1 Gate control system (modified after Melzack and Wall 1965, 1996).

Descending Inhibitory Mechanisms

The reticular formation and the periaqueductal gray in the medulla and mesencephalon contain the centers of the **descending inhibitory mechanisms**. These cause presynaptic inhibition using endogenous opiates at the spinal cord level.

Various systems, such as diffuse noxious inhibitory control (DNIC), use these inhibitory mechanisms. In DNIC, pain is inhibited by a "therapeutic pain stimulus" at a site distant from the original lesion. An important factor is the "biological dominance" of the administered pain stimulus. The brain determines what must be consciously sensed at that moment for survival, and whatever is unnecessary to survival may be repressed (Zusman and Moog-Egan 2003). The pain stimulus may be given using a slight prick with an acupuncture needle or by using painful stimuli such as counter irritation techniques. In counter irritation, a painful stimulus at a pain-free site relieves the original pain (Melzack and Wall 1996). Care must be taken to avoid further sensitization of the nervous system when administering "therapeutic pain." The pain must remain controllable and quickly disappear after removal of the stimulus.

Pain Management Strategies

There are a number of treatment procedures that influence pain perception and processing. If a boy falls down, his pain often quickly disappears if his mother gives him a hug and promises him an ice cream. **Influencing the emotional/affective experience** is more complex in adults undergoing physical therapy treatment. Various psychological methods such as cognitive, behavioral, operant, and other techniques for pain processing have a firm place in the realm of pain therapy (Huber and Winter 2006). This also applies to **use of the placebo effect** (Weiss 2003b) and **avoiding a nocebo effect** (Rölli 2004).

Explaining the nature of the pain and the possibilities for influencing it to the patient is a common approach in physical therapy and manual therapy treatment. Detailed strategies for pain management often require expert psychological guidance.

Desensitization of pain-processing systems to movement is a potential starting point for treatment and should be explained to the patient if it is a relevant option.

Summary

Physical therapy and manual therapy do not differ significantly in terms of pain management. A summary of options is provided below.

> **Note**
>
> **Pain therapy at the peripheral level:**
> - Reduce the noxious afferents (eliminate the cause of damage).
> - Reduce the excitability of the receptors using movements such as vibrations and oscillations, massage, thermotherapy, electrotherapy, etc.
> - Allow undisturbed wound healing (trophic conditions ↑, immobilization → dosed movement).
> - Increase the ability of the tissue to withstand stress in order to avoid overstress due to microtrauma/macrotrauma which could trigger pain (dosed training).
>
> **Pain therapy at the CNS level:**
> - Avoid central sensitization.
> - Inhibition ↑:
>   - Gate control
>   - Descending inhibitory mechanisms
> - Pain management strategies

7.2   Treatment of the Dysfunction

Along with treatment of pain, the dysfunction correlated with the pain or symptom can (and should) also be treated. In the view of manual therapy, the dysfunction is a **change in mobility** seen as limited movement or hypermobility and/or a **tissue change** such as atrophy, swelling, edema, etc.

It may be tempting to view the treatment of dysfunction **causally** rather than symptomatically, as for pain relief. Yet in everyday physical therapy practice, it is usually impossible to precisely identify the structural cause of the pain.

Indeed, it is difficult for the physical therapist to identify and treat the responsible structure given the relative lack of structure-specific techniques. It is difficult or even impossible, for instance, to determine clinically whether low back pain is coming from an intervertebral disk or from the zygapophyseal joints (Bogduk 2000). Often, pain is used to assess the effectiveness of a structure-specific treatment technique. Yet in reality, this only indicates the effect on the pain, while its origins remain unclear.

For practical reasons, the therapist must determine which type of tissue most correlates with the dysfunction. This helps with the choice of treatment techniques which vary significantly for articular, neural, or muscular problems or for other problems such as edema and tissue atrophy.

Difficulties can arise when physical therapists define a dysfunction as a "deviation from the norm" and wish to treat it. Different people may have seemingly unusual, yet physiological, ranges of motion, for instance, due to anatomical variation. The literature describes the "average anatomy," and thus while knowledge of anatomy helps to interpret test results, it does not directly determine their correct interpretation. If the clinical appearance does not correspond to the therapist's knowledge of anatomy, then the joint mechanics should be tested again. The end-feel is particularly useful for differentiating anatomical variation from pathological mobility (Kaltenborn 2005). If the end-feel is physiologically normal, then the range of motion for that individual person is normal—even if it differs from the average human being—and does not require treatment.

Note

A central aspect of manual therapy is the **correlation between symptoms and dysfunction**. This relationship should be understood as a phenomenon that helps with the treatment decision. A causal relationship between the symptoms and the dysfunction may be suspected at best, but in everyday practice it can rarely be proven.

In terms of physiology, any movement or manual treatment technique represents a stimulus that acts on the organism. The action potentials that are triggered are sent to the central nervous system (CNS), processed, and evoke the response, which is transmitted along efferent pathways. This results in an overall response of the organism to the stimulus.

Various models are used to explain what occurs in the organism as a result of stimulus processing. These are mainly founded on the knowledge from basic sciences such as physiology, neurology, and pathology. For the physical therapist, such processes are usually hidden in the individual patient. What a therapist usually sees are the effects caused by the efferents. These are evident on various levels:

- The symptoms are alleviated, especially pain.
- Mechanically, the range of motion increases, the muscles relax and/or get stronger, there is less resistance to movement, etc.
- Neurologically, the patient has improved coordination and neurovegetative reactions normalize such as secretion of sweat and skin color, etc.
- On a psychosocial level, the patients experience changes.

The mechanisms of these four effects are briefly explained in the following.

8.1   Effect on Symptoms—Especially Pain

The complex mode of action of individual physical therapy measures on pain-modulating mechanisms has already been discussed (see p. 34). There is also increasing evidence that passive joint mobilization in manual therapy can stimulate the pain relief system of the CNS (Schmid et al 2008; Nijs and van Houdenbove 2009; Nijs et al 2010). This could explain why different movement techniques lead to similar pain relief (e.g., Paatelma et al 2008; Powers et al 2008).

8.2   Effects on a Mechanical Level

In accordance with the concept of how pain originates, from a mechanical viewpoint the goal of manual therapy is **to reduce or avoid the tissue tension** that is causing the pain or symptom. This may be done by lengthening the tissue using **mobilization** of articular, muscular, and neural structures or by **limiting movement**.

8.2.1   Mobilization with Lengthening of Shortened Tissue Structures

When the tissue is "shortened" and is under tension during normal everyday movements, depending on the pathomechanics (see p. 32), pain may result. Movement may be limited by connective, muscle, or neural tissue. If the tissue is "lengthened," there is less tension at the end of the range of motion and thus symptoms are reduced.

"Lengthening" of shortened connective tissue may be accomplished by stretching stimuli, which trigger the corresponding physical and biological reactions. These biomechanical aspects of stretching are explained later under individual aspects of treatment (see p. 52).

The mobility of connective tissue structures may also be limited by **adhesions or attachments** to the surrounding area. This can happen, for instance, with scarring after surgery. Adhesions should be released—and, even better, avoided—using repeated end-range movements.

In "shortened" muscles, **muscle stretching** leads to a larger range of motion, mainly by increasing the tolerance to stretching (Zahnd 2005). Other effects such as injury prevention and reduction of muscle tension and shortening are controversially discussed (Kräutler 2003; Zahnd 2005). It is uncertain how long the stretch should be held in order to lengthen anatomically shortened muscles. Figures vary from about 15 seconds (Wilkinson 1992) to 2 minutes or longer (Evjenth and Hamberg 1984a and b) (see p. 44).

The **neural system** may also exhibit motion limitations compared with surrounding tissues. The responsible pathomechanism is either pressure, as in a herniated disk, or adhesions/"sticking together" of neural tissue with the surrounding tissue, such as after surgery near a nerve. The treatment is causal. If the problem is created by pressure, it must be promptly removed. When there are adhesions/"sticking together" of a nerve with the surrounding tissue, mobilization of the neural structures should be performed without much stretching of the actual neural structures (Coppieters and Butler 2008). Finally, neural

structures can be sensitized to movement/elongation (see p. 44).

Other causes of movement limitation should also be considered. These include **scars** and significant **lymphedema**. The appropriate examination and treatment modalities are taken from physical therapy; there are no approaches specific to orthopedic manual therapy.

> **Note**
>
> Perhaps the stretch mobilization just increases tissue tension, thereby stimulating afferences which might cause changes in the movement pattern and/or neutral output.

8.2.2 Movement Limitation, Movement Control, and Stabilization

Stabilization or control of movement can help avoid tension peaks or persistent tension in movement-limiting structures, which can occur when movement is not adequately controlled. This applies to joints with extreme ranges of rotatory motion. Examples are genu recurvatum or hypermobility of the lower lumbar spine in extension. With classic "postural control" and controlled movement, the patient can actively avoid these maximum positions. Hypermobility or clinical instability may also be present in joints/segments with physiological or even impaired rotatory movement. The patient is unable to hold the joint in the middle of the neutral zone and perform controlled movements. The neutral zone is the

region of high flexibility or laxity around the neutral position (Panjabi 1992).

The stabilizing system that ensures physiological limitation of movement is made up of **the combined action of three elements** (Panjabi 1992):

- Passive structures such as ligaments, capsules, intervertebral disks, etc.
- Active structures such as contractile muscles
- Regulating structures of the nervous system

Manual therapy analyzes the individual elements of this system in each patient. The result is used as the basis for deriving treatment (see p. 45).

8.3 Effects on a Neurological Level

The primary task of the nervous system is to receive information, process it, and respond to it. This requires the undisturbed conduction of electrical impulses and transport of chemical substances in the nervous system (Butler 1995). The network that makes up the nervous system passes through all of the body's tissues (except for cartilage) and thus is also subject to mechanical stress. Disruptions of the nervous system can effect impulse conduction, transport of chemical substances, and ability to withstand mechanical stress. The potential effects of movement therapy on the nervous system are similarly complex. If compression and adhesions have been ruled out as mechanical disturbances of the nervous system, yet neurodynamic tests are positive, the problem is presumably nervous system irritation of unknown cause. Treatment may be attempted by using movements which place the nervous system under longitudinal mechanical tension and then carefully increasing the dosage (Shacklock 2007).

It is still unclear to what degree **neurovegetative symptoms**—from headache to dizziness to complex regional pain syndrome (CRPS)—may be influenced by hypersensitivity of the nervous system. External and also mechanical influences, such as movements in normal or dysfunctional joints, are often described as triggering an extreme response by the neurovegetative system. Based on empirical evidence and anatomical considerations, it is mainly the segments C0–C1 and C2–C3 that are associated with symptoms such as headache, nausea, and dizziness (Cramer 1994; Biedermann 1997, 2000; Jull 1997; Huber and Winter 2006; Jull et al 2007).

Functional disorders affecting the thoracic spine have also been related to neurovegetative symptoms. This has been explained anatomically by the close proximity of the **sympathetic nuclei in the spinal cord from C8/T1 to L2/L3** to the nociceptive afferents of the thoracic spine. In neurovegetative symptoms, it is often worthwhile to perform a trial treatment of such dysfunction (Slater 2001).

8.4   Effects on Psychosocial, Cultural, and Economic Levels

As with any therapeutic intervention, orthopedic manual therapy also has various effects on the psychology of the patient and his or her social, cultural, and economic situation with which it interacts. This important aspect, which also includes the often-positive influence of the placebo effect (Weiss 2003b) and the negative influence of the nocebo effect (Rölli 2003), is an essential part of treatment success. The view of orthopedic manual therapy is the same as that of physical therapy and thus is not further elucidated here. It is important to recall the importance of such aspects in treatment.

8.5   Specificity of Treatment Techniques

One of the cornerstones of orthopedic manual therapy is the specificity of the treatment techniques used. Yet there is still uncertainty as to how specifically a joint may or should be moved (Schomacher 2008b).

Greater specificity of movement is achievable with passive rather than with active movements, and the specificity of movement is more obvious at the extremity joints such as the interphalangeal joints of the fingers. Yet, when the primary movement causes concomitant movements in adjacent joints, the specificity is not so clear. Thus, at what degree of hip joint movement does the lumbar spine begin to move with it or at what point is the movement of the glenohumeral joint transmitted to the acromioclavicular joint? The specificity of spinal mobilization is especially unclear. A few studies have shown, for instance, that posteroanterior mobilization by pushing against one spinal process can cause an increase in lordosis in the lumbar or cervical spine, but without selective movement in a single segment (Schomacher 2008b). Even manual fixation of a caudal cervical vertebra and passive mobilization of the cranial one did not result in movement of one single segment, thus questioning specificity of spinal mobilization (Schomacher and Learman 2010).

The question of the necessary specificity of movement treatments has been answered by studies showing, for instance, that in the cervical spine, even treatment of a site away from the symptom-altering segment can alleviate pain (Haas et al 2003; Cleland et al 2005, 2007; Krauss et al 2008; Aquino et al 2009; Schomacher 2009b).

Thus a large number of patients who are hoping for pain relief could probably be helped by general techniques. The specificity of manual therapy, that is, the movement of a single joint or vertebral segment, is probably only necessary in select patients with intractable dysfunction. This requires a significant amount of manual technical skill which can only be achieved through much practice and precise knowledge of functional anatomy.

Many physical therapists will initially only be able to approach this high level of specificity when attempting to bring about specific movements. Still, the movement primarily affects a joint region and thus for many patients is more helpful than general techniques. The specificity of techniques in manual therapy may be represented by a pyramid, with general measures at the bottom, semi-specific ones in the middle, and specific techniques at the top (**Fig. 8.1**).

- **Specific techniques** (primarily passive), which target a single joint or vertebral segment for mobilization or manipulation. Such techniques are only necessary in a small number of patients with specific dysfunctions.
- **Semi-specific techniques** such as active exercises and passive mobilizations, which are done with an emphasis on the region about a single joint or vertebral segment. Many patients will be better helped by such methods than by general techniques.
- **General techniques** such as exercise, massage, functional massage, etc. Every patient can benefit from these methods.

Note
According to Kaltenborn, specificity of treatment techniques is not necessary for pain relief (Schomacher 2005c). However, if the dysfunction correlates with the symptoms and must be examined and treated, then the technique would have to be specific for the joint (personal communication with F. Kaltenborn, 2007).

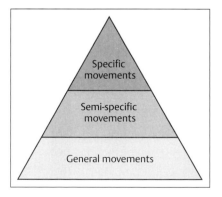

Fig. 8.1 Pyramid showing the specificity of various techniques.

8.6 Summary

Manual therapy has, first of all, a range of effects on various mechanisms in the pain-processing system. Second, it also has effects at a biomedical level on the mechanics of the locomotor system, including the neural system. Third, manual therapy takes into consideration important influences on the patient's experience of disease on psychosocio-cultural and economic levels.

Table 8.1 gives an overview of the therapeutic concepts underlying orthopedic manual therapy. Orthopedic manual therapy may be placed within the biopsychosocial model of disease, the predominant view in physical therapy.

Table 8.1 Overview of treatment models in orthopedic manual therapy

Model of disease		
Biomedical		**Psychosocial**
Mechanical model	**Model of the neural system**	**Psychosocio-cultural-economic model**
A "somatic dysfunction" in which the symptoms **correlate** with altered movement and tissue changes. This includes the mechanics of the neural system.	**Hypersensitivity** of the pain-modulating system and the neurovegetative nervous system influences the symptoms.	Influences from this area shape experience and management of symptoms
Treatment: ▪ Reduce or eliminate the somatic dysfunction, i. e., reduce tension.	Treatment: ▪ Reduce nociceptive afferents ▪ (= treatment of somatic dysfunction) ▪ Stimulation of the analgesic system ▪ Progressive desensitization	Treatment: ▪ Information: education ▪ Instruction: instruct the patient in effective self-treatment, also to enhance belief in self-efficacy. ▪ Further procedures
Specific movement techniques are useful for certain movement disorders (functional disorder with limited or hypermobile joint play).	Specific movement techniques are *probably* unnecessary. (exception: see somatic dysfunction)	Specific movements are not necessary.

Note

Treatment on a biomedical level:

Symptoms
Various possibilities for pain therapy based on pain physiology

Mechanics of the locomotor system:
Pathomechanism: Increased tissue tension correlates with symptoms such as pain.

Consequence for treatment: decrease tension by
▪ lengthening the tissue with stretching and mobilization, and
▪ avoiding end-range motions using control and stabilization of movement

This also applies to the mechanics of the neural system:
Pathomechanism: Neural mobility is limited by compression and/or adhesions/"sticking together" with surrounding tissues and/or irritation of the tissue.

Consequences for treatment:
▪ remove pressure = relief
▪ release adhesions/"sticky" tissues = repeated movement without tension on neural structures
▪ influence irritation = avoid tension and/or aim for adaptation with properly dosed tension

Treatment on psychosocio-cultural and economic levels:
Consideration of these aspects is integrated in the field of manual therapy.
There is no difference here between orthopedic manual therapy and physical therapy.

The examination process results in a description of the somatic dysfunction that correlates with the patient's symptoms as well as any additional causal or influencing factors. This is the physical therapy diagnosis which is based on the biopsychosocial model of disease.

At the level of the psychosocial model of the International Classification of Functioning, Disability and Health (ICF), the diagnosis also includes the interrelations between the patient's problem and his or her everyday activities as well as participation in social and professional life, including biographical and environmental factors. These factors are often crucial to the patient's perception of pain and disabilities. The aims of manual therapy are the same as of physical therapy in terms of influencing such factors. There are many opportunities for doing so, ranging from expressing empathy and acceptance in conversations with the patient to systematically planning consultations. Whenever necessary, the therapist should seek cooperation from a medical treatment team.

The goals of treatment should be formulated together with the patient during the assessment. The patient's expectations are not always the same as the goals of the therapist. Some patients may be resigned, and the therapist may be able to offer support, yet the therapist must also respect the patient's individual perception of his or her quality of life (Kool 2004).

The treatment may be divided into six areas which are devoted to the following points:

- Relief of symptoms including pain
- Movement restrictions (= hypomobility) with associated tissue changes
- Maintaining mobility
- Excessive and insufficiently controlled movement (= hypermobility) as well as bad posture with associated tissue changes
- Tissue changes
- Lacking knowledge about optimal movements and posture as well as other possible causes and influences

The treatment consists of the following measures, the selection of which depends on the affected structure. The same principle applies here as for the examination: much treatment does not always help much. Rather, the effects of a treatment should be controlled after the application of each specific measure. These control tests allow the therapist to respond at any time to developments in the treatment process by making appropriate adjustments. The treatment thus remains specific; thereby unnecessary or even counterproductive measures can be avoided.

The following section presents the six categories of treatment in detail.

Note

Results of Examination

Somatic dysfunction

Lacking knowledge and correct movements as well as optimal posture; additional causal and influencing factors

Symptoms — Mobility (hypomobility, hyper-mobility, or physiological mobility) and posture — Tissue changes

---

9.1 Symptom Relief Measures

The techniques available for pain relief are as varied as the possibilities in physical therapy (see p. 34). It is unclear which of these techniques is the most effective. The indication and dosage appear to be of greater importance than the choice of technique and application site. The indication refers to the decision as to whether or not pain relief measures are needed, either by use of temporary immobilization or repeated pain-relieving movements (Kaltenborn 2005). Alternatively, treatment of the dysfunction may have top priority. The dose refers to the intensity of the application: how long, how intense, and how often should the measure be performed for pain-relief?

In everyday practice, the success of symptom-relieving techniques may be measured with instruments such as the visual analogue scale (VAS). Still, it is unclear what actually causes a reduction in pain. Even natural progression, without treatment, can lead to fewer symptoms.

Ultimately, for the manual therapist the goal of pain relief is the patient's satisfaction as well as to provide a starting point for identifying the dysfunction which correlates with the symptoms and thus being able to treat them with lasting effectiveness.

Typical manual therapy approaches to pain relief include temporary immobilization and pain-relieving movements (Kaltenborn 2005).

> **Note**
>
> **Symptom-relieving measures**
>
> A: Immobilization:
> general: bed rest, etc.
> local: orthopedic corset, bandages, casts, orthopedic inlays, adhesive bandages, belts (sacroiliac belt), etc.
>
> B: General pain-relief measures:
> a. Thermotherapy
> b. Hydrotherapy
> c. Electrotherapy
>
> C: Specific symptom-relief measures:
> a. Intermittent traction (grades I and II) in the three-dimensionally pre-positioned joint (straight-lined translatoric separation of the joint partners),
> b. Vibrations, oscillations, etc.
> c. Rhythmic movements such as knee oscillations
> d. Functional massage as a combination of rhythmic movement and massage

9.2 Measures to Increase Mobility

The examination results indicate whether mobilization techniques or measures for control/stabilization of movement are needed.

The appropriate treatment of movement restriction is based on its cause, that is, whether it is articular, muscular, or neural in nature. Other problems, such as those caused by scarring after a burn injury or edema, are not discussed here in more detail; the treatment of these is based on classic physical therapy measures.

It is difficult to identify a movement restriction clinically as specifically and exclusively due to connective tissue shortening. Pain and other symptoms, in addition to the effects of limited use, also influence the patient's feeling of "stiffness." Patients with restricted mobility often protect the affected area, which further contributes to a feeling of stiffness. Thus patients must first cooperatively practice numerous movement repetitions on their own or with the help of the therapist or a device such as a sling table (Schomacher 2001a).

9.2.1 Treatment of Articular Limitations

The use of traction and gliding techniques to treat movement restrictions related to the joints was traditionally a defining characteristic of manual therapy and continues to be one today. These straight-lined and translatoric movements are intended to avoid point compression of joint surfaces which can occur during rotatory mobilization (Kaltenborn 2005).

Stretching the connective tissue surrounding a joint requires performing grade III movements beyond the first resistance for a sufficiently long period of time. Passive mobilizations/manipulations must always be complemented by active movements. Scientific studies on the cervical spine, for instance, have shown that mobilization alone has merely a placebo effect (Gross et al 2002a; Gross, Hoving et al 2004), while the combination of passive mobilization and self-exercises actually improves symptoms (Gross et al 2002b; Kay et al 2005). Self-exercises are thus

an integral part of manual therapy for the entire locomotor system (see p. 47).

Compression is not used for manual treatment in manual therapy. This is all the more important to recall when joint compression tests produce symptoms (Kaltenborn 2005). Without doubt, compression has stimulating effects on the bones and the cartilage. Yet the physical therapist cannot know or measure characteristics of these tissues. It would therefore be impossible to clinically control the needs and effects of a manual compression treatment on a specific tissue.

Nevertheless, compression as a trophic stimulus resulting from the physiological movements occurring during active exercise and progressive training is progressively increased until the tissue has normalized. Here too, clinical controls are lacking, yet the risk of tissue damage from active, gradually increasing movements performed by the patient is probably lower than it would be from passive movements performed manually by the therapist.

There are some physical therapists who perform compression as a joint treatment; its effects are measured by the influence on pain or on the limitation resulting from pain (e.g., van den Berg 2001). Compression in this case is thus one of an array of techniques for pain relief. Yet any conclusions on its tissue-changing effects are merely speculative.

9.2.2   Treatment of Muscular Limitations

Muscles may be affected by guarding/spasm and/or anatomical shortening. Treatment consists of muscle relaxation or stretching measures. Typical manual therapy treatments include movement repetitions, relaxing traction for mobilization, and specific muscle stretching techniques.

In a functional massage—movement repetitions plus massage—the therapist exerts pressure on the muscle, usually parallel to its fibers, while elongating it (Zahnd and Mühlemann 1998).

In relaxing traction, the therapist performs traction slowly and repeatedly to the end of grade II, that is, into the transition zone (Kaltenborn 2005). This technique primarily allows for reflexive relaxation.

A three-step procedure has been recommended for specific muscle stretching techniques (Evjenth and Hamberg 1984a and b):

- Prior to stretching, the patient contracts the targeted muscle painlessly. This fatigues the muscle and also make it easier to feel, which helps the patient relax it. Contraction is increased before the maximum range of motion and is repeated several times. Step by step the maximum range of motion is gradually approached during the relaxation phase.
- The patient should relax as much as possible and allow the maximum lengthening of the muscle to act as the actual stretch. The stretch is held for 12 to 18 seconds (Wilkinson 1992) or even 2 minutes or more (Evjenth and Hamberg 1984a and b).
- The patient repeatedly activates the muscle antagonists in order to use the increased range of motion caused by the stretching of the agonists. Activation of the antagonists can be promoted by training.

These three steps apply to stretching whether performed by the therapist or the patient. For long-term success, patients should also stretch regularly on their own (Evjenth and Hamberg 1990).

9.2.3   Treatment of Neural Limitations

The network of neural structures that passes through virtually all tissues in the body must adjust to movements in these tissues. As already described, neural mobility may be impaired by pressure and/or adhesions/"sticking to" the surrounding structures and/or irritation/hypersensitivity.

Pressure on the nervous system leads to diminished perfusion and thus oxygen insufficiency, which is quickly "life-threatening" for the nervous system. If involvement of neural structures in the patient's symptoms is suspected, the possibility of neural compression should be checked first and, if necessary, the pressure relieved (Shacklock and Studer 2007).

In **adhesions** or "**sticking together**" of neural structures and surrounding tissues, the therapist may try to repeatedly move the neural structures against the adjacent tissues to improve mobility. Optimally, this "**slider technique**" will separate the adhesions. In practical terms, the proximal portion of the neural structure is relaxed during distal movement and the distal portion during proximal movement (Konrad et al 2008). This largely avoids any tension on the neural structures (Coppieters and Butler 2008).

If neither pressure nor adhesions/"sticking together" of neural structures correlates with the symptoms, **hypersensitivity** of the nervous system may be considered. The corresponding pathomechanisms of pain physiology—peripheral and central neurogenic pain mechanisms as well as disease-induced hyperalgesia—have already been discussed elsewhere (see p. 9).

When there are inflammatory processes near a spinal nerve—an irritated zygapophyseal joint, for instance—the connective tissue of the affected nerve may also react painfully to mechanical stress. The release of inflammatory mediators may sensitize the nerve or its connective tissue. Patient repetition and tension-free movement of the nerve in the tissue ("slider technique") is intended to increase circulation and "wash out" the inflammatory substances.

If this does not relieve the symptoms, the therapist can try to progressively increase neural tension in order to improve tension tolerance. To do so, the nerve is pulled simultaneously on both ends, proximal and distal, until slight tension is felt (Hall et al 1998). This tension-producing movement is also known as the "**tensioner technique**."

> **Note**
>
> **Mobility-increasing measures**
>
> A. Joint mobilization
>   1. Joint mobilizations of only one joint or movement segment with traction and gliding in the (actual) resting position
>   2. Joint mobilizations outside the resting position
>   3. Translatoric mobilization grips with a rapid application of force: "high velocity thrust of small amplitude" (since its inclusion in 1978 by the IFOMPT in the WCPT, the technique has been a recognized OMT procedure for physical therapists)
>
> B. Soft-tissue mobilizations
>   1. Massage: functional massage, friction massage, etc.
>   2. Active muscle relaxation (using the PNF "hold-relax" technique, postisometric relaxation, reciprocal relaxation, dynamic activity of the antagonists, etc.)
>   3. Passive stretching of shortened muscles (connective tissue structures)
>
> C. Mobilization of neural tissues (dura mater, nerve roots, and nerves)
>   1. Relieve pressure
>   2. Carry out repeated tension-free movements
>   3. Carefully increase neural tension
>
> D. Exercises to promote and maintain the mobility of the soft tissues and joints

9.3 Measures to Maintain Mobility

People who are no longer able to move about normally, whether due to age, disease, or other circumstances, risk losing their mobility. To maintain mobility, regular (i.e., daily) movements must be performed through the entire range of motion for all joints. The most suitable movements are rotatory movements which patients can perform alone. If these are not possible, for instance, due to an external fixation device, translatoric movements should be used in order to maintain as much mobility as possible.

> **Note**
>
> **Measures to maintain mobility**
>
> A. Primarily self-exercises with active and passive movements
>
> B. Any technique from the section on "mobility-increasing measures" may be used

9.4 Mobility-Reducing Measures

As already described elsewhere, joint stability is ensured by a three-part system of passive elements (the connective tissues of the joints), active muscles, and regulating nerves (see p. 39).

9.4.1 Passive Stabilization

Physical therapy treatment does not have any directly strengthening or shortening effects on lax connective tissue structures that stabilize the joint. These passive structures can only be supported by external devices such as orthopedic inlays for instability of the arches of the foot, a lumbar support belt for patients with lumbar hypermobility, or supportive taping for poorly controlled ankle joints.

Concerns that passive stabilization devices will weaken the muscles are unwarranted as long as the appropriate indications are taken into account (**Table 9.1**), and only if the use of stabilizing devices is limited and thus without a risk of atrophy (Schomacher 2001a; Schomacher 2005d).

Certainly, it may be rather tempting for patients to completely and permanently rely on passive stabilization rather than active neuromuscular control. Yet the therapist can counteract this tendency through patient education.

Table 9.1 Indications for passive stabilization with arguments against atrophy risk

Indication	Arguments against risk of atrophy
Trial treatment	▪ Limited to several minutes or hours
Analgesia	▪ Pain inhibits muscle contraction and thus compromises the effects of training ▪ Use of passive aids can reduce pain and improve training ▪ Lumbar spine training in patients with low back pain, e.g., with a belt, yields better results than without in regard to mobility in flexion, pain, functional ability, etc. (Dalichau and Scheele 2004)
Learning movement	▪ Passive stabilizations can provide immediate kinesthetic feedback if the "ideal posture/movement" is lost
Prevention	▪ In high-stress situations (e.g., moving apartments), the use of supportive devices (e.g., belts) offers stabilizing protection and a better training effect

9.4.2 Active Stabilization

The active and guiding elements of the stabilizing system can be treated by **neuromuscular training**. The type of training seems to be unimportant regarding relief of pain and associated disability (Heymann 2002). Dysfunctions such as diminished activation of the deep cervical spine muscles, however, seem to require specific exercises (Falla et al 2008; Schomacher 2012). Whether classic, strength-building exercises based on training principles or a training program emphasizing muscle activation, coordination, and movement control is more appropriate, mainly depends on the patient's willingness to cooperate and on the rehabilitation phase. Initially, the patient is given low-load exercises with the goal of functional adaptation. Later, high-load exercises are given in order to stimulate morphological adaptation (Jull 2009).

Active training methods were established in manual therapy during the 1960s by a group of Scandinavian physical therapists working with Kaltenborn. Over the years, the group developed various techniques for stabilization and control of movement called "medical training therapy" which may be performed with or without training equipment (Jacobsen 1992; Grimsby 2000).

> **Note**
> The success of any active training program depends on the patient's motivation to participate (Richardson et al 1999). In addition to biomedical effects, there are also positive psychosocial effects from merely participating in an exercise program (Gibbons and Comerford 2002).

■ Static Stabilization Exercises

In static stabilization exercises, the therapist initially stimulates the joint or vertebral segment with joint play movements, asking the patient to resist (Schomacher 2001a). Depending on the possible joint play, the resistance may be to axial pull (traction) and pressure (compression) or to gliding. In addition, (the most) specific rotatory movements may be used. Variations include changing the degree of resistance or the starting position. Another variation is static or dynamic resistance using a short or long lever.

■ Dynamic Movement Control

Dynamic movement control typically begins with passive movements which allow the patient to perceive the kinesthetic sense or "feel of the movement" (Schomacher 2001a). Afterward, the patient should perform the movement with assistance, and finally should move alone and against resistance. Again, the therapist is free to vary treatment while adhering to basic principles. This includes adjusting the strength of resistance, speed or direction of movement, and changing the starting position. Also, the number of joints involved in the movement may be increased, or closed or open kinetic chains may be used.

"Functional exercises" may be used to adapt dynamic movement control to movements in the patient's occupation and everyday life (O'Sullivan 2000). Exercises such as selectively contracting the transversus abdominis and multifidus muscles to treat hypermobility of the lumbar spine (Richardson and Jull 1995; Richardson et al 1999) are readily incorporated into this type of training program. Mental training, or visualization of the "correct" movement, is another way to enhance perception and motor learning (Schomacher 2001a). After the patient has gained more control of movement, a systematic training program based on the physiology of training can follow with the aim of increasing the ability of the tissues to withstand stress, improving endurance, and increasing muscle volume (Evjenth and Schomacher 1997).

9.4.3 Treatment of Hypomobility in Adjacent Joints

"Stiff" joints or vertebral segments can increase the stress on adjacent joints, leading to hypermobility. Treatment of these movement restrictions reduces the stress on hypermobile joints (Kaltenborn 2004). A classic example is restricted hip joint mobility. This causes compensatory lumbar spine hypermobility to preserve the body's general functional mobility (Greenman 1998).

9.4.4 Avoidance of End-Range Movements

Any measure for stabilization or control is only effective as long as the patient is cooperating and avoids end-range movements or positions. If a patient with lumbar hypermobility in extension resumes his or her usual poor posture following physical therapy and training, with the pelvis pushed forward and thoracic spine backward, this can significant extend hypermobile lumbar spinal segments and erase the success of the treatment. Postural and movement control, that is, avoiding end-range movements, are thus a significant part of treating hypermobility.

> **Note**
> **Measures to reduce mobility**
> A. Passive stabilization: support and control measures (belts, tape, etc.)
> B. Active stabilization: exercises for better control and reduction of joint mobility
> C. Mobilization of hypomobile adjacent joints/segments
> D. Avoidance of end-range movements

9.5 Physical Therapy Tissue Treatments

Problems such as edema (e.g., in patients with venous or lymphatic disorders) and tissue atrophy (e.g., in complex regional pain syndrome or osteoporosis) are treatable by physical therapy. Targeted training may also be used as a tissue treatment. The tissue treatments used in manual therapy are taken from physical therapy.

9.6 Information, Instruction, and Training

The goal of pain-free, maximum functioning is nearly impossible to achieve without the cooperation of the patient. Providing information and possibilities for self-help as well as instruction are an essential part of manual therapy. Indeed, passive mobilization of a connective tissue limitation is only successful if the patient augments it with **active exercises**, **self-mobilizations**, and **positions**. The same applies to other areas of treatment as well. To ensure the patients' motivation and improve their management of pain and dysfunction, the therapist should offer a readily understandable explanation of the problem.

> **Note**
> **Information/instruction and training**
> A. Inform the patient about his or her symptoms, any additional causal or negative influences, and preventive measures; acquisition of behavior patterns that are adapted to the pathology during activities of daily living, e.g., improve static balance, postural education, back training exercises
> B. Exercises for mobility, coordination, muscle strength, endurance, and speed: medical training therapy

The following overview summarizes the six categories of treatment.

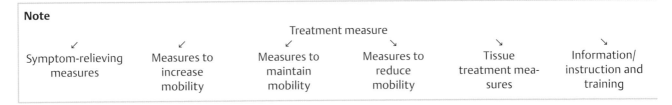

Note					
		Treatment measure			
↙	↙	↙	↘	↘	↘
Symptom-relieving measures	Measures to increase mobility	Measures to maintain mobility	Measures to reduce mobility	Tissue treatment measures	Information/ instruction and training

The manual therapy treatment is directed at the joint which correlates with the symptoms and demonstrates the dysfunction reported by the patient. Even (currently) asymptomatic joints may be treated if their malfunctioning (especially mechanical) has an effect on the symptomatic joint.

The results of the systematic examination should have shown:

- whether a joint changes the symptoms,
- whether there is joint dysfunction (i.e., hypomobility or hypermobility) or physiological mobility, and/or whether static stability problems (posture) are (also) responsible for symptoms,
- whether the symptoms are due to the capsuloligamentous unit, the articular surfaces and/or underlying bone, the surrounding soft tissues, or neural or other structures,
- whether the patient knows why he or she has symptoms, what influences them negatively, what can be done about them, and
- what the patient expects and hopes for from the physical therapist.

Joints that are physiologically mobile are not targeted for treatment. The treatment of hypermobility and static problems has already been discussed elsewhere (see pp. 45 and 47). For more information, interested readers are referred to further education and the literature. The following section addresses the treatment of dysfunction due to hypomobility caused by the capsuloligamentous structure.

The symptoms described are limited to pain from inflammation and irritation of the capsuloligamentous unit. The vast array of other causes of pain has already been dealt with in the discussion on pain physiology (see p. 34). Various treatment modalities are available (see p. 42). Further information on these is available in the literature or by attending further education.

This also applies to patient education. It should be emphasized that the patient's willingness to actively cooperate and perform self-exercises is often critical to a successful treatment outcome. While symptoms may be rather quickly alleviated, even without much effort from the patient, elimination of the actual dysfunction is often a lengthy process.

The following discussion addresses the treatment of hypomobility and pain due to capsuloligamentous causes. In orthopedic manual therapy, the suggested treatment for either cause is straight-lined translatoric traction and gliding. This is by no means the only possible approach, but it is characteristic of manual therapy.

10.1   Why Treatment with Translatoric Movements?

Movement restrictions often occur after prolonged joint immobilization, for example, trauma or inadequate end-range movements, which may be observed in people of all ages, not just older patients. Like any tissue, the hyaline cartilage of the joints responds according to the biological principles of adaptation: minimal stimulation diminishes life functions, a little stimululation enhance them, stronger stimulation inhibits them, and the strongest suspends them (see p. 10; Pschyrembel 2007). Inadequate stimulation of the cartilage results in atrophy and reduces its ability to withstand stress. This primarily affects those parts of the articular surfaces which are normally under stress during end-range movements and which, due to movement limitation, no longer receive these physiological stimuli. The tangential layer of cartilage, for instance, can already disappear after 60 days of immobilization (Akeson et al 1992).

Maximum joint rotation causes the surrounding structures to tighten and the pressure in the joint to increase.

If a patient, for example, attempts to actively use his or her muscles to move further against the limitation, or if he—or the therapist—presses against the bone to go slightly beyond the restriction, this further increases the joint pressure. At the end of the movement, gliding decreases due to increased joint pressure, and rolling predominates. This can ultimately result in impinging joint surfaces with point compression, possibly with very high peaks.

A useful comparison is with the pressure exerted by the heel of a shoe. For example, if a woman weighing 60 kg (130 lb) were to walk over a parquet floor wearing stilettos rather than flat-soled shoes, she would leave holes in the wood. It is not that she is too heavy, but rather the pressure exerted on a single point is too great. Similarly, rotatory mobilization need not be performed with excessive force, and yet, due to point-impinging joint surfaces, high-pressure points could damage the cartilage.

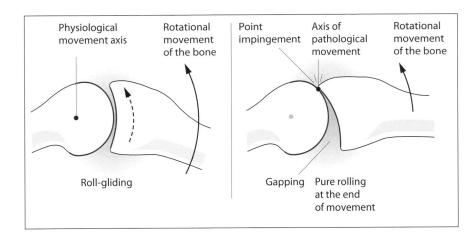

Fig. 10.1 Physiological roll-gliding as well as gaping and point-impinging of joint surfaces in a joint with reduced gliding.

The cartilage is "unfortunately" not innervated. If it were, the patient would quickly perceive the damage as pain. This means that damage may go initially undetected and only manifest clinically years later as a tendency toward arthritis. This has long been recognized in the field of orthopedics (Jordan 1963) (**Fig. 10.1**).

Kaltenborn sought to avoid this problem by using translatoric movements. In straight-lined translatoric traction, the joint partners are moved away from each other, which avoids increasing the pressure in the joint. The treatment of capsuloligamentous hypomobility should begin with this technique whenever possible.

Carrying out small translatoric gliding movements without significantly increasing joint pressure is more challenging. Thus, gliding techniques should not be performed until the end of treatment, with the aim of improving the last few degrees in the range of motion. These techniques should only be applied by therapists who can accurately control the dosage through precise motion palpation of the quantity and quality of gliding. For those joints for which gliding techniques are shown in this book—because effective traction is technically impossible—extra care must be taken in regard to the dosage.

In painful joints, increased pressure in the joint is often due to tension in the surrounding muscles. Muscle guarding is common and patients often avoid moving the affected joint. In these situations as well, the cartilage does not receive optimal physiological stimulation in the form of alternating pressure and relief. As a result of diminished gliding, along with increased rolling of the articulating surfaces, impinging of the capsule may occur during end-range movements. This is a common cause of capsuloligamentous pain (impingement syndrome) (Schomacher 2010).

Translatoric traction is a pain-relief movement that brings relief to the joint surfaces and avoids further impingement of the capsule. If performed intermittently, it nourishes the cartilage with alternating pressure and relief: the traction relieves the pressure while the intraarticular negative air pressure, adhesion forces, and muscle tension produce pressure. Repeated rotatory movements such as swinging the lower legs or walking are probably the simplest means of giving the knee joint cartilage the nourishing stimulus it needs. Changes to the cartilage after treatment unfortunately occur only very gradually, if at all.

10.2 Treatment of Capsuloligamentous Hypomobility

The articular cause of restricted movement is reduced gliding of the joint surfaces against one other. This may be due to changes in the synovial fluid or the smoothness of the joint cartilage. Or there may be shrinkage of the capsuloligamentous unit, with increased pressure which makes gliding more difficult. Treatment should aim to improve synovial fluid consistency and cartilage smoothness while also stretching the capsuloligamentous unit. The former may be achieved by repeated movements within the pain-free range. These should be performed before translatoric mobilization therapy in grade III to "warm

up" the joint prior to stretch mobilization. In highly painful joints, intermittent pain-free traction may be used.

Pain-free movements also increase circulation in the capsuloligamentous unit and reduce the viscosity of the synovial fluid, which are good conditions for effective stretching. The stretch is performed with straight-lined translatoric mobilization.

10.3   Treatment of Capsuloligamentous-Induced Pain

Pain caused by (post-)traumatic arthritis, either due to surgery or movement beyond the physiological limitations of the joint, results from inflammation of the joint capsule. The goals of treatment are to promote healing of the inflammatory process and stop the pain. Corresponding to pain management in the treatment model of manual therapy (see p. 34), the latter occurs, for example, by stimulating the mechanoreceptors in the joint capsule through repetitive movement. Movement also improves capsular circulation and transport of chemical pain mediators away from the site as well as healing the inflammation. As already explained, translatoric traction is one possibility for movement that avoids excessive stress to the joint surfaces and impinging of capsule parts. For maximum stimulation, traction is performed intermittently in the joint's actual resting position.

10.4   Dosage of Translatoric Movements

The use of translatoric traction to stretch the capsuloligamentous unit and relieve pain naturally leads to the question of dosage: how much traction is needed and for how long? To answer this question, the therapist relies on joint "slack" (see below), the patient's perception, and control tests.

10.4.1   Dosage of Traction and Gliding

The correct amount of traction or gliding cannot be given in Newtons because it depends on the individual ability of the capsuloligamentous unit to withstand stress. The classification proposed by Kaltenborn divides range of motion into three grades which can be perceived by palpation specifically in each joint (**Fig. 10.2**):

- **Grade I = loosen**: Sufficient traction is applied to neutralize the articular pressure which is normally present due to intraarticular negative air pressure, adhesion forces between joint surfaces, and tension from surrounding muscles. There is no separation of joint surfaces. This minimal amount of traction is also known as "piccolo traction."

- **Grade II = tighten**: The joint partners are moved until initial tension is felt in the capsuloligamentous unit. This tightening is easily palpable and serves as the most important guide for dosing translatoric movements. Tightening of the capsuloligamentous unit has been compared to tightening the ropes of a ship tied to its mooring in dock; in nautical terms the extra length of rope is known as "slack." When the rope is pulled taut, this is known as "taking up the slack." Similarly, one refers in orthopedic manual therapy to taking up the slack when tightening the capsuloligamentous unit.

- **Grade III = stretching**: After the capsuloligamentous unit has been tightened, the actual stretch may begin by moving the joint further. This is the start of passive stretching with the goal of increasing extensibility.

Because stretching places stress on the capsuloligamentous unit, it should be avoided in anyone with arthritis, as it causes pain. These patients should be treated with pain-relieving grade I–II intermittent traction, without stretching and within the slack.

The actual stretching of the capsuloligamentous unit using traction is a grade III mobilization. The mechanical aim is the plasticization—that is, permanent deformation—of the structure (see also note on p. 39). To avoid damaging the stretched tissue, it is advisable to go only slightly beyond the first resistance (**Fig. 10.3**). This is easily palpable, while the point at which the structure begins to tear is undetectable in actual practice. Thus the permanent (plastic) deformation of the structure is achieved by staying in the

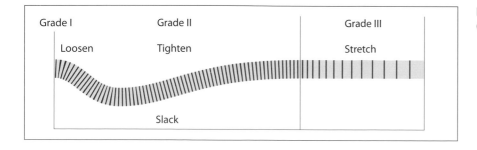

Fig. 10.2
Classification of range of motion.

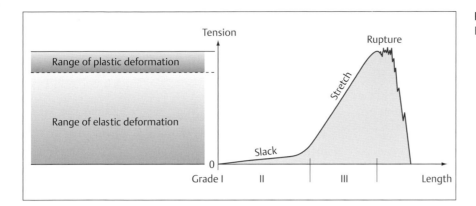

Fig. 10.3
Elastic and plastic deformation.

elastic range of elongation and is a result of various physical phenomena (see p. 52)

The dosages for gliding are the same as for traction. The only exception is grade I traction, which one tries to maintain during gliding. This is to minimize the virtually unavoidable increase in joint pressure which occurs during gliding, especially in grade III.

> **Note**
>
> Traction and gliding: Intensity:
> - For joint play   - Grades I, II, and III
> - For pain relief   - Grade I and within grade II
> - For stretch mobilization - Grade III
> - During gliding mobili-   - Grade I traction
>   zation

10.4.2 Duration of Traction and Gliding

There is a rather simple answer to the question of the duration of treatment application. Generally speaking, any measure should be performed for as long as it takes to achieve the desired goal. For pain-relieving traction or gliding, the absence of pain is a simple parameter: once the pain is gone, the measure may be ended.

Determining the length of a translatoric mobilization for stretching is more difficult, because any increase in the range of motion of shortened connective tissue is often only apparent after a longer period (several weeks).

The mobilization force must be sustained for at least a few seconds to overcome the viscosity of the capsuloligamentous tissue and exert pulling tension. Roughly speaking, mobilization should be held for more than 7 to 10 seconds after taking up the slack.

After a while, the patient will begin to feel some discomfort as a result of the stretching. At this point the therapist reduces the mobilization force to about grade II and returns after a brief "rest" lasting a few seconds to grade III mobilization. This is repeated a few times before the therapist completely stops the traction or gliding and re-tests mobility. A small change in mobility should be seen after 3 to 5 minutes of mobilization. If there is an increase in the range of motion, the mobilization should be repeated. Only if a control test fails to show increased mobility, should stretching/mobilization be ended for that day.

Ideally, both the patient and the therapist should feel the stretching. The patient should have a slight feeling of ten-

sion and the therapist should feel the first barrier of resistance and then go just beyond it in order to hold a grade III stretch. Often, however, only one person—either the patient or the therapist—notices something first. The mobilization should not go beyond this initial point, regardless of whom first feels it.

The goal of stretching is to elongate the connective tissue structures. This is a very time-consuming task which cannot be speeded up by applying greater force. On the contrary, pain occurring during treatment or even hours afterward indicates that the dosage was too high. Every hypomobile joint is unique and requires a new dosage for every session. This is why **Fig. 10.3** shows a stretching range rather than an individual point. This varies from "slight tension for a longer time" to "a lot of tension for a shorter time." One must be satisfied with gaining only a few degrees in the range of motion during each mobilization of capsuloligamentous hypomobility; it can take weeks or months until full mobility is restored if the cause is really connective tissue shortening. It is crucial that the patient supports treatment daily with appropriate positioning, repeated movements, and self-mobilizations. If a translatoric treatment significantly increases the range of motion within one treatment session, the cause of restriction was probably something other than capsuloligamentous shrinkage. Muscle tension, for example, might have decreased due to the reflexive effects of the mobilization.

Perhaps the issue of how long to stretch for may be illustrated by considering a piece of clothing that has shrunk in the laundry. Trying to forcefully stretch it out to its original size would probably just tear it. A more successful approach would be to take the wet fabric and stretch it out overnight, for instance, by hanging it over the back of a chair, and allow time rather than effort to take effect.

When adjusting the dosage for translatoric techniques to stretch connective tissue structures such as joint capsules, various variables must be taken into account. The parameters for adjusting the dosage are:

- Technique (traction or gliding)
- Starting position (in or outside of resting position)
- Strength and duration of stretching movement (from short to long and from less to more strength)
- Number and duration of stretching (self-)treatment sessions (per day/week)

To increase the intensity of the mobilization, the therapist should generally proceed

- from traction to gliding,
- from mobilization in the resting position to mobilization outside of the resting position, or
- from a shorter duration of stretching to a longer one.

As a final possibility, the therapist may slightly increase the stretching force at the beginning of grade III mobilization. In general, increasing the time spent stretching has priority over significantly increasing the force.

The treatment series ends when the range of motion and the movement quality with the end-feel have normalized or when there is a hard end-feel, preventing further mobilization (see p. 31)

(see p. 31)

Note

Dosage of translatoric movements

Pain-relieving movements	Stretching mobilization
- Intermittent grade I–II; - until pain is relieved.	- Static grade III, more than 7–10 seconds up to several/many minutes; - until the mild stretch begins to feel uncomfortable; - until control tests indicate no further improvement may be achieved today; - until a physiological range of motion and end-feel are reached—or a contraindication arises such as a hard end-feel.

In regard to practical application, it is important to recall the biomechanical characteristics of the capsule/ligament structure targeted by stretching techniques.

10.4.3 Biomechanical Aspects

In stretching mobilization, a distinction is made between physical and biological responses (Cunnings and Tillman 1992). The **physical response** occurs rapidly and immediately after treatment—for example, an increased range of motion. This may be explained by the physical phenomena related to stretching. These include reduced viscosity of tissue fluids, "creep," relaxation of structures, and the hysteresis effect. These terms are briefly explained in **Table 10.1**.

The **biological response** lasts longer than the physical one. It involves the re-structuring of the target structure in response to a stretching stimulus of sufficient duration and/or repetition. The capsule "grows" longer, hence the long-term effect. A control test done immediately after treatment would not show any significant quantitative functional improvement. Therapists should explain this to patients to ensure their cooperation over the long-term despite only very gradual improvement. The pa-

Table 10.1 Physical phenomena during "stretching"

Viscosity	Thickness or internal friction in gases and liquids (Brockhaus 1993) as a time-dependent mechanical property of a material (Panjabi and White 2001)
Creep	Viscoelastic phenomenon of deformation due to the effects of a constant force over a longer period of time (White and Panjabi 1990; Panjabi and White 2001)
Relaxation	Viscoelastic phenomenon of reduced tension (stress, force) in a structure due to constant elongation for a longer time (White and Panjabi 1990; Panjabi and White 2001)
Hysteresis	Viscoelastic phenomenon when viscoelastic materials do not regain their original length after stretching and the lost energy is transformed into heat (Panjabi and White 2001)

tients should also regularly place their hypomobile joint in a submaximal position for a period of time without a noticeable stretch sensation (Cunnings and Tillman 1992).

Considering the above-named biomechanical aspects, any stretching movement must be performed slowly (to reduce viscosity), increased incrementally or continuously (to allow for relaxation), and held at the end of the movement (to take advantage of creep).

Performance of stretching movements:

- stretch slowly,
- incrementally or continually increasing the stretch, and
- hold the stretch at the end of the movement.

! Grade III mobilization is a stretching stimulus. It is indicated for use in pathological shortening of joint structures. A healthy joint should not be treated with prolonged grade III mobilization to prevent hypermobility or exacerbation of possible mild hypermobility.

Note

10.5   Three-dimensional Traction and Three-dimensional Gliding

To increase the effectiveness of mobilization treatment, prior to performing the traction or gliding mobilization, the joint should be placed in a certain position which may be defined in all three anatomic planes. Hence one speaks of three-dimensional traction or three-dimensional gliding. The concept of three-dimensional positioning is well established and is also used to refer to biaxial and uniaxial joints. One "thinks" in three dimensions, even if a given joint allows for only one or two.

While learning joint mobilization techniques, the therapist should first select the resting position of the joint for the examination and treatment, which is also based on the three anatomical planes. This is where there is the greatest joint play and the entire joint capsule is lengthened or stretched.

For pain relief, the joint should be in the actual resting position; intermittent grade I–II traction or gliding may be performed.

When the stretching mobilization is performed with the joint in the resting position, the entire joint capsule will experience tension, although the shortened portions are stretched the most. In order to stretch these parts more, prior to the translatoric mobilization, the joint may be placed in a position outside of the resting position in order to produce pre-tension in the movement-limiting tissues. This enhances the effects of subsequent traction or gliding mobilization on these parts of the joint capsule. The effect of stretching is increased by the three-dimensional position of the joint.

For three-dimensional positioning outside of the resting position, the therapist must *feel* in which joint position and at which dosage the optimal amount of pre-tension is reached without point compression and without causing gaping of the joint surfaces. This book only shows techniques in the resting position to ensure optimal learning of these. For information on techniques applied outside of the (actual) resting position, the interested reader is referred to the literature (e.g., Kaltenborn 2011, 2012).

Note
Three-dimensional positioning for translatoric mobilization (traction and gliding)

For pain relief	■ in the resting position
For stretching mobilization	■ in the resting position (acts on the whole joint capsule and thus primarily on the shortened structures)
	■ outside of the resting position (emphasizes stretching of the shortened structures and requires a good sense of palpation for proper dosage)

11 Research

The demand for scientific studies on the efficacy of Orthopedic Manual Therapy (OMT) is closely connected with current political developments in the field and the need to meet quality assurance requirements.

The areas of research may be broadly divided into natural science/experimental studies and clinical studies. The former focuses on the individual factors, which explain why OMT is effective, while the latter analyzes individual and combined examination and treatment techniques.

The goal of clinical research is to determine the proper technique for the right patient at the right time and at the right dosage. This is a path that may be taken by any physical therapist during his or her everyday work with patients. Precise application of the techniques and a methodological analysis of recorded observations make scientific studies within a smaller framework possible.

The systematic procedure underlying the examination represents a learnable and controllable method of primary contact with the patient which is reimbursed by health insurance. For example in Norway, this was accomplished by physical therapists establishing a complete training program in Orthopedic Manual Therapy (Kalten-born 2007). It is thus essential for therapists to correctly recognize when physical therapy is indicated and when it is not. The therapist should also evaluate the indications and contraindications to treatment when it has been prescribed by a physician, as the patient's condition may have changed since the last visit to the doctor.

12.1 Indications

Joint mobility is examined to determine the indications or contraindications to translatoric movements for treatment. If the hypothesis based on the diagnostic summary suggests painful inflammation of the joint capsule (= arthritis) or capsuloligamentous hypomobility, then the therapist should perform a trial treatment. It consists of a function- and structure-specific measure that aims at proving or disproving the hypothesis.

In (post-traumatic) arthritis, the trial treatment consists of pain-relieving, grade I–II intermittent traction. In patients with capsuloligamentous hypomobility, grade III static traction is used. Sufficient time should be allowed for the trial treatment, as instantaneous improvement is not always to be expected. A treatment of approximately 3 to 5 minutes is advisable. The trial treatment may, of course, vary in length in individual patients.

! If the trial treatment both relieves the symptoms of the patient and improves the results of the functional tests, the hypothesis is confirmed. Treatment may then be continued along these lines. If not, the findings should be re-evaluated using the systematic examination with orienting questions.

To summarize, the manual translatoric examination and mobilization of the anatomical joint is indicated:

- To test joint mobility (joint play)
- To increase or maintain joint movement
- Whenever the beneficial effects of movement are indicated: trophic conditions ↑, circulation ↑, production and circulation of synovial fluid ↑, pressure and relief stimuli for cartilage metabolism, etc.
- To promote movement awareness and to increase or preserve the cortical image of movement when rotational movement is not possible, etc.

12.2 Contraindications

Contraindications in manual therapy are mainly related to the performance of movement. Throughout the examination and treatment procedure, the therapist should consistently be alert to signs that could contraindicate further movement. Right from the beginning of the session, the therapist should already consider whether or not a given movement may be performed.

12.2.1 Classification of the Condition

During the orienting examination, the physical therapist begins with the first key question (see p. 24): **Can and should I move the patient?** To determine this, the patient's condition may be classified as belonging to one of three categories: serious pathology, "life-threatening" compression for the nervous system, or a simple mechanical dysfunction with or without involvement of the nervous system (**Table 12.1**).

Table 12.1 Initial classification of the patient's condition during the examination

Category	Description
Serious pathology	▪ Rare in actual practice ▪ Physical therapy is ineffective ▪ **Red flags** (see **Table 12.2**) as warning signs of diseases such as **tumorous** and **systemic disorders** (Airaksinen et al 2006) ▪ Patient should be referred back to the physician
Compression which is "life-threatening" for the nervous system	▪ Rare in actual practice ▪ **Red flags** as warning signs of nervous system compression which could cause neural tissue damage ▪ Priority is given to immediate relief of compression ▪ Classic example: cauda equina syndrome as an emergency situation
Simple mechanical dysfunction with or without nervous system involvement	▪ **Majority of patients** ▪ **Main indication for physical therapy** ▪ No "red flags" ▪ Symptoms are "mechanosensitive": changes due to mechanical influences such as movement and posture ▪ Treatment consists primarily of movement and postural changes ▪ Also treatment of impaired neurodynamics ▪ Also therapy of radicular and peripheral compression symptoms which are not "acute, life-threatening" problems for the nervous system

12.2.2 Clinical Flags

Next are the questions (which are contained in the second orienting question) on the **acuteness of symptoms** (acute, subacute, or chronic) and the patient's **attitude toward pain management** (positive, negative, uncertain, or matter-of-fact, emotional, questionable). Other important questions relate to the **patient's perception of the cause of symptoms** and **the patient's expectations of physical therapy**. Unrealistic hopes and expectations for improvement can interfere with the treatment course and outcome. Signs of this include psychosocial risk factors (yellow flags) which the therapist should be aware of during the examination and treatment process. Therapists should also be alert to any work related negative socioeconomic (blue flags) and socio-professional factors (black flags) (**Table 12.2**).

Table 12.2 Clinical flags based on Main and de Williams (2002) and Waddell (1998)

Clinical flags	Significance
red flags	Biomedical signs of: ▪ Serious organ diseases ▪ Highly acute, "life-threatening" nervous system compression
yellow flags	Psychosocial or psychological indications of: ▪ Unrealistic hopes and opinions ▪ Negative coping strategies ▪ Distress = negative stress ▪ Negative behaviors toward the disease ▪ Unwillingness to change the condition ▪ Disease-exacerbating factors in the family and social environment
blue flags	Socioeconomic indications of: ▪ Negative effects on work status
black flags	Indications in the professional sphere of: ▪ Advantages from being sick and receiving health insurance compensation ▪ Workplace disputes ▪ Professional dissatisfaction ▪ Sense of inadequate working conditions ▪ Working factors ▪ Social insurance system

12.2.3 Contraindications to Movement

Next—as in the second orienting question **"Should I** exercise caution**?"**—the therapist must check whether **larger movements are contraindicated**. This may be the case in highly acute nervous system compression or in any other situation involving increased irritation.

The patient history or the results of inspection or active movements as demonstrated by the patient may suggest a larger lesion. The therapist should use specific tests for the neurovascular system and (passive) stability (bone fracture, ligament rupture, etc.) to rule out this possibility before repeated movements are performed actively or passively. This is crucial to avoid worsening the patient's condition with the examination.

The contraindications to movement may be divided into general contraindications, which also apply to other passive treatment techniques, and specific contraindications which apply in particular to grade III translatoric movements for mobilization (Kaltenborn 2004).

General Contraindications:

- Loss of stability, for example, due to trauma (fracture, sprain, etc.), inflammation, infection, or congenital bone anomalies
- Highly acute nervous system compression

- Massive degenerative changes affecting the vertebral column, for example, spondylosis, spondylarthrosis, and uncovertebral joint arthrosis
- Severe pathological bone changes, for example, due to neoplasms, inflammation, infection, osteoporosis, osteomalacia, etc.
- Anomalies or pathological vascular changes that may lead to abnormal blood flow
- Coagulation disorders, as may occur during anticoagulation therapy or in patients with hemophilia, which involve a risk of hemorrhage
- Patient compliance is lacking, which casts doubt on the patient's overall cooperation, as well as any situation in which common sense suggests that treatment would be inappropriate;

Specific Contraindications:

Specific contraindications to grade III translatoric movements for mobilization:

- Hypermobility of the target joint
- Hard end-feel, lacking elasticity (= bone-to-bone stop)
- Pain and/or muscle guarding during mobilization techniques
- Control tests showing no improvement after mobilization.

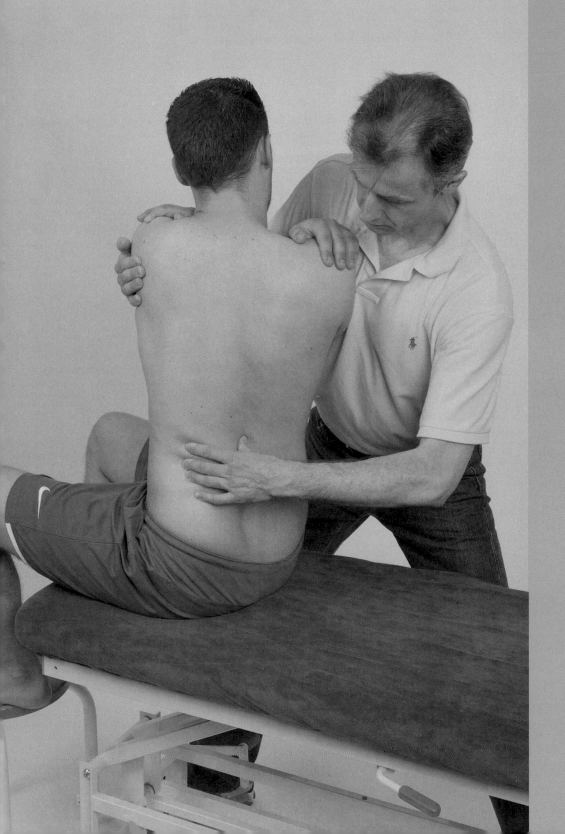

The examination and treatment techniques are shown on the following pages for each joint individually. Each section is structured in the same manner, beginning with the individual joint **anatomy** and the most important aspects for manual therapy (MT) followed by **general rotatory examinations** in the form of **active movements, comparing sides**. These tests give an initial impression of the extent of abnormal functioning and mobility. Even slight differences in range of motion, which are below the error of measurement of a classic two-arm angle goniometer of 5 to 10°, are visible. For evaluation of the spine, active movements in all directions are compared between adjacent sections of the spinal column.

Specific rotatory movement examinations test the quantity of movement. First, the patient actively moves the joint; then the therapist takes one joint partner and tests whether the movement continues passively. To evaluate the quality, the therapist first passively moves the joint from the zero position through the entire range of motion and then tests the end-feel. In certain joints, lateral stability is also tested.

> **Note**
> **Examination of rotatory movements**
> - Active movements, comparing sides
> - The patient moves actively
> - The therapist continues the movement passively
> - Passive movement through the entire range of motion and end-feel testing
> - Stability tests

The goals of this specific test of rotatory movements may be both symptom localization as well as an initial assessment of dysfunction. Depending on how acute the symptoms are, the examination may begin with the symptom-altering movement or with nonpainful movements.

■ Symptom Localization

First the patient should describe his or her **symptoms** and say in which **direction** of movement they occur. If the patient is unable to do so, the assessment must be primarily accomplished through active movements. If, rather than movement, staying in a certain position for a prolonged period influences the symptoms, then static posture should be analyzed. To ensure that the symptoms will not be exacerbated by movement testing, major **contraindications to movement** should be ruled out. This is especially important before larger passive movements, and when dealing with the spine, where compression and/or irritation of the nervous system or important vessels such as the vertebral artery can occur. In order to identify now the **area** or **joint** that correlates with the symptoms, each joint which is involved in the movement may be specifically moved in the symptom-altering direction without moving any others. The joint whose movement produces a change in symptoms probably allows symptoms to be (positively) influenced by optimal dosage of movement or control of movement.

The technique used for the patient interview is only presented in brief (see p. 26), and details concerning the inspection of the patient are not further elucidated given the limited scope of this book. The interview may be kept simple by asking where the pain is located and how it feels, how long the patient has had it, what triggers it, and with which other symptoms it is related. The inspection as well should be limited in this regard to simply observing the movements that alter the patient's symptoms. The movement examination for symptom localization is discussed in more detail for certain joints such as the shoulder girdle, after the technique for specific movements has already been practised on several other joints. For the spine, a search is made for the segment rather than the joint whose movement correlates with the symptoms. Moving a single segment is difficult, however, and also questionable (Schomacher and Learman 2010). Thus, in this book, symptom localization refers to specific regions rather than individual spinal segments.

■ Dysfunction

After identifying the joint that is responsible for the patient's symptoms, the therapist looks for the presence of dysfunction, that is, whether there is hypermobility, restricted mobility, or physiological mobility. It is advisable to continue the examination with nonpainful movements in order to obtain the most objective results of movement testing possible without the influence of painful irritation.

The examination of rotatory movements also serves for a **general assessment of adjacent joints**. The assessment is primarily done with general active movements. They also begin with the least painful in order to get an impression of possible dysfunction. This is especially important when testing the spine. Causal and influencing disorders and dysfunctions affecting other adjacent or even distant joints should also be taken into account.

> **Note**
>
> **Initial movement testing**
> - For symptom localization:
> Begin with the symptom-altering movement.
>
> - For an evaluation of joint function:
> Begin with the least painful movements.

After this initial portion of the examination comes the examination of translatoric movements. Tests of translation are limited to traction and compression techniques in this book. Gliding techniques are shown only for joints for which traction would be largely ineffective owing to technical reasons.

> **Note**
>
> **Examination of translatoric movements**
> - Traction (for certain joints, gliding techniques may be appropriate)
> - Compression

■ Documentation

In the **practice documentation scheme** found at the end of each section on the individual joints, specific aspects are listed which should be evaluated for that joint. At the end of the examination, the therapist should complete a **summary** of current findings. To facilitate this, a **formulation tool** is provided. With this, the **symptoms** are briefly described and the **direction** of movement in which they occur. Patients often also complain of symptoms that are related to sustaining a position for a longer period of time. In such instances, static posture must also be described and analyzed. Given that it is essential to manual therapy to check for any **contraindications**, their presence or absence must always be noted. Then the **area** or the **joint** must be identified which is in correlation with the symptoms. Finally, one must evaluate whether the joint is **hypomobile, hy-**

permobile, or **physiologically mobile**. Based on the end-feel, students of manual therapy should already be able to recognize whether it is more likely to be a capsuloligamentous or muscular **structure** which is changing the symptoms or movement. A positive translatoric test indicates that it is the joint. If the result is negative, other structures should be considered. Sometimes even **additional causal** and **influencing factors** may be identified.

A working hypothesis is formulated based on the symptom-altering dysfunction and potential causes or influences. The hypothesis is tested with a specific, targeted treatment known as the **trial treatment**. If a control test shows improvement of the function, and if there is improvement in the patient's symptoms, then the treatment measure is confirmed; if not, it is discarded.

If the examination results show (post-traumatic) arthritis of the joint or restricted mobility of the capsuloligamentous unit, translatoric traction in pain-relieving or stretching dosages is recommended as the trial treatment. If the initial hypothesis is confirmed, then treatment may continue with these techniques. This should be noted in the line which is labeled **treatment plan**.

The formulation of a **treatment goal** should be placed ahead of specific techniques in the treatment plan. The patient, physical therapist, and physician (as well as any other involved persons) should agree on a treatment goal which should be updated periodically—that is, the treatment goal should be adjusted according to the patient's recovery. The treatment goal also serves as a yardstick for measuring treatment success.

At the end of each chapter in the practical section is an **example** of a completed documentation scheme as an illustrative summary. Unfortunately, due to time and space considerations, this section on structuring the examination and treatment does not include important aspects

such as neuromuscular and vascular ones. Still, students should be able to recognize whether or not (posttraumatic) arthritis or capsuloligamentous hypomobility is present. If so, they should be able to treat it. If not, the advice of colleagues or teachers should be sought leading to attendance at further education courses. The missing parts of the examination, which are mentioned in Chapter 9, may be easily incorporated into the practice scheme shown here, allowing one to build on this basis without any significant changes. The documentation templates contained in the appendix give an example of this (see pp. 292 and 301, or go to the Thieme Media Center).

The recommended steps for the examination and the documentation templates may at first appear to be too lengthy and time-consuming for use in actual practice. "Finished" physical therapists may initially be critical of the procedure as "unrealistic." Still, the focus is on the acquisition of motor and cognitive skills which, as in sport or any other activity including physical therapy, requires a thorough and exact study of the processes involved. The more one practices, the more quickly one will be able to perform the examination and interpretation of findings. Development of these skills ultimately leads to economal use of time, as the most crucial examination steps can be more quickly identified and carried out while only the main findings have to be noted. A short report form, suitable for daily use, has been provided (see p. 301).

At the minimum, for each patient the physical therapist should complete a summary and treatment plan including the treatment goal. This is the only way to facilitate communication with physicians and colleagues as well as provide clinical proof of the effectiveness of physical therapy.

Together, these aspects form a solid foundation and practical basis for physical therapy in orthopedic manual therapy.

■ Ergonomics

The field of ergonomics is concerned with adjusting the workplace (conditions) to suit the characteristics of the human organism as well as with how the persons perform their work. A workplace design that corresponds to the work being done there, as well as useful ways of handling work processes, can reduce stress arising from working. Many orthopedic problems of the locomotor system are due to a discrepancy between stress and the ability to withstand it. In addition to progressively increasing the ability to withstand stress through targeted training, learning to avoid harmful stresses is another part of educating the patient in manual therapy.

The therapist also possesses a locomotor system and must take care to avoid excessive stress while performing manual therapy. Moreover, the efficiency of a technique often depends on proper positioning of the patient, optimal positioning of the therapist for application of the treatment, and the use of suitable aids. Hence, taking ergonomic principles into account is especially important in manual therapy.

One should pay attention to:

- an ergonomic position of the therapist,
- the use of an adjustable-height treatment table,
- placement of the patient in a relaxed position,
- good fixation of one joint partner using the hand or a device (wedge, belts, sandbags, etc.).
- a firm, comfortable grip for movement of the other joint partner, and
- movement of the joints without provocation of pain in either the patient or therapist.

Note
Practical procedure

Goal	Procedure
Determine the **symptoms** and the **triggering direction of movement** (or posture)	■ Interview, inspection, mainly active movement tests
Identify potential **contraindications to movement**	■ Interview, inspection, mainly active movement tests
Locate the **symptom-changing region** or joint	■ Rotatory testing, first actively, then assisted and, if necessary, passively
General evaluation of **adjacent joints**	■ Rotatory testing of adjacent joints, primarily active
Test the physiological joint using specific **rotatory testing**	■ Active movements performed during a comparison of both sides in the extremity joints, or, for the spine, compared with adjacent joints (e.g., hips, shoulders) and spinal regions ■ The patient moves actively out of the zero position. ■ The therapist takes over and tests whether the movement continues passively. ■ The therapist moves the joint passively from the zero position through the entire range of motion, and tests the end-feel. ■ If indicated for that joint type, the therapist also tests joint stability.
Test the anatomical joint with **Translatoric movement testing**	■ Traction and compression (gliding movements instead of traction for some joints)
Summary	*Formulation aid:* ■ Symptoms ↓ ■ Direction ↓ ■ Contraindications ↓ ■ Region (joint/segment) ↓ ■ Mobility: hypomobility, hypermobility, or physiologically mobile ↓ ■ Structure: muscle or joint, etc.
Trial treatment	■ Pain-relieving grade I–II intermittent traction for a painfully inflamed and irritated joint capsule ■ Static grade III traction (stretching) for capsuloligamentous hypomobility **Note**: The trial treatment should be sufficiently long, lasting 3–5 min or more.
Current physical therapy diagnosis	Brief summary of the previous summary (if confirmed by the trial treatment).
Treatment plan with treatment goal	Continue with techniques from the trial treatment or from further education.

14.1 Interphalangeal Joints of the Toes

(Articulationes interphalangeales pedis)

14.1.1 Anatomy

Joint type:	ginglymus (= hinge joint), modified sellar joint
Distal joint surface:	concave
Resting position:	slight flexion
Close packed position:	maximum extension
Capsular sign:	limitation in both directions; greater restriction of flexion

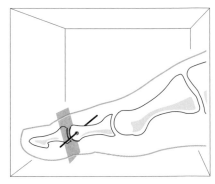

Fig. 14.1

14.1.2 Rotatory Tests

■ **Active Movements, Comparing Sides**

The patient moves all toes on both feet in flexion and then extension.

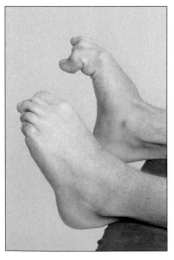

Fig. 14.2

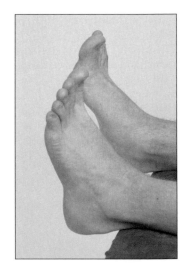

Fig. 14.3

■ Specific Tests for Active and Passive Movements (Quantity and Quality)

a) **Flexion** from the zero position:

- The therapist fixates the proximal phalanx and asks the patient to actively flex the toes.
- Then the therapist takes the distal phalanx and tests whether the movement continues passively further.
- Lastly, the therapist moves the distal phalanx passively out of the zero position and through the entire range of motion and then tests the end-feel.

Physiological end-feel:
firm and elastic

b) **Extension** from the zero position:

- The therapist fixates the proximal phalanx and asks the patient to actively extend the toes.
- Then the therapist takes the distal phalanx and tests whether the movement continues passively further.
- Finally, the therapist moves the distal phalanx passively out of the zero position through the entire range of motion and tests the end-feel.

Physiological end-feel:
firm and elastic

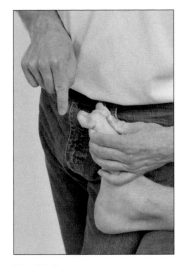

Fig. 14.4

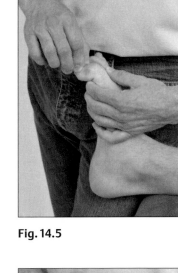

Fig. 14.5

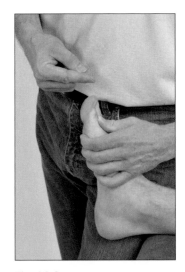

Fig. 14.6

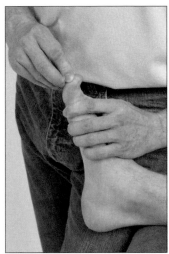

Fig. 14.7

■ Stability Tests in the Zero Position:

The therapist fixates the proximal and takes the distalphalanx from lateral and tests the gaping of the joint on the tibial and fibular sides.

> **!** The stability tests may be performed with the joints in any position.

Physiological end-feel:
very firm and elastic

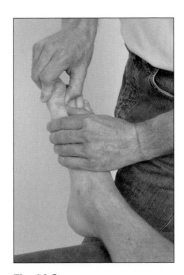

Fig. 14.8

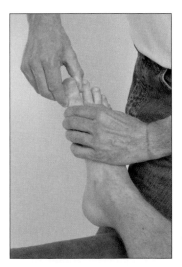

Fig. 14.9

14.1.3   Translatoric movement tests

a) **Traction** in the resting position:

The therapist holds the proximal phalanx and grasps the head of the distal phalanx, which he pulls at a right angle away from the treatment plane. The dorsally located thumb can be used to palpate the movement in the joint space.

Physiological end-feel: firm and elastic

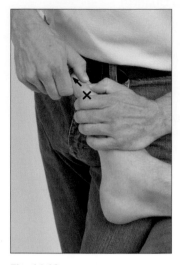

Fig. 14.10

b) **Compression** in the resting position:

The therapist fixates the proximal phalanx and grasps the distal phalanx, which he presses at a right angle to the treatment plane.

Physiological end-feel: hard

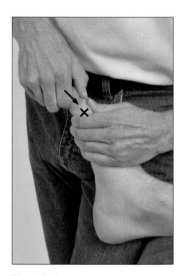

Fig. 14.11

◼ Treatment of Capsuloligamentous Hypomobility

The head piece of the table is slightly elevated with a wedge placed on top of it. The patient's foot is resting on the wedge. The proximal phalanx is hanging over the end of the wedge with the joint space over the edge. The therapist uses the thenar eminence of his proximal hand to hold the proximal phalanx against the wedge. Using his distal hand, he applies traction to the head of the distal phalanx.

❗ To prevent slippage due to sweating of the toes, a single layer of paper tissue may be placed between the toe and the therapist's hand.

❗ Pain-relieving traction may also be performed using the test version (see **Fig. 14.10**).

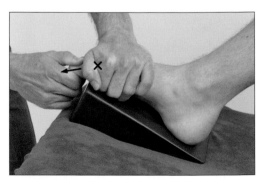

Fig. 14.12

Documentation Template: Practice Scheme

Interphalangeal Joints of the Toes					
Symptoms					
Symptom-altering direction					
Contraindications?	Nervous system: Other:				
Symptom-altering joint					
General assessment of adjacent joints					
Active movements, comparing sides					

Specific rotatory tests	Active	Continues passively?	Passive	End-feel	Symptoms/pain	Comments
Flexion						
Extension						

Stability tests	Quantity	Quality	End-feel	Symptoms/pain	Comments
Tibial gaping					
Fibular gaping					

Translatoric movement tests	Quantity	Quality	End-feel	Symptoms/pain	Comments
Traction					
Compression					

Summary Formulation aid: ■ Symptoms ■ Direction ■ Contraindications ■ Site (joint) ■ Restricted mobility, hypermobility, or physiological mobility ■ Structure: muscle, joint, etc.	*Text:*
Trial treatment	
Physical therapy diagnosis	
Treatment plan with treatment goal and prognosis	
Treatment progress	
Final examination	

Documentation: Practice Example

Interphalangeal joint (PIP of the second toe on the right foot in a patient with claw toe)	
Symptoms	*Limited extension of the toe with mild pain*
Symptom-altering direction	*Extension*
Contraindications?	Nervous system: *No findings* Other: *No findings*
Symptom-altering joint	*Proximal interphalangeal joint (PIP) of the second toe on the right foot*
General assessment of adjacent joints	*Mild clawing of the other toes as well*
Active movements, comparing sides	*Limited extension of the interphalangeal joints affecting all toes, especially the second toe on the right foot*

Specific rotatory tests	Active	Continues passively?	Passive	End-feel	Symptoms/pain	Comments
▪ Flexion	*ca. 30°*	*ca. 5°*	*Gradually increasing resistance*	*Firm and elastic*	*Almost no pain*	
▪ Extension	*ca. –20°*	*<5°*	*Difficult to move*	*Very firm and elastic and slightly painful*	*End-range pulling pain*	*Patient fears pain with movement*

Stability tests	Quantity	Quality	End-feel	Symptoms/pain	Comments
▪ Tibial gaping	*No findings*	*No findings*	*Firm and elastic*	*No findings*	
▪ Fibular gaping	*No findings*	*No findings*	*Firm and elastic*	*No findings*	

Translatoric movement tests	Quantity	Quality	End-feel	Symptoms/pain	Comments
▪ Traction	*Hypo 2*	*First resistance occurs earlier*	*Very firm and elastic*	*Some pain at end-range*	
▪ Compression	*No findings*	*No findings*	*Hard*	*No findings*	

Summary Formulation aid: ▪ Symptoms ▪ Direction ▪ Contraindications ▪ Site (joint) ▪ Restricted mobility, hypermobility, or physiological mobility ▪ Structure: muscle, joint, etc.	*Text:* ▪ *Mild end-range pain in the second toe of the right foot* ▪ *during extension.* ▪ *There are no contraindications today to further movement testing.* ▪ *Pain is correlated with movement in the proximal interphalangeal joint,* ▪ *which has restricted mobility (extension – 20 degrees).* ▪ *Symptoms are due to the capsuloligamentous unit which causes mild pain with end-range tension.*
Trial treatment	▪ *Pain-relieving intermittent grade I–II traction. After trial treatment for 5 minutes, the patient reported a significant reduction in pain.* ▪ *This was followed by grade III traction for 5 minutes, which resulted in decreased resistance at end-range and a slight increase in range of motion.*
Physical therapy diagnosis	*see summary*

Continued ▶

Documentation: Practice Example *(Continued)*

Interphalangeal joint
(PIP of the second toe on the right foot in a patient with claw toe)

Treatment plan with treatment goal and prognosis	▪ *Continue pain-relieving traction until a firm and elastic end-feel is achieved; then grade III mobilizing traction.* ▪ *Treatment goal: pain-free physiological mobility.* **(Further information on examination and treatment techniques may be obtained through further education.)**
Treatment progress	
Final examination	

14.2   Metatarsophalangeal Joints of the Foot

(Articulationes metatarsophalangeales pedis)

14.2.1   Anatomy

Joint type: condylar joint, modified ovoid

Distal joint surface: concave

Resting position: ca. 10° extension

Close packed position: MTP I maximum extension

MTP II–V maximum flexion

Capsular sign: restriction in all directions; flexion is most limited

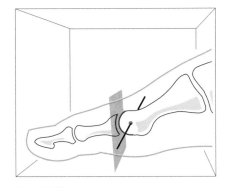

Fig. 14.13

14.2.2 Rotatory Tests

■ Active movements, Comparing sides

The patient is asked to move all the toes on both feet at the same time, first in flexion and then extension. Then the patient should try to spread the toes apart (= abduction) and bring them close together (= adduction).

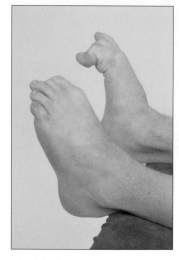

Fig. 14.14

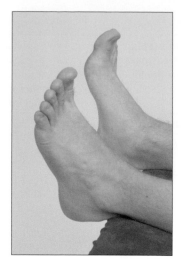

Fig. 14.15

> **Note**
> The therapist demonstrates the movements of toe abduction and adduction with the fingers for better comprehension.

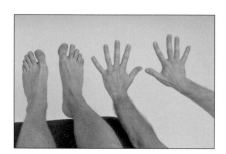

Fig. 14.16

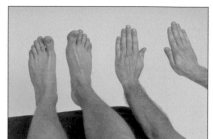

Fig. 14.17

■ Specific Active and Passive Movement Testing (Quantity and Quality)

a) **Flexion** from the zero position:

- The therapist fixates the metatarsal bone and asks the patient to actively flex the toes.
- Then the therapist takes the phalanx and tests whether the movement continues passively.
- Finally, the therapist moves the phalanx passively from the zero position through the entire range of motion and tests the end-feel.

Physiological end-feel:
firm and elastic

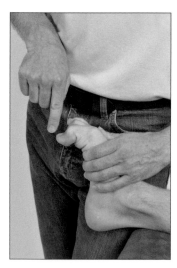

Fig. 14.18

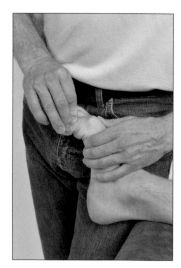

Fig. 14.19

b) **Extension** from the zero position:

- The therapist fixates the metatarsal bone and asks the patient to actively extend the toes.
- Then the therapist takes the phalanx and tests whether the movement continues passively.
- Finally, the therapist moves the phalanx passively from the zero position through the entire range of motion and tests the end-feel.

Physiological end-feel:
firm and elastic.

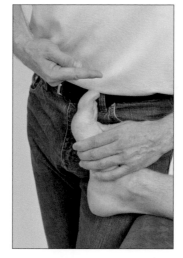 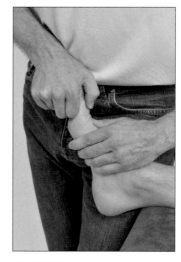

Fig. 14.20   **Fig. 14.21**

c) **Abduction** from the zero position:

- The therapist fixates the metatarsal bone and asks the patient to actively spread the toes.
- Then the therapist takes the phalanx and tests whether the movement continues passively.
- Finally, the therapist moves the phalanx passively from the zero position through the entire range of motion and tests the end-feel.

Physiological end-feel:
firm and elastic

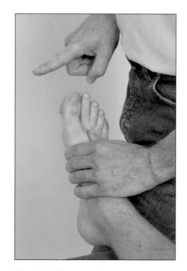 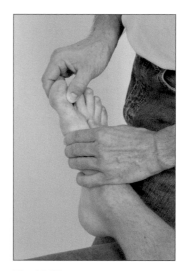

Fig. 14.22   **Fig. 14.23**

d) **Adduction** from the zero position:

- The therapist fixates the metatarsal bone and asks the patient to actively move the toes toward the center of the foot (= second ray) in the direction of adduction.
- Then the therapist takes the phalanx and tests whether the movement continues passively.
- Finally, the therapist moves the phalanx passively from the zero position through the entire range of motion and tests the end-feel.

Physiological end-feel:
firm and elastic.

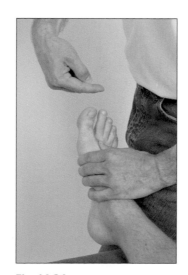 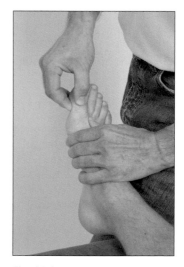

Fig. 14.24   **Fig. 14.25**

14.2.3 Translatoric movement tests

a) **Traction** from the resting position:

The therapist fixates the metatarsal bone and grasps the head of the phalanx, which he moves at a right angle away from the treatment plane. The dorsally located thumb may be used to palpate the motion in the joint space.

Physiological end-feel:
firm and elastic

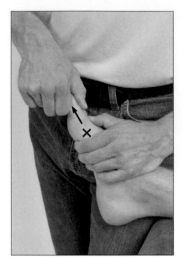

Fig. 14.26

b) **Compression** in the resting position:

The therapist fixates the metatarsal bone and grasps the distal phalanx, which he presses toward the plane of treatment at a right angle.

Physiological end-feel: hard

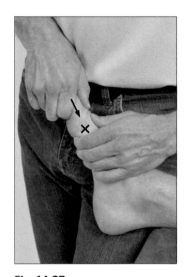

Fig. 14.27

14.2.4 Treatment of Capsuloligamentous Hypomobility

The patient's foot is placed on the head piece of the treatment table on top of a wedge. The metatarsal bone is lying on the end of the wedge with the joint space protruding over the edge. Using the thenar eminence on the proximal hand, the therapist fixates the metatarsal bone against the wedge. The distal hand pulls on the head of the phalanx to perform traction.

! To prevent slippage due to sweating fingers, a single layer of paper tissue may be placed between the metatarsal bone and the therapist's hand.

! Pain-relieving traction may also be performed in the test version (see **Fig. 14.26**).

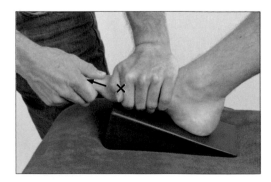

Fig. 14.28

Metatarsophalangeal joints						
Symptoms						
Symptom-altering direction						
Contraindications?	Nervous system: Other:					
Symptom-altering joint						
General assessment of adjacent joints						
Active movements, comparing sides						

Specific rotatory tests	**Active**	**Continues passively?**	**Passive**	**End-feel**	**Symptoms/pain**	**Comments**
▪ Flexion						
▪ Extension						
▪ Abduction						
▪ Adduction						

Translatoric movement tests	**Quantity**	**Quality**	**End-feel**	**Symptoms/pain**	**Comments**
▪ Traction					
▪ Compression					

Summary Formulation aid: ▪ Symptoms ▪ Direction ▪ Contraindications ▪ Site (joint) ▪ Restricted mobility, hypermobility, or physiological mobility ▪ Structure: muscle, joint, etc.	*Text:*
Trial treatment	
Physical therapy diagnosis	
Treatment plan with treatment goal and prognosis	
Treatment progress	
Final examination	

Documentation: Practice Example

Metatarsophalangeal joint of the great toe (Hallux valgus of right foot)	
Symptoms	*Pain affecting the great toe during walking*
Symptom-altering direction	*Extension, slight change with abduction or adduction*
Contraindications?	Nervous system: *No findings* Other: *No findings*
Symptom-altering joint	*Metatarsophalangeal joint of the great toe of the right foot*
General assessment of adjacent joints	*The remaining toes are in a slight clawing position and there is hallux valgus of the great toe of the left foot as well.*
Active movements, comparing sides	*The great toe of the right foot is in a position of adduction; active abduction is impossible.*

Specific rotatory tests	Active	Continues passively?	Passive	End-feel	Symptoms/pain	Comments
▪ Flexion	*ca. 30°*	*< 5°*	*Slight friction*	*Firm and elastic*		
▪ Extension	*ca. 30°*	*< 5°*	*Slight friction*	*Firm and elastic*	*Mild pain at end range*	
▪ Abduction	*ca. –20°*	*< 5°*	*Slight friction first stop is earlier*	*Very firm and elastic*	*Mild pain at end range*	
▪ Adduction	*0°*	*ca. 30°*	*Slight friction*	*Firm and elastic*	*Mild pain at end range*	

Translatoric movement tests	Quantity	Quality	End-feel	Symptoms/pain	Comments
▪ Traction	*Clearly hypo-mobile 2*	*Strong resistance to movement*	*Very firm and elastic*	*Mild pain at end range*	
▪ Compression	*No findings*	*No findings*	*No findings*	*No findings*	

Summary Formulation aid: ▪ Symptoms ▪ Direction ▪ Contraindictions ▪ Site (joint) ▪ Restricted mobility, hypermobility, or physiological mobility ▪ Structure: muscle, joint, etc.	*Text:* ▪ *Malalignment of the great toe of the right foot with hallux valgus and –20° movement limitation; mild pain at end range* ▪ *The limitation mainly affects abduction, but extension and adduction are also affected. Extension is the most painful direction.* ▪ *There are no contraindications today to further movement testing.* ▪ *The pain is coming from the metatarsophalangeal joint,* ▪ *due to hypomobility of the capsuloligamentous unit* ▪ *The feeling of friction in the joint suggests early cartilage degeneration.*
Trial treatment	*After initial pain-relieving intermittent grade I–II traction, mobilizing grade III traction was performed for 5 minutes. The patient reported a feeling of lightness in the great toe afterward and the current end of motion is passively reachable with less resistance to movement.*

Continued ▶

Metatarsophalangeal joint of the great toe (Hallux valgus of right foot)	
Physical therapy diagnosis	*see summary*
Treatment plan with treatment goal and prognosis	■ *Continue grade III mobilizing traction after brief initial pain-relieving traction.* ■ *Treatment goal: pain-free physiological mobility.* **(Further information on examination and treatment techniques may be obtained through further education.)**
Treatment progress	
Final examination	

14.3 Intermetatarsal and Tarsometatarsal Joints

(Articulationes intermetatarsales and tarsometatarsales)

14.3.1 Anatomy

Joint type:
- Distal intermetatarsal joint: syndesmosis
  Joint surfaces: no true joint surfaces
- Proximal intermetatarsal joints II–V: amphiarthroses
  Joint surfaces: irregular small curvature, considered concave in manual therapy
- Tarsometatarsal joints I–V: amphiarthroses
  Distal joint surface: irregular small curvature, considered concave in manual therapy

Resting position: not described

Close packed position: not described

Capsular sign: not described with the exception of the tarsometatarsal joint, with equal limitation in all directions

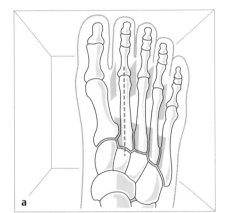

❗ Movements always occur in all three joints simultaneously. General movements of the forefoot in relation to the hindfoot are referred to as pronation and supination. In pronation, the lateral border of the foot lifts and in supination the medial border of the foot lifts. These movements occur in the tarsal and metatarsal joints and may occur passively, e.g., when walking on an uneven surface. During active motion, pronation occurs together with eversion in the subtalar joint and supination occurs with inversion. Clinical usage differs from usage in anatomy texts, in which pronation and supination also refer to movements in the subtalar joint (Rauber and Kopsch 1987). Together with the tarsal joints and the subtalar joint, the intermetatarsal and tarsometatarsal joints form the arches of the foot. Arch stability is essential. Grade III mobilizations to stretch the intermetatarsal and tarsometatarsal joints and increase the range of motion are seldom indicated.

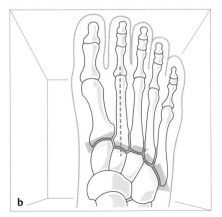

Fig. 14.29 a, b

Note
The planes of treatment are each approximately perpendicular to the dorsum of the foot.

14.3.2 Rotatory Tests

■ Active Movements, Comparing Sides

Active arching and flattening of the arch are so unusual for many people that therapists rarely see a significant range of motion (hence no figures are included). The therapist should ask the patient to do so and compare the movements of the feet if possible. If the patient is unable to actively perform the movement, then the examination proceeds with passive movements.

■ Specific Active and Passive Movement Testing (Quantity and Quality)

a) **Increasing** the vault of the foot:

■ The therapist asks the patient to actively increase the vault of the foot.
■ Then using both middle fingers, the therapist supports the second metatarsal from plantar and presses the first and fifth metatarsals with the thumbs from dorsal plantarly (toward the sole of the foot), thus testing whether the movement continues passively.
■ Finally, the therapist moves the vault of the foot passively in the same way from the zero position through the entire range of motion and tests the end-feel.

Physiological end-feel: firm and elastic.

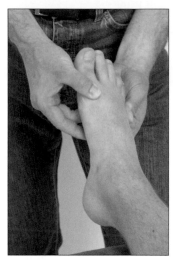

Fig. 14.30

b) **Flattening** the vault of the foot:

■ The therapist asks the patient to actively flatten the vault of the foot.
■ Then using both thumbs, the therapist supports the second metatarsal from dorsal and presses the first and fifth metatarsals with the middle fingers from plantar dorsally (toward the dorsum of the foot), thus testing whether the movement continues passively.
■ Finally, the therapist moves the vault of the foot passively in the same way from the zero position through the entire range of motion and tests the end-feel.

Physiological end-feel: firm and elastic.

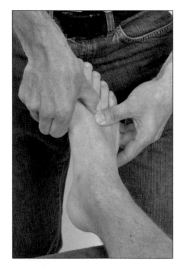

Fig. 14.31

c) **Individual movements** of the intermetatarsal joints:

The therapist kneels on one knee at the end of the bench. Fixating the second metatarsal with the fibular hand, he moves the first metatarsal passively with the tibial hand plantarly and dorsally and tests in each case the end-feel.

Then, with the tibial hand he fixates the second metatarsal, which forms the stable longitudinal axis of the foot, while the fibular hand moves the third metatarsal plantarly and dorsally and tests in each case the end-feel. The fourth metatarsal is moved against the third, and the fifth against the fourth in the same way.

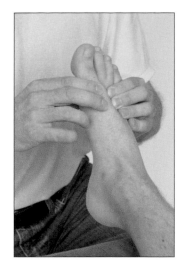

Fig. 14.32

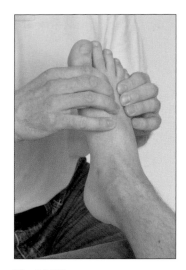

Fig. 14.33

Gripping the distal metatarsal head, the therapist tests the syndesmosis. A proximal grip at the base of the metatarsal bones produces translatoric gliding in the proximal intermetatarsal joints. For practical reasons, this test is also done here.

All of these movements also cause related movements of the tarsometatarsal joints in the direction of flexion or extension.

Physiological end-feel:
firm and elastic

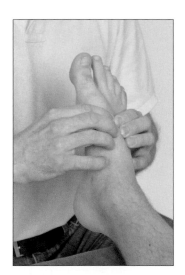

Fig. 14.34

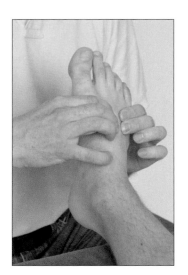

Fig. 14.35

d) **Flexion** and **Extension** in the tarsometatarsal joints:

The therapist fixates one of the tarsal bones (first, second, or third cuneiform or the cuboid bone) and moves the corresponding metatarsal bone passively plantarly in flexion and then dorsally in extension, also testing the end-feel each time. The associated movement is gliding in the intermetatarsal joints.

Physiological end-feel:
firm and elastic

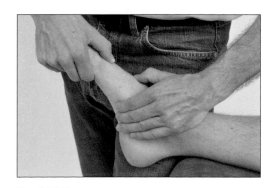

Fig. 14.36

14.3.3 Translatoric movement tests

a) **Traction** of the tarsometatarsal joint:

With the thumb and index finger of the proximal hand, the therapist fixates the corresponding tarsal bones (first, second, or third cuneiform or the cuboid bone). The thumb and index finger of the distal hand hold the head of the corresponding metatarsal bone, which the therapist pulls at a right angle away from the treatment plane. The dorsally located thumb may be used to palpate the movement in the joint space.

Physiological end-feel:
firm and elastic

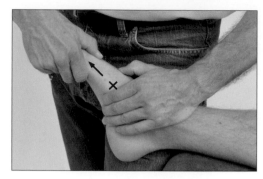

Fig. 14.37

b) **Compression** of the tarsometatarsal joint:

The therapist uses the thumb and index finger of the proximal hand to hold the corresponding tarsal bones (first, second or third cuneiform or the cuboid bone). The thumb and index finger of the distal hand hold the corresponding metatarsal bone, which the therapist presses at a right angle toward the treatment plane.

Physiological end-feel: hard

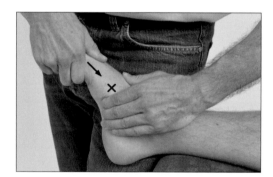

Fig. 14.38

c) **Compression** of the intermetatarsal joints:

The therapist grasps the midfoot with both hands from tibial and fibular and presses the first through fifth metatarsals at a right angle to the treatment plane. The compression may be applied either more distally or proximally. If there is pain provocation, compression between the individual metatarsals may be performed for more precise localization.

For translatoric gliding in the proximal intermetatarsal joints, the reader is referred to the individual movements of these joints described above.

Physiological end-feel: hard

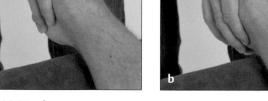

Fig. 14.39 a, b

Note

The gliding in the tarsometatarsal joints is described in the section on the ankle joint (p.90) as part of the Translatoric movement testing of the intertarsal joints.

14.3.3 Treatment of Capsuloligamentous Hypomobility

◼ Mobilization of the Tarsometatarsal Joint

The foot of the patient is placed on a wedge resting on the head piece of the table. The tarsal bone (e.g., first cuneiform) that will not be moved is lying on the edge of the wedge so that the tarsometatarsal joint space is hanging over the end. Using the thenar eminence, the therapist fix- ates the first cuneiform against the wedge. The therapist uses the thumb and index finger of the distal hand to grasp the first metatarsal head and pull it at a right angle away from the treatment plane.

> **!** Pain-relieving traction may also be performed using the test version (see **Fig. 14.37**).

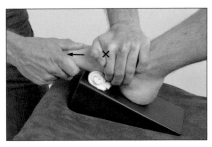

Fig. 14.40

◼ Mobilization of the Intermetatarsal Joints

The foot of the patient is placed on a wedge on the head piece of the table. The metatarsal (e.g., second) that will be fixated is lying on the edge of the wedge so that the metatarsal (first in the example) that will be mobilized is protruding over the end. The therapist fixates the second metatarsal against the wedge with the thenar eminence of his fibular hand. His tibial hand is wrapped around the first metatarsal which he mobilizes by pressing it with the thenar eminence toward the plantar surface.

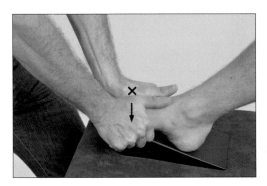

Fig. 14.41

> **!** For dorsal mobilization, the patient is in a supine position, the dorsum of the foot is similarly fixated on the wedge and the corresponding metatarsal bone is mobilized dorsally with the same technique. For the proximal joint, the therapist uses both hands, placing the thenar eminence at the level of the metatarsal bases; for the distal joint the placement is at the height of the head. If there is any uncertainty, the proximal joint should first be mobilized.

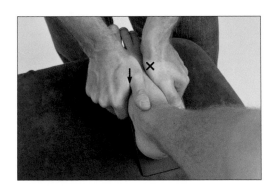

Fig. 14.42

> **!** For pain relief, specific movements within the slack (laxity) of the joint capsule (= grade I–II) may also be performed using the test version (see **Figs. 14.32–14.35**).

Within the intertarsal joints, the individual bones may be moved against each other with translatoric movements (see p. 90).

Tarsometatarsal and intermetatarsal joints						
Symptoms						
Symptom-altering direction						
Contraindications?	Nervous system: Other:					
Symptom-altering joint						
General assessment of adjacent joints						
Active movements, comparing sides						
Specific rotatory tests	**Active**	**Continues passively?**	**Passive**	**End-feel**	**End-feel**	**Comments**
▪ Increasing the vault of the foot						
▪ Flattening of the vault of the foot						
▪ Specific movements of the intermetatarsal joints						
▪ Flexion of the tarsometatarsal joint						
▪ Extension of the tarsometatarsal joint						
Translatoric movement tests	**Quantity**		**Quality**	**End-feel**	**Symptoms/pain**	**Comments**
▪ Traction on the tarsometatarsal joint						
▪ Compression of the tarsometatarsal joint						
▪ Compression of the intermetatarsal joints						
Summary Formulation aid: ▪ Symptoms ▪ Direction ▪ Contraindications ▪ Site (joint) ▪ Restricted mobility, hypermobility, or physiological mobility ▪ Structure: muscle, joint, etc.	*Text:*					

Continued ▶

Tarsometatarsal and intermetatarsal joints	
Trial treatment	
Physical therapy diagnosis	
Treatment plan with treatment goal and prognosis	
Treatment progress	
Final examination	

Documentation: Practice Example

Tarsometatarsal and intermetatarsal joints (Pain when walking, following 4-week long cast immobilization for second metatarsal fracture, right foot)	
Symptoms	*Pain in right midfoot when walking*
Symptom-altering direction	*Flattening of the arch of the foot*
Contraindications?	Nervous system: *No findings* Other: *No findings*
Symptom-altering joint	*Tarsometatarsal joint 1, right*
General assessment of adjacent joints	*The entire right foot appears "stiff" and less mobile than the left.*
Active movements, comparing sides	*The arch of the foot on the left has greater passive mobility than the right; active movements of the arches are not possible on either side.*

Specific rotatory tests	**Active**	**Continues passively?**	**Passive**	**End-feel**	**Symptoms/ pain**	**Comments**
▪ Raising of the vault of the foot	*Barely possible*	*Slight*	*Increased resistance to movement*	*Firm and only slightly elastic*		
▪ Flattening of the vault of the foot	*Barely possible*	*Slight*	*Increased resistance to movement*	*Firm, hardly elastic*	*Somewhat painful*	
▪ Specific movements of the intermetatarsal joints	*Barely possible*	*Slight*	*Slight increased resistance to movement*	*Somewhat more firm than physiologically*		
▪ Flexion of the 1st tarsometatarsal joint	*Slight*	*Slight*	*Increased resistance to movement*	*Very firm, hardly elastic*		
▪ Extension of the 1st tarsometatarsal joint	*Slight*	*Slight end-range pain*	*Increased resistance to movement*	*Very firm, hardly elastic*	*End-range pain*	

Translatoric movement tests	**Quantity**	**Quality**	**End-feel**	**Symptoms/pain**	**Comments**
▪ Traction on the 1st tarsometatarsal joint	*Hypo 2*	*Increased resistance to movement*	*Very firm, hardly elastic*	*Slight end-range pain*	
▪ Compression of the 1st tarsometatarsal joint	*No findings*	*No findings*	*Hard*	*No findings*	
▪ Compression of the intermetatarsal joints	*No findings*	*No findings*	*Hard*	*No findings*	

| **Summary**
Formulation aid:
▪ Symptoms
▪ Direction
▪ Contraindications
▪ Site (joint)
▪ Restricted mobility, hypermobility, or physiological mobility
▪ Structure: muscle, joint, etc. | *Text:*
▪ *Pain in the right midfoot when walking*
▪ *with flattening of the arch and extension of the tarsometatarsal joints.*
▪ *There are no contraindications today to further movement testing*

▪ *The symptoms correlate with the first tarsometatarsal joint, arising from mildly painful restriction*

▪ *of capsuloligamentous structures.* |

Continued ▶

Tarsometatarsal and intermetatarsal joints (Pain when walking, following 4-week long cast immobilization for second metatarsal fracture, right foot)	
Trial treatment	▪ *Approximately 5-minute long grade I–II pain-relieving intermittent traction, after which the patient reported less pain when walking.* ▪ *This was followed by approximately 5-minute long grade III mobilizing traction, which led to a further decrease in pain when walking. Resistance also appeared to decrease during passive movements.*
Physical therapy diagnosis	*See above*
Treatment plan with treatment goal and prognosis	▪ *Continue pain-relieving traction; after reducing pain, grade III mobilizing traction.* ▪ *Treatment goal: pain-free physiological mobility* **(Further information on examination and treatment techniques may be obtained through further education.)**
Treatment progress	
Final examination	

14.4　Subtalar Joint

(Talocalcaneal joint: articulatio subtalaris and posterior part of the articulatio talocalcaneonavicularis)

14.4.1　Anatomy

Joint type:
- articulatio subtalaris: ginglymus
  Distal joint surface: convex
- articulatio talocalcaneonavicularis: spheroidal joint
  Distal joint surface: concave

Resting position:　　　mid-position between eversion and inversion

Close packed position:　maximum inversion

Capsular sign:　　　　not described

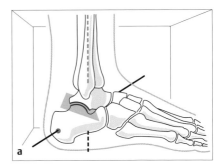

> **Note**
> In clinical practice, one refers to a common treatment plane that is between the planes of the posterior and anterior joint spaces.

! The subtalar joint must be actively stabilized in the frontal plane when standing. Insufficient stability leads to valgus or varus of the foot.

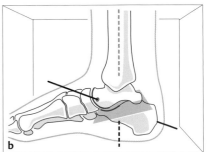

Fig. 14.43 a, b

14.4.2 Rotatory Tests

■ Active Movements, Comparing Sides

The patient moves both feet in the direction of inversion and eversion (the therapist may show the direction of movement with his index finger).

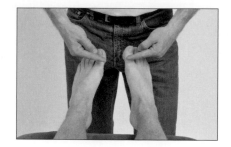

Fig. 14.44

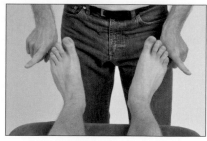

Fig. 14.45

■ Specific Active and Passive Movement Testing (Quantity and Quality)

a) **Inversion** from the zero position:

■ The therapist fixates the talus in the ankle mortise and also the bones of the lower leg. The patient is asked to actively move the foot toward the therapist's index finger in the direction of inversion.

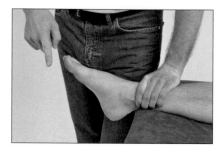

Fig. 14.46

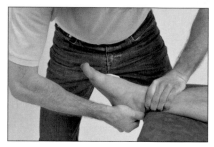

Fig. 14.47

■ Then the therapist takes the calcaneus and tests whether the movement continues passively.
■ Finally, the therapist moves the calcaneus passively from the zero position through the entire range of motion and tests the end-feel.

Physiological end-feel:
firm and elastic

b) **Eversion** from the zero position:

■ The therapist fixates the talus in the ankle mortise and asks the patient to actively move the foot toward the therapist's index finger in the direction of eversion.
■ Then the therapist takes the calcaneus and tests whether the movement continues passively.
■ Finally, the therapist moves the calcaneus passively from the zero position through the entire range of motion and tests the end-feel.

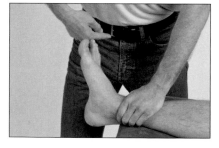

Fig. 14.48

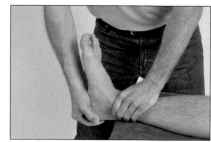

Fig. 14.49

Physiological end-feel:
firm and elastic

14.4.3 Translatoric movement tests

a) **Traction** from the resting position:

The therapist fixates the talus in the ankle mortise, places his hand around the calcaneus and moves it at a right angle away from the <u>treatment plane</u>. The index finger of the proximal hand may be used to palpate the movement between the medial tubercle of the posterior talar process and the calcaneus.

Physiological end-feel: firm and elastic

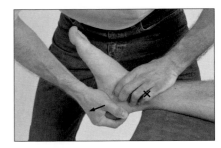

Fig. 14.50

b) **Compression** in the resting position:

The therapist fixates the lower leg against the bench, which also stabilizes the talus, and presses the calcaneus at a <u>right angle toward the treatment plane</u>.

> **!** Isolated fixation of the talus is not possible without fixation of the lower leg. During compression, the ankle joint is also tested. This compression test in lying is indicated only if standing (= compression) produces symptoms.

Physiological end-feel: hard

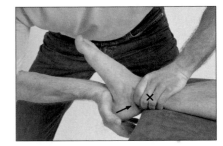

Fig. 14.51

14.4.4 Treatment of Capsuloligamentous Hypomobility

With the patient lying in the prone position, the therapist fixates the talus with the lateral hand on the collum tali. Using the medial hand, he pushes the calcaneus at a <u>right angle away from the treatment plane</u>.

> **!** Pain-relieving traction may also be performed using the test version.

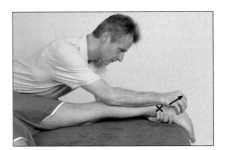

Fig. 14.52

Documentation Template: Practice Scheme

Subtalar joint						
Symptoms						
Symptom-altering direction						
Contraindications?	Nervous system: Other:					
Symptom-altering joint						
General assessment of adjacent joints						

Active movements, comparing sides						
Specific rotatory tests	**Active**	**Continues passively?**	**Passive**	**End-feel**	**Symptoms/ pain**	**Comments**
▪ Inversion						
▪ Eversion						

Translatoric movement tests	**Quantity**	**Quality**	**End-feel**	**Symptoms/pain**	**Comments**
▪ Inversion					
▪ Eversion					

Summary Formulation aid: ▪ Symptoms ▪ Direction ▪ Contraindications ▪ Site (joint) ▪ Restricted mobility, hypermobility, or physiological mobility ▪ Structure: muscle, joint, etc.	*Text:*
Trial treatment	
Physical therapy diagnosis	
Treatment plan with treatment goal and prognosis	
Treatment progress	
Final examination	

Documentation: Practice Example

Subtalar joint (Pain 5 weeks after 2-week long immobilization for an inversion sprain, right foot)	
Symptoms	*Pain in the subtalar joint of the right foot*
Symptom-altering direction	*Inversion*
Contraindications?	Nervous system: *No findings* Other: *No findings*
Symptom-altering joint	*Subtalar joint of the right foot*
General assessment of adjacent joints	*Overall diminished mobility in the right ankle joint*
Active movements, comparing sides	*Inversion is significantly more restricted in the subtalar joint of the right foot than in the left; there is also diminished eversion in comparison.*

Specific rotatory tests	**Active**	**Continues passively?**	**Passive**	**End-feel**	**Symptoms/ pain**	**Comments**
▪ Inversion	*20°*	*ca. 10°*	*Soft resistance to movement*	*Firm*	*Mild end-range pain*	
▪ Eversion	*10°*	*ca. 10°*	*No findings*	*Firm and elastic*		

Translatoric movement tests	**Quantity**	**Quality**	**End-feel**	**Symptoms/pain**	**Comments**
▪ Inversion	*Hypo 2*	*Soft resistance to movement*	*Slightly firm*	*Mild end-range pain*	
▪ Eversion	*No findings*	*No findings*	*Hard*	*No findings*	

Summary Formulation aid: ▪ Symptoms ▪ Direction ▪ Contraindications ▪ Site (joint) ▪ Restricted mobility, hypermobility, or physiological mobility ▪ Structure: muscle, joint, etc.	*Text:* ▪ *Pain* ▪ *with inversion* ▪ *There are no contraindications today to further movement tests.* ▪ *The symptoms are located in the subtalar joint* ▪ *which is hypomobile (passive: 30°)* ▪ *due to a restricted and painfull joint capsule.*
Trial treatment	▪ *Pain-relieving grade I–II intermittent traction. After 5 minutes, pain subsided.* ▪ *Afterward further trial treatment consisting of ca. 5-minute-long grade III traction, after which the range increased slightly.*
Physical therapy diagnosis	*See above*
Treatment plan with treatment goal and prognosis	▪ *Continue pain-relieving grade I–II traction and then grade III mobilizing traction.* ▪ *Treatment goal: pain-free physiological mobility* **(Further information on examination and treatment techniques may be obtained through further education.)**
Treatment progress	
Final examination	

14.5　Ankle Joint

(Articulatio talocruralis)

14.5.1　Anatomy

Joint type:	ginglymus (= hinge joint), modified sellar joint
Distal joint surface:	convex
Resting position:	10° plantar flexion
Close packed position:	maximum dorsiflexion
Capsular sign:	plantar flexion > dorsiflexion

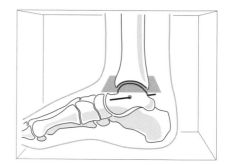

Fig. 14.53

14.5.2　Rotatory Tests

■ Active movements, Comparing Sides

The patient moves both feet in maximum plantar flexion and dorsiflexion.

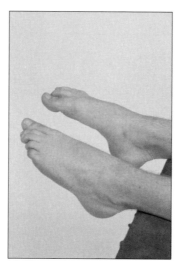

Fig. 14.54

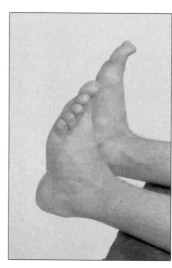

Fig. 14.55

■ Specific Active and Passive Movement Testing (Quantity and Quality)

a) **Plantar flexion** from the zero position:

- The therapist fixates the lower leg against the bench and asks the patient to actively point the foot (plantar flexion) downward as far as possible.
- Then from dorsal, the therapist grasps the collum tali and tests whether the movement continues passively.

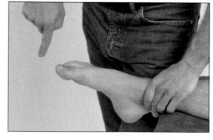

Fig. 14.56

- Finally, the therapist moves the talus passively out of the neutral position through the entire range of motion and tests the end-feel.

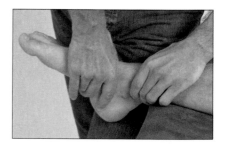

Fig. 14.57

Physiological end-feel:
firm and elastic

b) **Dorsiflexion** from the zero position:

- The therapist fixates the lower leg against the bench and asks the patient to <u>actively</u> flex the foot (dorsiflexion).
- Then from plantar, the therapist places his hand on the sustentaculum tali and the plantar talonavicular ligament, pressing the caput tali dorsally and thereby testing whether the movement <u>continues</u> <u>passively</u>. The therapist may rest his elbow against his pelvis in order to achieve more strength.
- Finally, the therapist moves the talus <u>passively</u> out of the zero position and through the entire range of motion and tests the <u>end-feel</u>.

Physiological end-feel:
firm and elastic

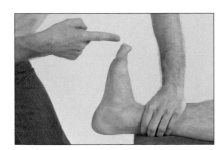

Fig. 14.58

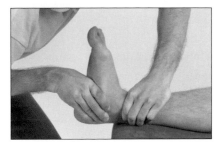

Fig. 14.59

Stability tests in the Zero Position

The therapist fixates the lower leg against the bench and with the second metacarpal head of the distal hand grasps the caput tali from tibial or fibular in order to <u>passively</u> gap the joint on the tibial or fibular side. The <u>end-feel</u> is also assessed.

> **!** Stability tests may be performed with the joint in any position. They provide information in particular about the stability of the ankle mortise formed by the lateral and medial malleoli into which the talus fits. See also the stability tests for the distal tibiofibular syndesmosis in the section on the lower leg (see p. 96).

Physiological end-feel:
very firm and elastic

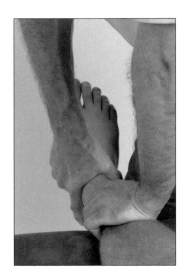

Fig. 14.60

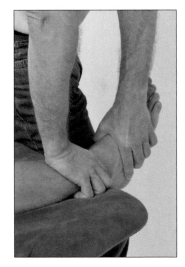

Fig. 14.61

14.5.3 Translatoric movement tests

a) **Traction** from the resting position:

The therapist fixates the lower leg against the bench with his lateral hand. Then, he places his medial hand on the foot, grasping the collum tali from dorsal with the little finger. The thumb of the medial hand rests on the sole of the foot and holds the ankle joint in the resting position. The forearm of the medial hand forms the extension of the lower leg axis and pulls the talus at a right angle away from the treatment plane. The index finger of the lateral hand can palpate the movement between the tibial malleolus and the medial tubercle of the posterior talar process.

Physiological end-feel: firm and elastic

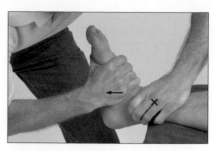

Fig. 14.62

b) **Compression** in the resting position:

The therapist fixates the lower leg against the bench and applies pressure to the calcaneus at a right angle to the treatment plane.

> **!** In this technique, the subtalar joint is simultaneously compressed. This test should be performed with the patient lying down if standing produces symptoms.

Physiological end-feel: hard

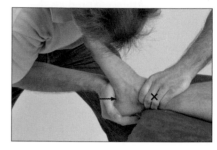

Fig. 14.63

14.5.4 Translatoric movement testing of the Intertarsal Joints

The hindfoot forms a functional unit consisting of the ankle joint, the subtalar joint, and the intertarsal joints. Together with the joints of the midfoot, the subtalar joint and the intertarsal joints form the three arches of the foot: the longitudinal medial and lateral arches, and the transversal anterior arch. It is essential for the intertarsal joints to be stable in order to allow for functioning of the hindfoot and the arches of the foot (especially the medial arch). Rotatory tests of the intertarsal joints are done along with the movements of the hindfoot and midfoot. Translatoric traction does not allow for an adequate evaluation of mobility, because technically specific traction is nearly impossible. So too are specific compression tests. Tests of translatoric gliding, however, do allow a quite specific evaluation of the mobility of the intertarsal joints. Their treatment plane is roughly perpendicular to the dorsum of the foot. The proximal bone is fixated and the distal one is moved. The order may be chosen as the therapist wishes, but the use of a system, such as the one suggested here, is recommended so as not to neglect an important test and to keep one's head clear for sensing the movements. Given that the intertarsal joints should be mainly stable, only the tests for mobility are shown here. If there is only minimal movement, the intertarsal joint is probably stable rather than hypomobile. Mobilization is rarely indicated and hence is not shown here. If there is a high degree of mobility, the joint may be hypermobile. The patient should be advised to use stabilizing measures such as wearing sole inlays and stable shoes.

a) **Gliding between the talus and navicular bone in the resting position** (Test 1):

The therapist stands next to the patient and supports the lateral margin of the foot against his own thigh. With his proximal hand, he grasps the neck of the talus with his thumb and the calcaneus with his fingers. The thumb and index finger of his distal hand wrap around the navicular bone and move it dorsally and plantarly, parallel to the treatment plane which is roughly at a right angle to the dorsum of the foot.

Physiological end-feel: firm and elastic

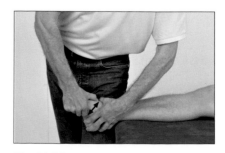

Fig. 14.64

Alternative grip:

If the therapist's hand is small and the patient's foot is large, the foot may be placed on the head piece of the bench while the therapist uses his arm to stabilize the lower leg against his own body. His proximal hand presses the neck of the talus against the calcaneus plantarly against the bench, thereby fixating the talus. His proxi-mal hand and forearm should ensure that the patient's foot and lower leg are stable; this may be tested by us-ing the distal hand to loosely move the forefoot back and forth. This should be possible without tension. Next, the therapist wraps the thumb and index finger of his distal hand around the navicular bone which he moves dorsally and plantarly, parallel to the treatment plane.

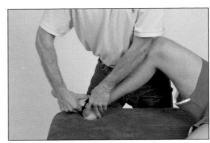

Fig. 14.65

b) **Gliding between the navicular and first to third cuneiform bones in the resting position** (Test 2).

The therapist stands as in the previous example and fixates the navicular bone with the thumb and index finger of his proximal hand. The thumb and index finger of his distal hand grasp the first cuneiform (then the second and the third or all three together) and moves it (or them) dorsally and plantarly, parallel to the treatment plane.

Physiological end-feel:
firm and elastic

c) **Gliding between the first to third cuneiforms and the corresponding metatarsals in the resting position** (Tests 3 to 5).

With the same grip as before, but 1 to 2 cm further distally, the therapist's proximal hand fixates the first, second, or third cuneiform and his distal hand moves the base of the opposing metatarsal bone dorsally and plantarly, parallel to the treatment plane (see **Fig. 14.66** for tests 2 to 5).

Physiological end-feel:
firm and elasti

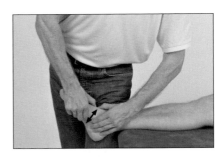

Fig. 14.66

d) **Gliding between the cuboid and fourth and fifth metatarsals in the resting position** (Test 6).

The therapist kneels on one knee at the distal end of the bench. The patient's leg is positioned so that there is slight hip adduction. The index and middle fingers of the therapist's proximal hand grasp the dorsal surface of the cuboid from the fibular side of the patient's leg while his thumb grasps it from plantar and fixates it. The index and middle fingers of his distal hand grasp the dorsal aspect of the fourth and fifth metatarsal bones from the fibular side. His thumb is placed on the plantar surface around the bases of the fourth and fifth metatarsals (or around each individual one) and moves them dorsally and plantarly, parallel to the treatment plane.

Physiological end-feel:
firm and elastic

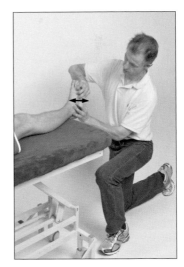

Fig. 14.67

e) **Gliding between the cuboid, and navicular and cuneiform bones in the resting position** (Test 7):

Still kneeling on one knee at the distal end of the bench, the therapist now has the patient's leg positioned with slight hip abduction. The index and middle fingers of his tibial hand grasp the dorsal aspect of the navicular and cuneiform bones from the tibial side while his thumb is placed on plantar aspect of the navicular and cuneiform bones to fixate them. As before, the index and middle fingers of his fibular hand grasp the dorsal aspect of the cuboid bone and his thumb grasps the plantar aspect, moving it dorsally and plantarly, parallel to the treatment plane.

Physiological end-feel:
firm and elastic

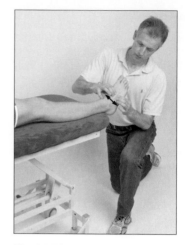

Fig. 14.68

f) **Gliding between the cuboid and calcaneus in the resting position** (Test 8):

Still kneeling on one knee at the distal end of the bench, the therapist continues to fixate the patient's leg in a position of slight hip abduction. From the tibial side of the patient's leg, his tibial hand is wrapped flat around the calcaneus and fixates it. Pulling it slightly distally makes fixation easier. As before, he uses the index and middle fingers of his fibular hand to grasp the dorsal surface of the cuboid from the fibular side, while his thumb wraps around the cuboid on the plantar aspect and moves it dorsally and plantarly, parallel to the treatment plane.

Physiological end-feel:
firm and elastic

Including the tests of the subtalar joint (Test 9) and the ankle joint (Test 10), there are a total of 10 Translatoric movement tests with which the entire hindfoot may be examined.

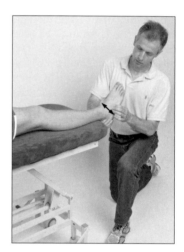

Fig. 14.69

14.5.5 Treatment of Capsuloligamentous Hypomobility

The lower leg of the patient is fixed to the head of the bench with a belt. The therapist grasps the foot with the medial hand as in the traction test and places the lateral hand on top of it for support. The forearms are parallel to one another and form the prolongation of the lower leg axis, moving the talus at a right angle away from the treatment plane.

Alternatively, a belt may be placed around the collum tali and around the pelvis of the therapist. By leaning backward, the therapist can increase the force of traction.

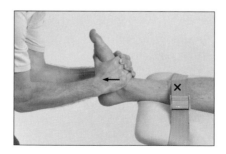

Fig. 14.70

! Pain-relieving traction may also be performed using the test version.

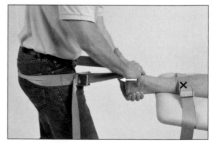

Fig. 14.71

! The ankle joint is closely connected to the tibiofibular syndesmosis. Restricted mobility in the ankle joint can lead to hypermobility in the syndesmosis, especially with mobilization in end-range rotation, which therefore should be avoided.

Documentation template: Practice Scheme

Ankle joint	
Symptoms	
Symptom-altering direction	
Contraindications?	Nervous system: Other:
Symptom-altering joint	
General assessment of adjacent joints	

Active movements, comparing sides						
Specific rotatory tests	**Active**	**Continues passively?**	**Passive**	**End-feel**	**Symptoms/ pain**	**Comments**
▪ Plantar flexion						
▪ Dorsiflexion						

Stability tests	**Quantity**	**Quality**	**End-feel**	**Symptoms/pain**	**Comments**
▪ Fibular gaping					
▪ Tibial gaping					
Translatoric movement tests	**Quantity**	**Quality**	**End-feel**	**Symptoms/pain**	**Comments**
▪ Traction					
▪ Compression					

Summary Formulation aid: ▪ Symptoms ▪ Direction ▪ Contraindications ▪ Site (joint) ▪ Restricted mobility, hypermobility, or physiological mobility ▪ Structure: muscle, joint, etc.	*Text:*
Trial treatment	
Physical therapy diagnosis	
Treatment plan with treatment goal and prognosis	
Treatment progress	
Final examination	

Documentation: Practice Example

<table>
<tr><th colspan="7" style="text-align:center">Ankle joint
(Pes equinus in a bed-ridden patient)</th></tr>
<tr><td>Symptoms</td><td colspan="6">Difficulty standing and walking related to pain in the feet</td></tr>
<tr><td>Symptom-altering direction</td><td colspan="6">Dorsiflexion</td></tr>
<tr><td>Contraindications?</td><td colspan="6">Nervous system: No findings
Other: No findings</td></tr>
<tr><td>Symptom-altering joint</td><td colspan="6">Ankle joints, both sides</td></tr>
<tr><td>General assessment of adjacent joints</td><td colspan="6">All joints of the lower extremities begin with the limitations typically seen in bed-ridden patients (flexion contractures).</td></tr>
<tr><td>Active movements, comparing sides</td><td colspan="6">Dorsiflexion limited by ca. – 10° on both sides</td></tr>
</table>

Specific rotatory tests	Active	Continues passively?	Passive	End-feel	Symptoms/pain	Comments
▪ Plantar flexion	40°	ca. 10°	No findings	Firm and elastic		
▪ Dorsiflexion	– 10°	< 5°	Increased resistance to movement	Initial soft resistance, then very firm and elastic	Pain at maximum end-rage	Knee slightly bent during testing

Stability tests	Quantity	Quality	End-feel	Symptoms/pain	Comments
▪ Fibular gaping	No findings	No findings	Firm and elastic	No findings	
▪ Tibial gaping	No findings	No findings	Firm and elastic	No findings	

Translatoric movement tests	Quantity	Quality	End-feel	Symptoms/pain	Comments
▪ Traction	Hypo 2	Firm resistance to movement	Very firm and elastic	No findings	Tested in actual resting position ca. 20°
▪ Compression	No findings	No findings	Hard	No findings	

<table>
<tr><td>Summary
Formulation aid:
▪ Symptoms
▪ Direction
▪ Contraindications
▪ Site (joint)
▪ Restricted mobility, hypermobility, or physiological mobility
▪ Structure: muscle, joint, etc.</td><td>Text:
▪ Difficulty standing and walking
▪ with dorsiflexion of both feet.
▪ No contraindications today to further movement testing.
▪ Symptoms are localized in both ankle joints
▪ and are correlated to restricted mobility,

▪ caused by shortening of the plantar flexors (the initial soft and elastic end-feel) and shrinkage of the capsuloligamentous unit (then very firm and less elastic end-feel).</td></tr>
<tr><td>Trial treatment</td><td>Mobilizing grade III traction of the ankle joint. After ca. 5-minute-long trial treatment, the end-feel seems to be slightly less firm.</td></tr>
<tr><td>Physical therapy diagnosis</td><td>See above</td></tr>
</table>

Ankle joint	
(Pes equinus in a bed-ridden patient)	
Treatment plan with treatment goal and prognosis	▪ *Continue grade III mobilizing traction of the ankle joint followed by relaxation and stretching of the plantar flexors.* ▪ *Treatment goal: pain-free physiological mobility* **(Further information on examination and treatment techniques may be obtained through further education.)**
Treatment progress	
Final examination	

14.6 Lower Leg

(Syndesmosis tibiofibularis distalis and articulatio tibiofibularis proximalis)

14.6.1 Anatomy

Joint type: syndesmosis tibiofibularis: syndesmosis, unmodified sellar joint
  ▪ Joint surface: the fibular malleolus is concave.

Articulatio tibiofibularis: amphiarthrosis
  ▪ Joint surface: anatomical variants are common; in manual therapy the head of the fibula is considered concave.

Resting position: 10° plantar flexion of the ankle joint

Close packed position: maximum dorsiflexion of the ankle joint

Capsular sign: not described.

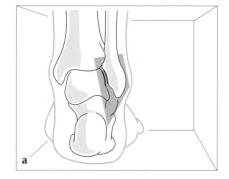
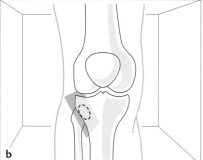

Fig. 14.72 a, b

> **!** Lower leg joints with little motion are considered stable. They usually do not restrict movement of the knee and ankle joints. Stretching grade III mobilizations to increase the range of motion are rarely indicated.

Note
An axis of rotation lies horizontally between the lower third and the upper two thirds of the fibula. During dorsiflexion of the ankle joint, the fibular malleolus moves slightly posteriorly and the head of the fibula slightly anteriorly (Lazannec et al., 1994).

14.6.2   Rotatory Tests

■ Active Movements, Comparing Sides

The patient moves both feet in maximum plantar flexion and dorsiflexion as in the test of the ankle joint. It is not possible to actively isolate the movements of the fibula and tibia. However, they do move relative to one another during ankle joint motion.

■ Specific Active and Passive Movement Testing (Quantity and Quality)

Given that rotatory movements of the fibula in relation to the tibia can only occur with ankle joint motions, movement testing is the same as for the ankle joint (see p. 88).

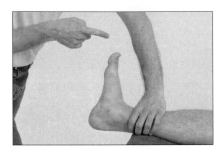

Fig. 14.73

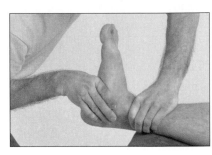

Fig. 14.74

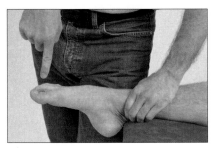

Fig. 14.75

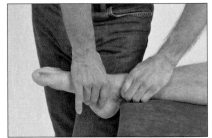

Fig. 14.76

■ Stability Tests in the Zero Position

The stability of the distal tibiofibular syndesmosis is essential for the stability of the ankle joint because the talus is fixated as far as possible by the malleoli. Tibiofibular joint stability may be tested using the ankle joint stability tests (see p. 99). The stability of the tibiofibular joints may also be tested with translatoric gliding movements (see below).

14.6.3   Translatoric movement tests

■ Tibiofibular Syndesmosis

a) **Traction** from the resting position:

Separation of the two bones is technically impossible.

b) **Compression** in the resting position:

The therapist fixates the lower leg against the bench and presses the fibular malleolus against the tibia.

Physiological end-feel: hard

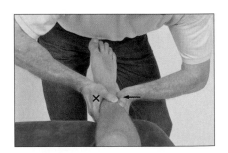

Fig. 14.77

c) **Gliding** in the tibiofibular joint from the resting position:

The therapist fixates the tibia against the bench with his medial hand. Next he places the thumb and index finger of his lateral hand around the fibular malleolus and moves it anteriorly and posteriorly. The therapeut can palpate either with the index finger or the thumb of his fixating hand.

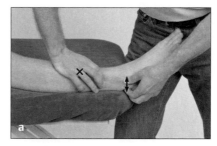
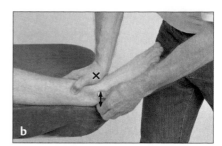

Fig. 14.78

Physiological end-feel:
very firm and elastic

■ Tibiofibular Articulation

a) **Traction** from the resting position:

Separation of the two bones is technically impossible.

b) **Compression** of the tibiofibular joint in the resting position:

The patient's foot is resting on the raised head piece of the bench with the knee in about 90° flexion. The therapist fixates the proximal tibia with his medial hand. He then presses the head of the fibula against the tibia with the lateral hand anteriorly and medially.

Physiological end-feel: hard

c) **Gliding** in the tibiofibular joint, from the resting position:

The patient's foot is resting on the raised head piece of the bench with the knee in about 90° flexion. The therapist fixates the proximal tibia with his medial hand. Using the thumb and index finger or middle finger of his lateral hand, he holds the head of the fibula from posterolateral and moves it anterolaterally and posteromedially.

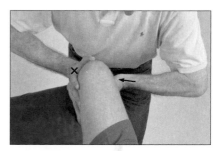

Fig. 14.79

Physiological end-feel:
very firm and elastic

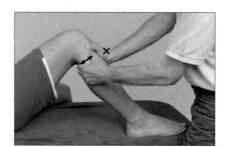

Fig. 14.80

14.6.4 Treatment of Capsuloligamentous Hypomobility

Traction therapy is not possible in either joint due to technical reasons.

■ Tibiofibular Syndesmosis

The therapist fixates the tibia against the bench with his medial hand. Using the lateral hand, he places the thenar eminence on the fibular malleolus, which he moves posteriorly. For anterior mobilization of the fibular malleolus, the patient is lying prone and the therapist uses the same grip.

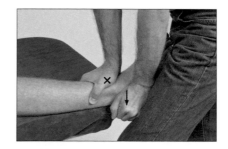

Fig. 14.81

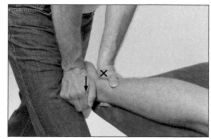

Fig. 14.82

> **!** For pain relief, grade I–II intermittent gliding mobilization may be used. It may also be done with the test version. Grade III mobilization may be indicated if ankle joint dorsiflexion is restricted by tibiofibular joint hypomobility which, however, is quite seldom.

■ Tibiofibular Articulation

a) Gliding anteriorly

The patient is lying in the prone position with the lower leg resting on the raised head piece of the bench. The therapist first locates the fibular head from posterior with the thumb of the distal hand. Next he places his proximal hand (the area over the pisiform) over it, holds the tibia with the distal hand, and moves the fibular head anterolaterally. This technique may also be done with the patient on all fours.

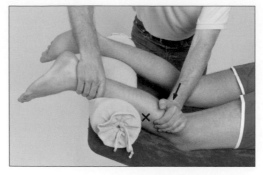

Fig. 14.83

b) Gliding posteriorly

The patient is lying on his or her side with the affected leg on top. The therapist first uses the thumb of his distal hand to find the head of the fibula from anterior, places the pisiform of the proximal hand on it, holds the tibia distally, and then moves the fibular head posteromedially.

> **!** For pain relief, grade I–II intermittent gliding mobilization may be performed, also in the test version.
> Grade III stretching mobilization is rarely indicated.

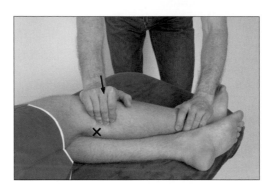

Fig. 14.84

Documentation template: Practice Scheme

Lower leg	
Symptoms	
Symptom-altering direction	
Contraindications?	Nervous system: Other:
Symptom-altering joint	
General evaluation of adjacent joints	

Continued ▶

Documentation template: Practice Scheme *(Continued)*

Lower leg						
Active movements, comparing sides						
Specific rotatory tests	**Active**	**Continues passively?**	**Passive**	**End-feel**	**Symptoms/ pain**	**Comments**
▪ Plantar flexion, ankle joint						
▪ Dorsiflexion, ankle joint						
Stability tests	**Quantity**	**Quality**	**End-feel**	**Symptoms/pain**	**Comments**	
▪ Fibular gaping ankle joint						
▪ Tibial gaping ankle joint						
Translatoric movement tests	**Quantity**	**Quality**	**End-feel**	**Symptoms/pain**	**Comments**	
Syndesmosis: ▪ Compression						
Syndesmosis: ▪ Gliding						
Articulation: ▪ Compression						
Articulation: ▪ Gliding						
▪ Ankle joint: traction						
▪ Ankle joint: compression						
Summary Formulation aid: ▪ Symptoms ▪ Direction ▪ Contraindications ▪ Site (joint) ▪ Restricted mobility, hypermobility, or physiological mobility ▪ Structure: muscle, joint, etc. ▪ Additional causal or influencing factors:	*Text:*					
Trial treatment						
Physical therapy diagnosis						
Treatment plan with treatment goal and prognosis						
Treatment progress						
Final examination						

Documentation template: Practice Example

<table>
<tr><td colspan="7">Lower leg
(Some pain with dorsiflexion of the right ankle joint 3 months after fracture of the fibular malleolus with lesion of the tibiofibular ligaments)</td></tr>
<tr><td>Symptoms</td><td colspan="6">Pain in the right foot when standing or walking</td></tr>
<tr><td>Symptom-altering direction</td><td colspan="6">Dorsiflexion</td></tr>
<tr><td>Contraindications?</td><td colspan="6">Nervous system: No findings
Other: No findings</td></tr>
<tr><td>Symptom-altering joint</td><td colspan="6">Ankle joint, right</td></tr>
<tr><td>General evaluation of adjacent joints</td><td colspan="6">The right tarsal joints appear to be slightly hypermobile.</td></tr>
<tr><td>Active movements, comparing sides</td><td colspan="6">Dorsiflexion of the right foot is limited by –10°</td></tr>
</table>

Specific rotatory tests	Active	Continues passively?	Passive	End-feel	Symptoms/pain	Comments
▪ Plantar flexion, ankle joint	*Nearly 30°*	*< 5°*	*Increased resistance to movement*	*Very firm and elastic*		
▪ Dorsiflexion, ankle joint	*–10°*	*< 5°*	*Increased resistance to movement*	*Very firm and elastic*	*Mild pain at end-range*	

Stability tests	Quantity	Quality	End-feel	Symptoms/pain	Comments
▪ Fibular gaping	*Hyper 4*	*Little resistance to movement*	*Slightly firm and elastic*	*Minimal pain*	
▪ Tibial gaping	*Hyper 4*	*Little resistance to movement*	*Slightly firm and elastic*	*Minimal pain*	

Translatoric tests	Quantity	Quality	End-feel	Symptoms/pain	Comments
Syndesmosis: ▪ Compression	*No findings*	*No findings*	*Hard*	*No findings*	
Syndesmosis: ▪ Gliding	*Hyper 4*	*Moves easily*	*Slightly firm and elastic*	*Mild pain at end-range*	
Articulation: ▪ Compression	*No findings*	*No findings*	*Hard*	*No findings*	
Articulation: ▪ Gliding	*No findings*	*No findings*	*Firm and elastic*	*No findings*	
▪ Ankle joint: traction	*hypo 2*	*Increased resistance to movement*	*Very firm and elastic*	*No findings*	
▪ Ankle joint: compression	*No findings*	*No findings*	*Hard*	*No findings*	

Continued ▶

Lower leg (Some pain with dorsiflexion of the right ankle joint 3 months after fracture of the fibular malleolus with lesion of the tibiofibular ligaments)	
Summary Formulation aid: ■ Symptoms ■ Direction ■ Contraindications ■ Site (joint) ■ Restricted mobility, hypermobility, or physiological mobility ■ Structure: muscle, joint, etc. ■ Additional causal or influencing factors:	*Text:* ■ *Pain in the right foot when standing or walking* ■ *during dorsiflexion.* ■ *There are no contraindications today for further movement tests.* ■ *The symptoms appear in the ankle joint and are correlated with the tibiofibular syndesmosis.* ■ *which is hypermobile* ■ *due to laxity of the syndesmosis causing instability of the ankle joint in the frontal plane.* ■ *Hypomobility of the ankle joint in the sagittal plane due to capsuloligamentous shrinkage (–10° dorsiflexion and 30° planarflexion) is worsening the situation by exacerbating the hypermobility of the tibiofibular syndesmosis during rotatory movements into dorsiflexion by the therapist and the patient himself.*
Trial treatment	■ *5-minute long pain-relieving grade I–II intermittent gliding mobilization of the tibiofibular joint. This relieves the pain during dorsiflexion.* ■ *This was followed by 10-minute long grade III traction mobilization of the ankle joint. This led to reduced resistance to movement during dorsiflexion and end-range movement was less painful.*
Physical therapy diagnosis	*See above*
Treatment plan with treatment goal and prognosis	■ *After initial pain-relieving gliding mobilization of the tibiofibular syndesmosis, continue grade III traction mobilization of the ankle joint. No rotatory end-range movements in dorsiflexion by the patient and by the physical therapist, which cause further separation of the ankle mortise and would exacerbate the hypermobility of the joint.* ■ *Treatment goal: pain-free physiological mobility.* **(Further information on examination and treatment techniques may be obtained through further education.)**
Treatment progress	
Final examination	

14.7   Knee Joint

(Articulatio genu: articulationes femoropatellaris et femorotibialis)

14.7.1   Anatomy

Joint type:
- Patellofemoral joint: gliding joint
  Joint surface: three concave facets of the patella
- Femorotibial joint: trocho-ginglymus
  Joint surface: the tibial plateau is concave except for the lateral half which is slightly convex in the sagittal plane. Given that the rotatory axis for flexion/extension is located in the femoral condyles, the tibia is considered concave in manual therapy.

Resting position:
- Patellofemoral joint: extension of the knee joint
- Femorotibial joint: 25–35° flexion

Close packed position:
- Patellofemoral joint: maximum flexion

- Femorotibial joint: maximum extension and external rotation

Capsular sign:
flexion > extension

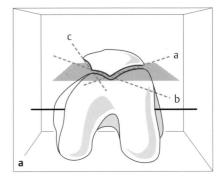

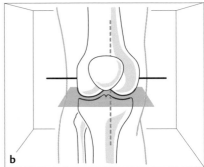

Fig. 14.85 a, b

14.7.2   Rotatory Tests

■ Active Movements, Comparing Sides

The patient moves both knees toward maximum flexion ("heels to buttocks"), then maximum extension ("with the backs of the knees pressing against the bench, lift the heels"). Finally, with approximately 90° flexion, the patient performs maximum external and internal rotation.

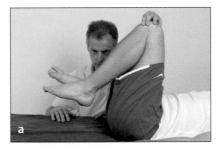

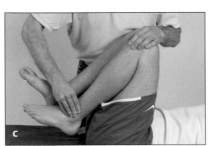

Fig. 14.86 a–c

! After the patient has performed bilateral flexion, the therapist can hold the thighs with his proximal hand and with the distal hand press against the patient's lower legs to increase the flexion. During this, the thumb and index finger of the proximal hand palpate the tibial border at the anterior joint space. This makes it easier to detect differences between sides in flexion as well as any gaping of the joint space.

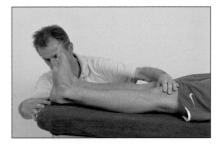

Fig. 14.87

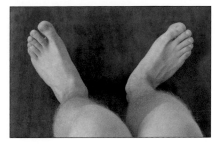

Fig. 14.88

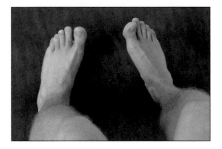

Fig. 14.89

Specific Active and Passive Movement Testing (Quantity and Quality)

a) **Flexion** from the zero position:

- The therapist asks the patient to maximally bend the knee.
- Next, the therapist fixates the thigh, and with the thumb and index finger of the proximal hand he palpates the anterior joint space and tests whether the movement of the lower leg continues passively.
- Finally, he moves the lower leg passively from the zero position in maximum flexion and tests the end-feel.

Physiological end-feel:
soft and elastic

! The thumb and index finger of the proximal hand palpate the anterior joint space to sense the movement of the tibia. Often there is gaping of the joint space at the end of passive flexion. This indicates restricted posterior gliding of the tibia.

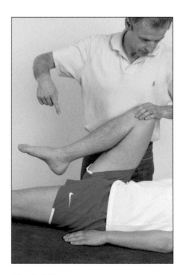

Fig. 14.90

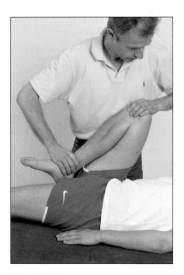

Fig. 14.91

b) **Extension** from the zero position:

- The therapist fixates the patient's thigh against the bench, allowing the lower leg to hang over the end with the knee flexed. Next he asks the patient to extend the knee to its maximum.
- Then the therapist takes the distal lower leg and tests whether the movement continues passively.
- Finally, the therapist moves the lower leg passively out of the zero position (or slightly flexed position), through the entire range of motion, and tests the end-feel.

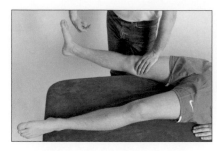

Fig. 14.92

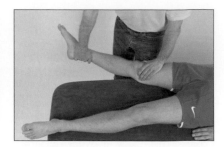

Fig. 14.93

Physiological end-feel:
firm and elastic

c) **External rotation** from the zero position:

- The knee is in approximately 90° flexion with the heel on the bench. The tip of the foot is raised as high as possible so that the ankle joint is locked in dorsiflexion. The therapist fixates the distal thigh and asks the patient to rotate the tip of the foot externally.
- Then the therapist takes the foot at the height of the collum tali, holds the maximum dorsiflexion in the ankle joint and tests whether the movement continues passively in the direction of external rotation.
- Finally, he moves the knee passively from the zero position with the same grip in the direction of external rotation and tests the end-feel.

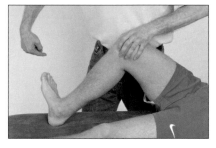

Fig. 14.94

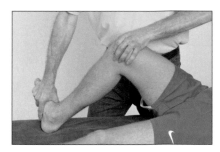

Fig. 14.95

> **!** The thumb and index finger of the proximal hand can be used to feel the movement of the tibia in the anterior joint space.

Physiological end-feel:
firm and elastic

d) **Internal rotation** from the zero position:

- The knee is in approximately 90° flexion with the heel on the bench. The tip of the foot is raised as high as possible so that the ankle joint is locked in dorsiflexion. The therapist fixates the distal thigh and asks the patient to rotate the tip of the foot internally.
- Then the therapist takes the foot at the height of the collum tali, holds the maximum dorsiflexion in the ankle joint and tests whether the movement continues passively in the direction of internal rotation. For support, the therapist may rest his hand and forearm on the bench.
- Finally, with the same grip he moves the knee from the zero position passively in the direction of internal rotation and tests the end-feel.

Physiological end-feel:
firm and elastic

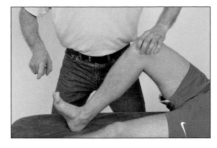
Fig. 14.96

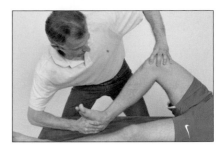
Fig. 14.97

! The thumb and index finger of the proximal hand can be used to feel the movement of the tibia in the anterior joint space.

▣ Stability Tests in the Zero Position

- The therapist places his proximal hand on the lateral side of the knee and his distal hand on the medial side of the distal lower leg. The therapist rotates his body slightly to test the medial gaping of the knee joint.
- To test lateral stability, the therapist places his proximal hand on the medial side of the knee and the distal hand from lateral around the distal lower leg. He then rotates his body to exert stress on the lateral joint space.

Physiological end-feel:
very firm and elastic

! The stability tests may be performed with the joint in any position. The therapist may also use his abdomen to help support the patient's leg during the test.

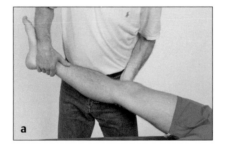
Fig. 14.98 a, b

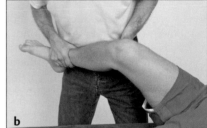

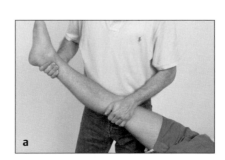
Fig. 14.99 a, b

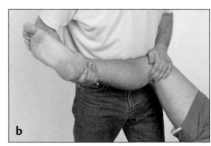

14.7.3 Translatoric Test

■ Patellofemoral Joint

a) **Traction** in the resting position:

The back of the knee is supported by a firm cushion or sandbag to prevent hyperextension of the knee joint. With the thumb and index finger, the therapist places both hands around the patella and tries to raise it at a right angle from the treatment plane.

! The range of motion is minimal and an evaluation of hypomobility/hypermobility is impossible. If there is severe compression pain, however, the test provides relief. In this case it is also suitable as a pain-relief treatment.

Physiological end-feel:
very firm and elastic

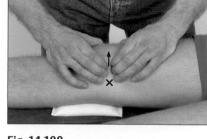

Fig. 14.100

b) **Compression** in the resting position:

The back of the knee is again supported by a firm cushion or sandbag to prevent hyperextension of the knee joint. With one hand, the therapist

stabilizes the femur or tibia lying on the sandbag and with the other he presses the patella at a right angle toward the treatment plane.

Physiological end-feel: hard

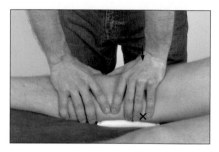

Fig. 14.101

c) **Gliding** in the resting position:

The back of the knee is supported as described above. The therapist uses the thumbs and index fingers of both his hands to move the patella medially, laterally, distally, and proximally, parallel to the plane of treatment. The patellar distal gliding test yields the most information if done with the knee prepositioned in flexion, directly comparing sides.

Physiological end-feel:
firm and elastic; very firm and elastic with proximal gliding due to the patellar ligament.

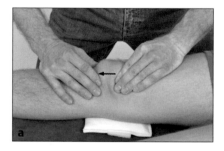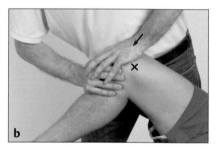

Fig. 14.102 a, b

! **Fig. 14.102 b** shows distal gliding in prepositioned flexion of the knee. This allows better assessment of mobility of the patella which is limited in the resting position not only by the joint's capsule but mainly by the femoro-patellar ligaments.

■ Femorotibial Joint

a) **Traction** in the resting position:

The patient is lying in the prone position. The therapist uses his proximal hand to hold the distal thigh against the bench. Using his distal hand, the therapist holds the distal lower leg, which he stabilizes against his abdomen, and pulls the tibia at a right angle away from the treatment plane. With the index finger of the proximal

hand, he can palpate the movement in the anteromedial joint space.

Physiological end-feel:
firm and elastic

! The amount of femorotibial traction is primarily limited by the tightening of the cruciate and lateral ligaments. It therefore says little about the length and flexibility of the joint capsule.

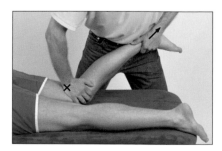

Fig. 14.103

b) **Compression** in the resting position:

The patient is in the prone position. The therapist uses his proximal hand to fixate the distal thigh against the bench. With his distal hand, the therapist holds the distal lower leg, which is stabilized against his abdomen, and pushes the tibia <u>at a right angle toward the treatment plane</u>.

Physiological end-feel: hard

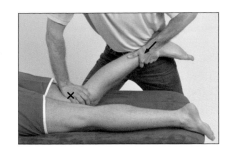

Fig. 14.104

14.7.4 | Treatment of Capsuloligamentous Hypomobility

■ **Patellofemoral Joint**

Gliding distally:

The back of the knee is supported by a firm cushion or sandbag to prevent hyperextension of the knee joint. With his medial hand, the therapist grips the patella and tries to raise it slightly (grade I traction). Then with the thenar eminence he moves the patella distally.

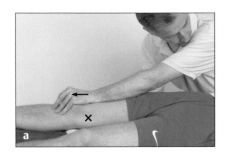

> ❗ For pain relief, intermittent gliding or, in case of very strong pain, even traction may also be performed in the test version (see **Figs. 14.100 and 14.102**).

> ❗ Distal gliding can improve restricted flexion. It is much more effective if done with the knees prepositioned in flexion.

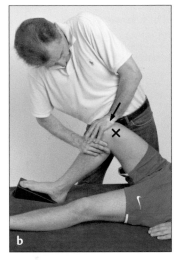

Fig. 14.105 a, b

■ **Femorotibial Joint**

Traction in the resting position:

The patient is lying in the prone position with his or her distal thigh secured to the bench with a belt. The therapist places his hands on the distal thigh and pulls the tibia <u>at a right angle away from the treatment plane</u>. To facilitate traction, the therapist may place a belt around his hands and pelvis.

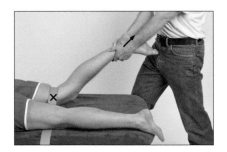

Fig. 14.106

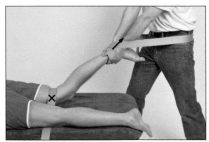

Fig. 14.107

> ❗ Pain-relieving traction may also be performed in the test version.

> ❗ Positioning the knee joint with slight external rotation prior to traction reduces the tension on the cruciate ligaments.

Documentation template: Practice Scheme

Knee joint						
Symptoms						
Symptom-altering direction						
Contraindications?	Nervous system: Other:					
Symptom-altering joint						
General assessment of adjacent joints						
General assessment of adjacent joints						

Specific rotatory tests	**Active**	**Continues passively?**	**Passive**	**End-feel**	**Symptoms/ pain**	**Comments**
▪ Flexion						
▪ Extension						
▪ External rotation						
▪ Internal rotation						

Stability tests	**Quantity**	**Quality**	**End-feel**	**Symptoms/pain**	**Comments**
▪ Tibial gaping					
▪ Fibular gaping					

Translatoric movement tests	**Quantity**	**Quality**	**End-feel**	**Symptoms/pain**	**Comments**
Patellofemoral joint: ▪ Traction					
▪ Compression					
▪ Distal gliding					
▪ Medial gliding					
▪ Lateral gliding					
▪ Proximal gliding					
Femorotibial joint: ▪ Traction					
▪ Compression					

Summary Formulation aid: ▪ Symptoms ▪ Direction ▪ Contraindications ▪ Site (joint) ▪ Restricted mobility, hypermobility, or physiological mobility	*Text:*

Continued ▶

Documentation template: Practice Scheme *(Continued)*

Knee joint	
Summary Formulation aid (confirmed): ▪ Structure: muscle, joint, etc.	
Trial treatment	
Physical therapy diagnosis	
Treatment plan with treatment goal and prognosis	
Treatment progress	
Final examination	

Documentation: Practice Example

Knee joint (Painfully restricted movement, day 1 after arthroscopic control of right knee)						
Symptoms	*Pain with movement, right knee joint*					
Symptom-altering direction	*All directions trigger pain, especially flexion and extension, less severe with internal and external rotation.*					
Contraindications?	Nervous system: *No findings* Other: *No findings*					
Symptom-altering joint	*The knee joint with the patellofemoral and femorotibial joints*					
General assessment of adjacent joints	*No findings*					
Active movements, comparing sides	*Extension and flexion of the right knee significantly restricted compared with left side, both rotations minimal*					
Specific rotatory tests	**Active**	**Continues passively?**	**Passive**	**End-feel**	**Symptoms/ pain**	**Comments**
▪ Flexion	*80°*	*< 5°*	*Muscle guarding*	*Soft and elastic*	*Pain at end range*	*Patient is anxious about pain occurring*
▪ Extension	*– 20°*	*< 5°*	*Muscle guarding*	*Soft and elastic*	*Pain at end range*	*Ditto*
▪ External rotation	*30°*	*< 5°*	*Muscle guarding*	*Soft and elastic*	*Pain at end range*	*Ditto*
▪ Internal rotation	*10°*	*< 5°*	*Muscle guarding*	*Soft and elastic*	*Pain at end range*	*Ditto*

Stability tests	**Quantity**	**Quality**	**End-feel**	**Symptoms/pain**	**Comments**
▪ Fibular gaping	*Not testable*				*Did not test due to pain*
▪ Tibial gaping	*Not testable*				*Ditto*

Continued ▶

Knee joint (Painfully restricted movement, first day after arthroscopic control of right knee)					
Translatoric movement tests	**Quantity**	**Quality**	**End-feel**	**Symptoms/pain**	**Comments**
Patellofemoral joint: ▪ Traction	*No findings*	*No findings*	*Firm*	*No relief of pain symptoms*	*Perceived as pleasant*
▪ Compression	*No findings*	*No findings*	*Hard*	*No findings*	
▪ Distal gliding	*Hypo 2*	*Increased, soft resistance to movement*	*Soft and elastic*		
▪ Medial gliding	*Barely hypo*	*No findings*	*Firm and elastic*	*No findings*	
▪ Lateral gliding	*Barely hypo*	*No findings*	*Firm and elastic*	*No findings*	
▪ Proximal gliding	*No findings*	*No findings*	*Very firm and little elastic*	*No findings*	
Femorotibial joint: ▪ Traction	*No findings*	*No findings*	*Firm and elastic*	*No relief of pain symptoms*	*Perceived as pleasant*
▪ Compression	*No findings*	*No findings*	*Hard*	*No findings*	

Summary Formulation aid: ▪ Symptoms ▪ Direction ▪ Contraindications ▪ Site (joint) ▪ Restricted mobility, hypermobility, or physiological mobility ▪ Structure: muscle, joint, etc.	*Text:* ▪ *Pain in the knee joint* ▪ *with flexion (80°) and extension (–20°) and to a lesser degree with internal rotation (10°) and external rotation (30°)* ▪ *There are no contraindications to further movement testing except of increased caution because of high pain and irritability.* ▪ *The pain is located in the knee joint* ▪ *and is due to anxious tension* ▪ *in the periarticular muscles as a result of postoperative muscle guarding. The patellofemoral and tibiofemoral joints are not directly affected.*
Trial treatment	*10-minute long relaxation techniques for painful muscle tension. These may be performed, for instance, reflexively by careful, pain-relieving grade I–II traction or repeated nonpainful, rotatory movements. Afterward the patient reports relief of pain; the range of motion is improved by a few degrees in all directions.*
Physical therapy diagnosis	*See above*
Treatment plan with treatment goal and prognosis	▪ *Continue relaxation techniques for the muscles surrounding the joint which are also pain relieving. After pain subsides, re-examination of the joints (stability tests could not be performed today).* ▪ *Treatment goal: pain-free physiological mobility.* **(Further information on examination and treatment techniques may be obtained through further education.)**
Treatment progress	
Final examination	

14.8 | Hip Joint

(Articulatio coxae)

14.8.1 | Anatomy

Joint type:	enarthrosis, unmodified ovoid joint
Distal joint surface:	convex
Resting position:	30° flexion, 30° abduction, slight external rotation
Close packed position:	maximum extension, internal rotation, and abduction
Capsular sign:	internal rotation > extension > abduction > external rotation

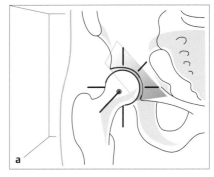

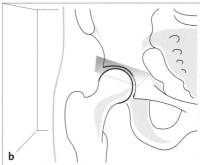

Fig. 14.108 a, b

14.8.2 | Rotatory Tests

■ Active Movements, Comparing Sides

The patient is lying in the supine position. To produce flexion, he or she is asked to bring both knees as close to the chest as possible; for abduction, the feet are placed on the bench with the knees upright, and the patient is asked to move the knees as far laterally as possible; and for adduction, the patient is asked to cross their legs as far as they will go. The test for adduction should be done once with the right leg over the left, and once with the left over the right. In the prone position, the patient should bend the knees to about 90° and for internal rotation should move both feet as far laterally as possible.

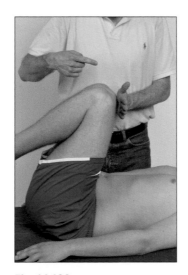

Fig. 14.109

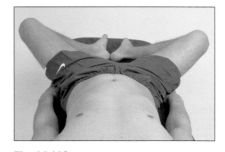

Fig. 14.110

To test external rotation, the patient should cross their lower legs. Given potential differences, the right lower leg should cross on top once and the left on top once. To test extension, the patient should lie face down with the pelvis on the edge of the bench.

The hip joints are flexed and both forefeet are on the floor. Fixating the ischial tuberosity with his proximal hand, the therapist asks the patient to extend the right leg backward and upward. The therapist extends the index finger of his distal hand, placing the finger tip on the posterior aspect of the thigh. The therapist maintains the level of the hand by resting it against his leg. Next the patient extends their left leg in the same manner. The therapist can now observe how far the left leg extends relative to the position of his index finger, which marks the height of right leg extension.

! The order of active movements, comparing sides, deviates from the usual order due to practical considerations.

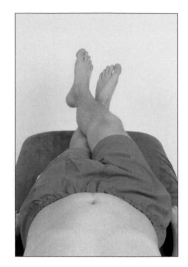

Fig. 14.111

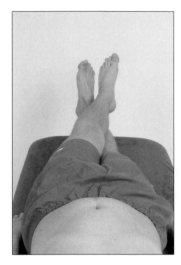

Fig. 14.112

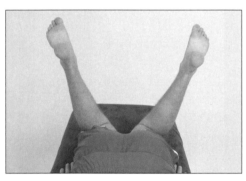

Fig. 14.113

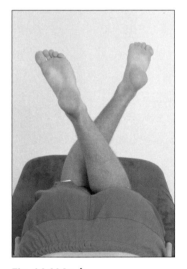
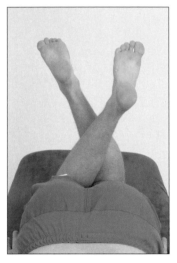

Fig. 14.114 a, b

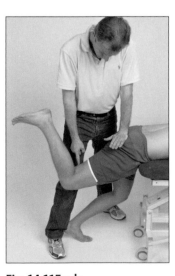
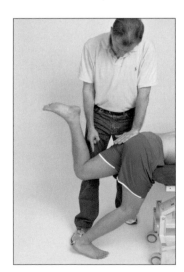

Fig. 14.115 a, b

Specific Active and Passive Movement Testing (Quantity and Quality)

a) **Flexion** from the zero position:

- With the lateral hand, the therapist palpates between the patient's ilium and sacrum to sense the initial movement of the pelvis as it is pulled along during flexion. He then asks the patient to raise the knee as close to the chest as possible to flex the hip joint.
- Then the therapist places his hand from posterior around the thigh and presses it perpendicularly toward the bench. This limits additional movement of the lumbar spine which would otherwise occur as the knee approaches the patient's chest. The therapist then tests whether the movement continues passively.
- Finally, the therapist moves the thigh passively from the zero position to maximum flexion. Lastly, he presses the femur perpendicu-

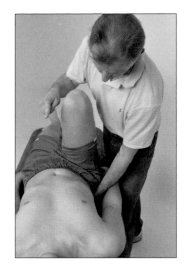

Fig. 14.116

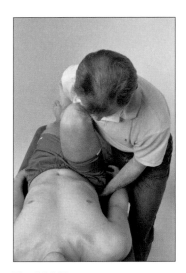

Fig. 14.117

larly toward the bench and with the lateral hand controls the beginning movement of the ilium. Then he tests the end-feel.

Physiological end-feel:
firm and elastic

> **!** During passive movements of about 90–110° flexion, there is often also beginning movement of the ilium. At this point, the therapist applies pressure on the femur perpendicularly to the bench.

b) **Extension** from the zero position:

- The patient is lying prone with the pelvis on the edge of the bench. The hip joints are flexed and the tips of the feet are on the floor. The therapist fixates the ischial tuberosity with the proximal hand and asks the patient to extend the right leg backward and upward.
- Then the therapist takes the distal thigh and tests whether the movement continues passively.
- Finally, the therapist moves the leg out of the zero position through the entire range of motion and tests the end-feel.

Physiological end-feel:
firm and elastic

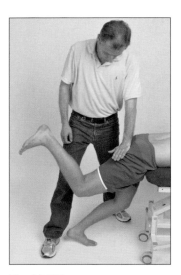

Fig. 14.118

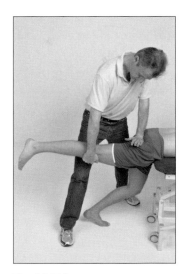

Fig. 14.119

> **Note**
> Maximum hip joint flexion of the other leg prevents further movement in lumbar spine extension. The therapist must nevertheless observe the lumbar spine, as movement cannot always be completely avoided.

c) **Abduction** from the zero position:

- With his proximal forearm on the ASIS (anterior superior iliac spine) of the pelvis or stabilizing the ipsilateral iliac crest with his cranial hand, the therapist asks the supine patient to move his or her leg on the bench externally in abduction. If necessary, the therapist can support the leg to relieve its weight.
- Then the therapist takes the leg and tests whether the movement continues passively. To protect the knee joint, a cradle grip may be used. If the knee is stable, the therapist may hold the distal lower leg. The common deviation in external rotation may be more easily controlled by holding the lower leg from lateral with the distal hand.
- Finally, the therapist moves the leg from the zero position through the entire range of motion and tests the end-feel.

Physiological end-feel:
firm and elastic, sometimes soft and elastic due to the adductors

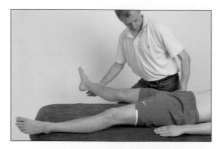

Fig. 14.120

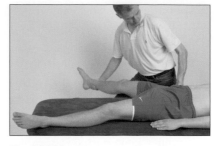

Fig. 14.121

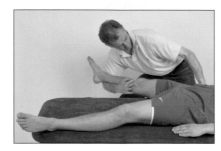

Fig. 14.122

d) **Adduction** from the zero position:

- The patient has bent the contralateral leg and placed the foot alongside the knee. Fixating the pelvis, the therapist asks the patient to move the nonsupporting leg further medially on the bench.
- Then the therapist takes the leg and checks whether the movement continues passively.
- Finally, the therapist moves the leg out of the zero position through the entire range of motion and tests the end-feel.

Physiological end-feel:
firm and elastic

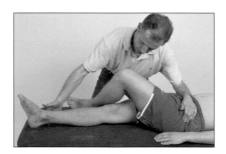

Fig. 14.123

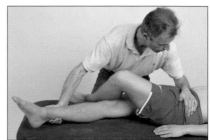

Fig. 14.124

> **Note**
> Given that restricted adduction is very rare, tests of adduction are often left out in everyday practice.

e) **External rotation** from the zero position:

- The patient is lying in the prone position with the knee joint flexed by about 90°. The therapist stabilizes the pelvis on the same side with the proximal hand and asks the patient to move the foot medially to produce external rotation.
- Then the therapist takes the lower leg and tests whether the movement continues passively. If the knee joint is stable, the therapist can hold the distal lower leg. If there is hypermobility, it is advisable to control separation in the joint space with palpation. If the knee is unstable, it should be ex-

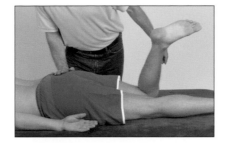

Fig. 14.125

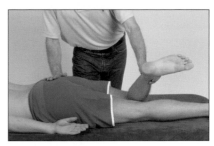

Fig. 14.126

tended and the therapist should use a bimanual grip around the femoral condyles.
- Lastly, the therapist moves the leg from the zero position through the entire range of motion and tests the end-feel.

Alternatively, testing may be done with the patient in the supine position with the knee and hip joints in approximately 90° flexion.

Physiological end-feel:
firm and elastic

f) **Internal rotation** from the zero position:

- The patient is lying in the prone position with the knee bent about 90°. With his proximal hand, the therapist stabilizes the pelvis on the same side and asks the patient to move the foot laterally to test internal rotation.
- Then the therapist takes the lower leg and tests whether the movement continues passively. If the knee joint is stable, the therapist may hold the distal lower leg. In patients with hypermobile knee joints, it is advisable to palpate the opening of the joint space; to do so, the therapist stands on the opposite side. If the knee is unstable, it should be extended and the therapist should use a bimanual grip around the femoral condyles.
- Finally, the therapist moves the leg from the zero position through the entire range of motion and tests the end-feel.

Alternatively, testing may be done with the patient in the supine position with the knee and hip joints in approximately 90° flexion.

Physiological end-feel:
firm and elastic

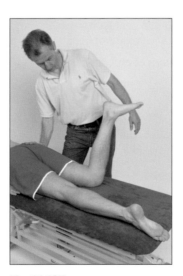

Fig. 14.127

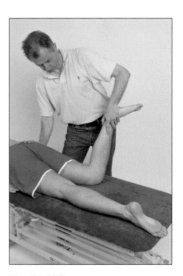

Fig. 14.128

14.8.3 Translatoric movement tests

a) **Traction** in the resting position:

The patient is lying in the supine position. The therapist graps the distal lower leg and pulls it distally. This causes the femur to move at a right angle away from the treatment plane. The knee joint is locked in a position of extension and external rotation (= stable). If the knee joint is unstable, the therapist can hold the femoral condyles during traction.

Physiological end-feel:
firm and elastic

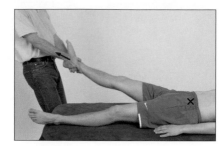

Fig. 14.129

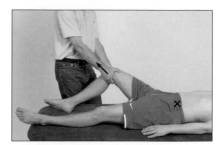

Fig. 14.130

> **Note**
>
> For a quick comparison of sides, the pelvis is generally not fixated for the traction test. This means, however, that only the "give" or "relaxation" of the joint may be palpated because the effective traction without fixation of the pelvix is small (Llopis et al 2008). The end-feel can only be palpated if the pelvis is fixated firmly—as described for treatment.

b) **Compression** in the resting position:

The therapist places his lateral hand from dorsal on the patient's innominate (hip) bone and controls its stable position. He places his medial hand on the distal end of the femur and presses the femur at a right angle toward the treatment plane. To increase the pressure, the therapist may place his abdomen against his medial hand and use the weight of his upper body.

Physiological end-feel: hard

> **Note**
>
> The compression test should be performed with the patient lying down if standing produces symptoms.

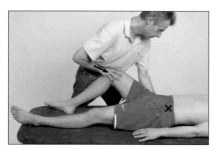

Fig. 14.131

14.8.4 Treatment of Capsuloligamentous Hypomobility

The patient is in the supine position. The pubis on the side being treated is fixated with a belt (with a hand towel wrapped around it for cushioning) or a special hip traction system. A second belt is used to fixate the ASIS from ventral. The therapist uses both hands to grasp the distal end of the lower leg and using the locked knee pulls the femur at a right angle away from the treatment plane. The therapist can facilitate traction by placing the belt around his hands and pelvis and using the weight of his body. Alternatively, traction may be performed as in the test, grasping the femoral condyles and using a belt.

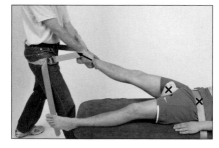

Fig. 14.132

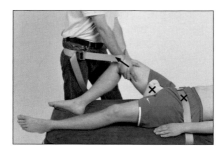

Fig. 14.133

> **!** To relieve pain, intermittent traction may also be performed as in the test version.

Documentation template: Practice Scheme

Hip joint	
Symptoms	
Symptom-altering direction	
Contraindications?	Nervous system: Other:
Symptom-altering joint	
General assessment of adjacent joints	
Active movements, comparing sides	

Specific rotatory tests	Active	Continues passively?	Passive	End-feel	Symptoms/pain	Comments
▪ Flexion						
▪ Extension						
▪ Abduction						
▪ Adduction						
▪ External rotation						
▪ Internal rotation						

Translatoric movement tests	Quantity	Quality	End-feel	Symptoms/pain	Comments
▪ Traction					
▪ Compression					

Summary Formulation aid: ▪ Symptoms ▪ Direction ▪ Contraindications ▪ Site (joint) ▪ Restricted mobility, hypermobility, or physiological mobility ▪ Structure: muscle, joint, etc.	*Text:*
Trial treatment	
Physical therapy diagnosis	
Treatment plan with treatment goal and prognosis	
Treatment progress	
Final examination	

Documentation: Practice Example

Hip joint	
(Patient diagnosed with coxarthrosis)	
Symptoms	*Mild pain in the right hip at the end of the stance phase on the right*
Symptom-altering direction	*Internal rotation and extension*
Contraindications?	Nervous system: *No findings* Other: *No findings*
Symptom-altering joint	*Right hip joint*
General assessment of adjacent joints	*No findings except for increased lumbar hyperlordosis; patient also reports frequent low back pain.*
Active movements, comparing sides	*Internal rotation and extension are markedly restricted in the right hip, abduction to a lesser degree.*

Specific rotatory tests	Active	Continues passively?	Passive	End-feel	Symptoms/ Pain	Comments
▪ Flexion	*100°*	*< 5°*	*No findings*	*Firm to hard and elastic*		
▪ Extension	*0°*	*< 5°*	*Increased resistance to movement*	*Very firm and elastic*		
▪ Abduction	*30°*	*ca. 10°*	*Earlier first stop*	*Soft and elastic*		
▪ Adduction	*20°*	*ca. 10°*	*No findings*	*Firm and elastic*		
▪ External rotation	*40°*	*ca. 10°*	*No findings*	*Firm and elastic*		
▪ Internal rotation	*20°*	*< 5°*	*Increased resistance to movement*	*Very firm and elastic*	*Mild pain at end-range*	

Translatoric movement tests	Quantity	Quality	End-feel	Symptoms/pain	Comments
▪ Traction	*Hypo 2*	*Increased resistance to movement*	*Very firm and elastic and slightly painful*		
▪ Compression	*No findings*	*No findings*	*Hard*	*No findings*	

Summary	
Formulation aid: ▪ Symptoms ▪ Direction ▪ Contraindications ▪ Site (joint) ▪ Restricted mobility, hypermobility, or physiological mobility ▪ Structure: muscle or joint, etc.	*Text:* ▪ *Mild end-range pain in the right hip at the end of the stance phase as well as* ▪ *with internal rotation (20°), extension (0°), and abduction (30°).* ▪ *There are no contraindications today to further movement testing.* ▪ *The symptoms are located in the right hip joint,* ▪ *which has restricted mobility* ▪ *due to capsuloligamentous shrinkage (positive capsular sign) and for abduction due to tension in the adductor muscles (soft and elastic end-feel on abduction).*

Continued ▶

Documentation: Practice Example *(Continued)*

Hip joint (Patient diagnosed with coxarthrosis)	
Trial treatment	▪ *5-minute long pain-relieving grade I–II traction, after which there was a slight reduction in end-range pain.* ▪ *Then 5-minute long grade III traction mobilization with significant reduction in end-range pain and less resistance to movement.*
Physical therapy diagnosis	*See above*
Treatment plan with treatment goal and prognosis	▪ *After initial pain-relieving traction, grade III traction mobilization. Additional soft-tissue techniques for the adductor muscles.* ▪ *Treatment goal: pain-free physiological mobility* **(Further information on examination and treatment techniques may be obtained through further education.)**
Treatment progress	
Final examination	

14.9 Interphalangeal Joints of the Fingers

(Articulationes interphalangeae manus proximales et distales)

14.9.1 Anatomy

Joint type:	ginglymus (= hinge joint), modified sellar joint
Distal joint surface:	concave
Resting position:	slight flexion
Close packed position:	maximum extension
Capsular sign:	restriction in both directions, mainly affecting flexion

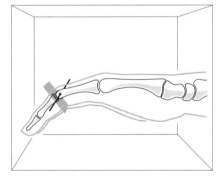

Fig. 14.134

14.9.2 Rotatory Tests

■ **Active Movements, Comparing Sides**

The patient is asked to move all the fingers on both hands at the same time, first flexing and then extending them. The therapist may demonstrate the movement if necessary.

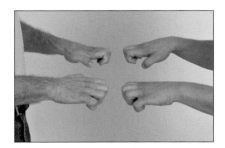

Fig. 14.135

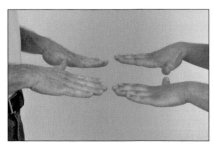

Fig. 14.136

■ Specific Active and Passive Movement Testing (Quantity and Quality)

a) **Flexion** from the zero position:

- The therapist fixates the proximal phalanx and asks the patient to actively flex the finger.
- Then the therapist takes the distal phalanx and tests whether the movement continues passively.
- Finally, the therapist moves the distal phalanx passively from the zero position through the entire range of motion and tests the end-feel.

Physiological end-feel:
firm and elastic

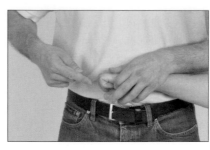

Fig. 14.137

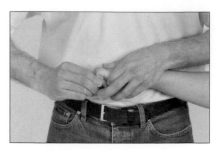

Fig. 14.138

b) **Extension** from the zero position:

- The therapist fixates the proximal phalanx and asks the patient to actively extend the finger.
- Then the therapist takes the distal phalanx and tests whether the movement continues passively.
- Finally, the therapist moves the distal phalanx passively from the zero position through the entire range of motion and tests the end-feel.

Physiological end-feel:
firm and elastic

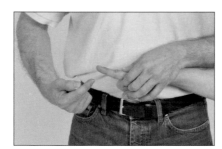

Fig. 14.139

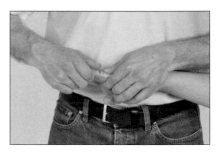

Fig. 14.140

■ Stability Tests in the Zero Position

The therapist fixates the proximal and distal phalanges and passively tests the opening of the joint on the radial and ulnar sides and tests the end-feel.

> **!** Stability tests may be performed in any joint position.

Physiological end-feel:
very firm and elastic

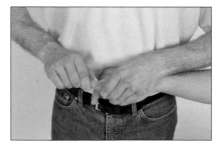

Fig. 14.141

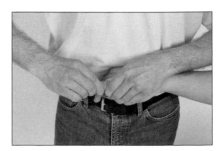

Fig. 14.142

14.9.3 Translatoric movement tests

a) **Traction** in the resting position:

The therapist fixates the proximal phalanx and grasps the head of the distal phalanx, which he pulls at a right angle away from the treatment plane. The thumb of the dorsal hand may be used to palpate the motion in the joint space.

Physiological end-feel: firm and elastic.

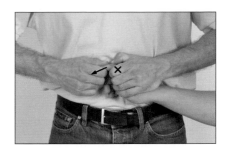

Fig. 14.143

b) **Compression** in the resting position:

The therapist fixates the proximal phalanx and grasps the distal phalanx which he presses at a right angle toward the treatment plane.

Physiological end-feel: hard.

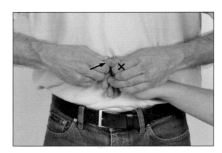

Fig. 14.144

14.9.4 Treatment of Capsuloligamentous Hypomobility

The patient's forearm is resting on the head piece of the table. The dorsum of his or her hand is on a wedge. The proximal phalanx is near the end of the wedge with the joint space hanging over the edge. The therapist fixates the patient's proximal phalanx against the wedge with the thenar eminence of his proximal hand. With his distal hand he grasps the head of the distal phalanx and performs traction.

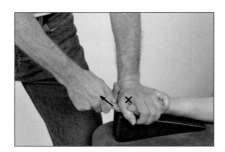

Fig. 14.145

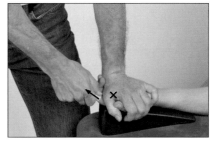

Fig. 14.146

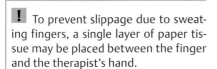
! To prevent slippage due to sweating fingers, a single layer of paper tissue may be placed between the finger and the therapist's hand.

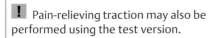
! Pain-relieving traction may also be performed using the test version.

Documentation template: Practice Scheme

Interphalangeal joint of the finger					
Symptoms					
Symptom-altering direction					
Contraindications?	Nervous system: Other:				
Symptom-altering joint					
General assessment of adjacent joints					
Active movements, comparing sides					

Specific rotatory tests	Active	Continues passively?	Passive	End-feel	Symptoms/pain	Comments
Flexion						
Extension						

Stability tests	Quantity	Quality	End-feel	Symptoms/pain	Comments
Radial gaping					
Ulnar gaping					

Translatoric movement tests	Quantity	Quality	End-feel	Symptoms/pain	Comments
Traction					
Compression					

Summary Formulation aid: ■ Symptoms ■ Direction ■ Contraindications ■ Site (joint) ■ Restricted mobility, hypermobility, or physiological mobility ■ Structure: muscle, joint, etc.	*Text:*
Trial treatment	
Physical therapy diagnosis	
Treatment plan with treatment goal and prognosis	
Treatment progress	
Final examination	

Documentation: Practice Example

<table>
<tr><td colspan="7" align="center">

Interphalangeal joint of the finger
(Pain with movement of the middle finger after volleyball injury, without hematoma;
this initial examination was done by a physical therapist at the volleyball court)

</td></tr>
<tr><td>**Symptoms**</td><td colspan="6">*Pain in the middle finger of right hand*</td></tr>
<tr><td>**Symptom-altering direction**</td><td colspan="6">*Flexion and extension*</td></tr>
<tr><td>**Contraindications?**</td><td colspan="6">Nervous system: *no findings*
Other: *no findings*</td></tr>
<tr><td>**Symptom-altering joint**</td><td colspan="6">*Testing distal (DIP) and proximal interphalangeal (PIP) joints with active flexion and extension while fixating the proximal phalanx shows that the pain is in correlation with the PIP of the middle finger.*</td></tr>
<tr><td>**General assessment of adjacent joints**</td><td colspan="6">*Limited active flexion and extension of all fingers of the right hand due to fear of pain; they are freely movable with passive motion, however.*</td></tr>
<tr><td>**Active movements, comparing sides**</td><td colspan="6">*Restricted movement of the right middle finger (flexion and extension) compared to the left.*</td></tr>
<tr>
<td>**Specific rotatory tests**</td>
<td>**Active**</td>
<td>**Continues passively?**</td>
<td>**Passive**</td>
<td>**End-feel**</td>
<td>**Symptoms/ pain**</td>
<td>**Comments**</td>
</tr>
<tr>
<td>▪ Flexion</td>
<td>*ca. 60°*</td>
<td>*< 5°*</td>
<td>*Gradually increasing resistance*</td>
<td>*Empty*</td>
<td>*Provokes reported pain*</td>
<td>*Patient fears pain with movement*</td>
</tr>
<tr>
<td>▪ Extension</td>
<td>*ca. –20°*</td>
<td>*< 5°*</td>
<td>*Gradually increasing resistance*</td>
<td>*Empty*</td>
<td>*Provokes reported pain*</td>
<td>*Patient fears pain with movement*</td>
</tr>
<tr>
<td>**Stability tests**</td>
<td>**Quantity**</td>
<td>**Quality**</td>
<td>**End-feel**</td>
<td colspan="2">**Symptoms/pain**</td>
<td>**Comments**</td>
</tr>
<tr>
<td>▪ Radial gaping</td>
<td>*Uncertain*</td>
<td>*Increased resistance to movement*</td>
<td>*Empty*</td>
<td colspan="2">*Early provocation of reported pain*</td>
<td></td>
</tr>
<tr>
<td>▪ Ulnar gaping</td>
<td>*No findings*</td>
<td>*No findings*</td>
<td></td>
<td colspan="2">*No findings*</td>
<td>*Patient fears pain with movement*</td>
</tr>
<tr>
<td>**Translatoric movement tests**</td>
<td>**Quantity**</td>
<td>**Quality**</td>
<td>**End-feel**</td>
<td colspan="2">**Symptoms/pain**</td>
<td>**Comments**</td>
</tr>
<tr>
<td>▪ Traction</td>
<td>*Uncertain*</td>
<td>*Early first resistance*</td>
<td>*Empty*</td>
<td colspan="2"></td>
<td></td>
</tr>
<tr>
<td>▪ Compression</td>
<td>*No findings*</td>
<td>*No findings*</td>
<td></td>
<td colspan="2">*Slight provocation of reported pain*</td>
<td></td>
</tr>
<tr>
<td>**Summary**
Formulation aid:
▪ Symptoms
▪ Direction
▪ Contraindications</td>
<td colspan="6">*Text:*
▪ *Pain in the right middle finger with movement following a sports injury (volleyball hit finger)*
▪ *with flexion (ca. 60°) and extension (ca. –20°).*
▪ *There are no contraindications today for further movement testing except increased caution due to the pain after trauma.*</td>
</tr>
</table>

Continued ▶

Interphalangeal joint of the finger **(Pain with movement of the middle finger after volleyball injury, without hematoma;** **this initial examination was done by a physical therapist at the volleyball court)**	
Summary Formulation aid: ▪ Site (joint) ▪ Restricted mobility, hypermobility, or physiological mobility ▪ Structure: muscle, joint, etc.	*Text:* ▪ *The pain is located in the PIP joint* ▪ *and is caused by painfully restricted mobility,* ▪ *especially of the radial collateral ligament (sprain?).*
Trial treatment	▪ *Refer patient to physician to determine the extent of injury (osseous involvement, etc.?), need for medical care, and possible legalities (accident insurance, sick leave, etc.).* ▪ *If there is a mild sprain, the doctor will prescribe physical therapy (PT) after a brief period of immobilization. Then a new PT examination must be done.*
Physical therapy diagnosis	*See summary*
Treatment plan **with treatment goal** **and prognosis**	▪ *Await physician response.* ▪ *Treatment goal: physician decides necessary treatment of the injury.* **(Further information on examination and treatment techniques may be obtained through further education.)**
Treatment progress	
Final examination	

14.10 Metacarpophalangeal Joints

(Articulationes metacarpophalangeales manus)

14.10.1 Anatomy

Joint type:	condylar joints, modified ovoid
Distal joint surface:	concave
Resting position:	slightly flexed, additional slight ulnar abduction for MCP II–V
Close packed position:	MCP I in maximum extension, MCP II–V in maximum flexion
Capsular sign:	limitations in all directions; restriction of flexion is the greatest

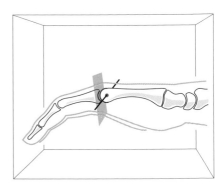

Fig. 14.147

14.10.2 Rotatory Tests

■ Active Movements, Comparing Sides

The patient moves all fingers on both hands in flexion, then extension, then spreads the fingers (= abduction), and finally brings them close together (= adduction). The therapist may demonstrate to help the patient's understanding.

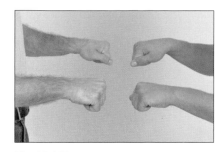

Fig. 14.148

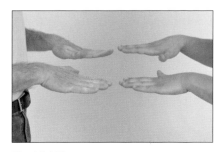

Fig. 14.149

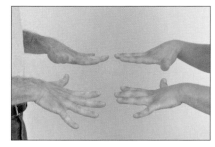

Fig. 14.150

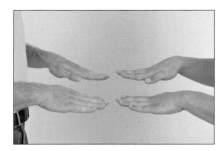

Fig. 14.151

■ Specific Active and Passive Movement Testing (Quantity and Quality)

a) **Flexion** from the zero position:

- The therapist fixates the metacarpal bone and asks the patient to actively flex the finger.
- Then the therapist takes the first phalanx and tests whether the movement continues passively.
- Finally, the therapist moves the phalanx passively from the zero position through the entire range of motion and tests the end-feel.

Physiological end-feel:
firm and elastic

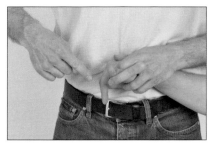

Fig. 14.152

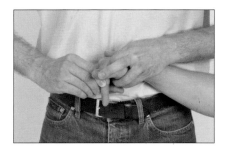

Fig. 14.153

b) **Extension** from the zero position:

- The therapist fixates the metacarpal bone and asks the patient to actively extend the finger.
- Then the therapist takes the first phalanx and tests whether the movement continues passively.

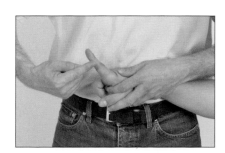

Fig. 14.154

- Finally, the therapist moves the phalanx <u>passively</u> from the zero position through the entire range of motion and tests the <u>end-feel</u>.

Physiological end-feel:
firm and elastic

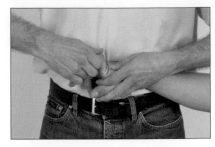

Fig. 14.155

c) **Abduction** from the zero position:

- The therapist fixates the metacarpal bone and asks the patient to <u>actively</u> spread the finger apart.
- Then the therapist takes the first phalanx and tests whether the movement <u>continues passively</u>.
- Finally, the therapist moves the phalanx <u>passively</u> from the zero position through the entire range of motion and tests the <u>end-feel</u>.

Physiological end-feel:
firm and elastic

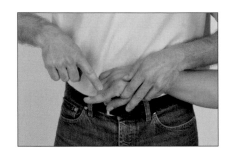

Fig. 14.156

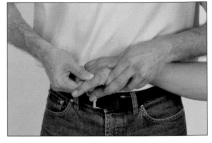

Fig. 14.157

d) **Adduction** from the zero position:

- The therapist fixates the metacarpal bone and asks the patient to <u>actively</u> adduct the finger toward the center of the hand (= third ray).
- Then the therapist takes the first phalanx and tests whether the movement <u>continues passively</u>.
- Finally, the therapist moves the phalanx <u>passively</u> from the zero position through the entire range of motion and tests the <u>end-feel</u>.

Physiological end-feel:
firm and elastic

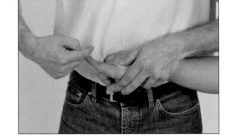

Fig. 14.158

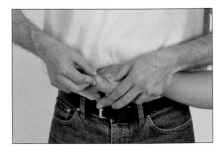

Fig. 14.159

14.10.3 Translatoric movement tests

a) **Traction** in the resting position:

The therapist fixates the metacarpal bone and grasps the head of the first phalanx, which he pulls at a right angle away from the treatment plane.

The thumb of the dorsal hand may be used to palpate the movement in the joint space.

Physiological end-feel: firm and elastic

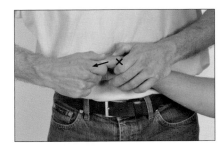

Fig. 14.160

b) **Compression** in the resting position:

The therapist fixates the metacarpal bone and grasps the first phalanx,

which he presses at a right angle toward the treatment plane.

Physiological end-feel: hard

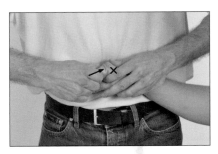

Fig. 14.161

14.10.4 Treatment of Capsuloligamentous Hypomobility

The patient's forearm is lying on the head piece of the table. The back of his or her hand is resting on the wedge. The metacarpal bone is on the end of the wedge with the joint space protruding over the edge. The therapist fixates the metacarpal bone against the wedge with the thenar eminence of his proximal hand. Using his distal hand, he grasps the head of the first phalanx and applies traction.

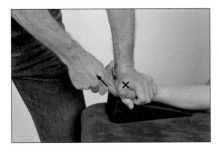

Fig. 14.162

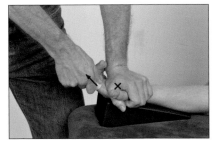

Fig. 14.163

! To prevent slippage due to sweating fingers, a single layer of paper tissue may be placed between the finger and the therapist's hand.

! Pain-relieving traction may also be performed using the test version.

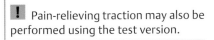

Metacarpophalangeal joints

Symptoms	
Symptom-altering direction	
Contraindications?	Nervous system: Other:
Symptom-altering joint	
General assessment of adjacent joints	
Active movements, comparing sides	

Specific rotatory tests	Active	Continues passively?	Passive	End-feel	Symptoms/pain	Comments
▪ Flexion						
▪ Extension						
▪ Abduction						
▪ Adduction						

Translatoric movement tests	Quantity	Quality	End-feel	Symptoms/pain	Comments
▪ Traction					
▪ Compression					

Summary Formulation aid: ▪ Symptoms ▪ Direction ▪ Contraindications ▪ Site (joint) ▪ Restricted mobility, hypermobility, or physiological mobility ▪ Structure: muscle, joint, etc.	Text:
Trial treatment	
Physical therapy diagnosis	
Treatment plan with treatment goal and prognosis	
Treatment progress	
Final examination	

Documentation: Practice Example

Metacarpophalangeal joints
(Movement limitation following 5-week long immobilization after complex diaphyseal fracture of the second metacarpal on the right hand. The fracture has healed sufficiently for weight bearing.)

Symptoms	*Feeling of stiffness in right index finger*
Symptom-altering direction	*Flexion is more strongly limited than extension*
Contraindications?	Nervous system: *no findings* Other: *no findings*
Symptom-altering joint	*Metacarpophalangeal joint (MCP) of the index finger*
General assessment of adjacent joints	*All joints of the right hand are somewhat "stiff" with limited mobility due to immobilization and protection.*

Active movements, comparing sides	*The right index finger is significantly less mobile than the left.*				
Specific rotatory tests	**Active**	**Continues passively?**	**Passive**	**End-feel**	**Symptoms/ pain**	**Comments**
▪ Flexion	*ca. 60°*	*< 5°*	*Increased resistance to movement*	*Very firm and less elastic*	*None; slight pulling feeling at end-range*	
▪ Extension	*ca. –20°*	*< 5°*	*Increased resistance to movement*	*Very firm and less elastic*	*None; slight pulling feeling at end-range*	
▪ Abduction	*Nearly 0°*	*< 5°*	*Increased resistance to movement*	*Very firm and less elastic*	*None; slight pulling feeling at end-range*	
▪ Adduction	*ca. 10°*	*< 5°*	*Increased resistance to movement*	*Very firm and less elastic*	*None; slight pulling feeling at end-range*	

Translatoric movement tests	**Quantity**	**Quality**	**End-feel**	**Symptoms/pain**	**Comments**
▪ Traction	*Hypo 2*	*Increased resistance to movement*	*Very firm and less elastic*		
▪ Compression	*No findings*	*No findings*	*Hard*		

| **Summary**
Formulation aid:
▪ Symptoms
▪ Direction

▪ Contraindications
▪ Site (joint)
▪ Restricted mobility, hypermobility, or physiological mobility
▪ Structure: muscle, joint, etc. | *Text:*
▪ *Feeling of stiffness in the MCP of the index finger.*
▪ *with active and passive movements in all directions (flexion ca. 60°), extension (ca. – 20°), abduction (nearly 0°) and adduction (ca. 10°).*
▪ *There are no contraindications today to further movement testing.*
▪ *The symptoms are located in the MCP of the index finger,*
▪ *which has limited mobility (see above)*

▪ *due to shrinkage of the capsuloligamentous unit.* |

Continued ▶

Metacarpophalangeal joints (Movement limitation following 5-week long immobilization after complex diaphyseal fracture of the second metacarpal on the right hand. The fracture has healed sufficiently for weight	
Trial treatment	*5-minute long grade III traction after which the patient said that movement was easier and the therapist felt less resistance.*
Physical therapy diagnosis	*See above*
Treatment plan with treatment goal and prognosis	▪ *Continue grade III traction therapy.* ▪ *Treatment goal: pain-free physiological mobility* **(Further information on examination and treatment techniques may be obtained through further education.)**
Treatment progress	
Final examination	

14.11   Metacarpal Joints II–V

(Articulationes intermetacarpales and carpometacarpales II–V)

14.11.1   Anatomy

Joint type:
- Distal intermetacarpal joint: syndesmosis
  Joint surfaces: no true joint surfaces
- Proximal intermetacarpal joints II–V: amphiarthroses
  Joint surfaces: irregular, small curvature, considered concave in manual therapy
- Carpometacarpal joints II–V: amphiarthroses
  Distal joint surface: irregular, small curvature, considered concave in manual therapy

Resting position: not described

Close packed position: not described

Capsular sign: not described except for carpometacarpal joints II–V, with uniform limitation in all directions

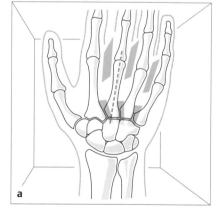

a

! Movements always occur simultaneously in all three joints. Active movements are often accompanied by movements in the wrist and fingers. Restricted mobility only occurs after prolonged immobilization and then usually is more significant in the other hand joints. The metacarpal joints should mainly be stable. Grade III stretching mobilization, to increase the range of motion, is thus rarely indicated.

Note
The treatment planes are each approximately perpendicular to the dorsum of the hand.

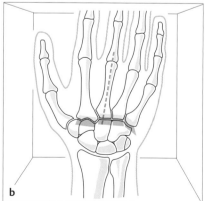

b

Fig. 14.164 a, b

14.11.2 Rotatory Tests

◼ Active Movements, Comparing Sides

The therapist asks the patient to actively increase the concavity of the hand and then to flatten it. The therapist may demonstrate the movement to help the patient's understanding.

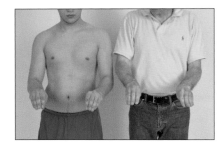

Fig. 14.165

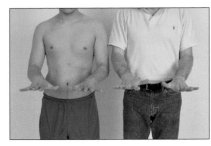

Fig. 14.166

◼ Specific Active and Passive Movement Testing (Quantity and Quality)

a) **Increase** the hollow of the palm:

- The therapist asks the patient to actively hollow out the palm.
- Next, the therapist supports the third metacarpal from palmar with his two middle fingers. His thumbs press the dorsal surfaces of the second and fifth metacarpals in palmar direction to test whether the movement continues passively.
- Finally, in the same manner the therapist moves the hollow of the palm passively from the zero position through the entire range of motion and tests the end-feel.

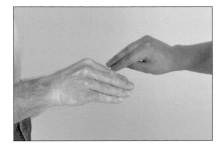

Fig. 14.167

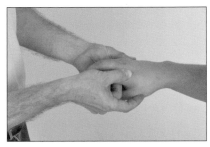

Fig. 14.168

Physiological end-feel:
firm and elastic

b) **Flattening** of the hand:

- The therapist asks the patient to actively flatten out the hand.
- Next, he supports the third metacarpal from dorsal with both thumbs and uses his middle fingers to press the second and fifth metacarpals from palmar to dorsal to test whether the movement continues passively.
- Finally, in the same manner he moves the joints of the palm passively from the zero position through the entire range of motion and tests the end-feel.

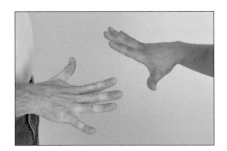

Fig. 14.169

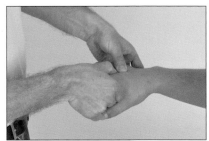

Fig. 14.170

Physiological end-feel:
firm and elastic

c) **Individual movements** of the metacarpal joints II–V:

The therapist fixates the third metacarpal with his ulnar hand, and with his radial hand he moves the second metacarpal passively toward the palm and then the back of the hand and tests the end-feel. This causes gliding motion in the intermetacarpal joints as well flexion and extension of the carpometacarpal joints. The third metacarpal forms the stable longitudinal axis of the hand. Thus the therapist next fixates the third metacarpal with his radial hand while his ulnar hand moves the fourth metacarpal against the third

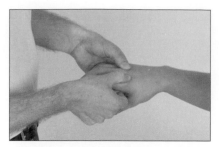

Fig. 14.171

and then the fifth against the fourth. Fixating the distal metacarpal heads emphasizes testing of the syndesmosis, while a proximal grip around the bases of the metacarpals tests the proximal true intermetacarpal joint.

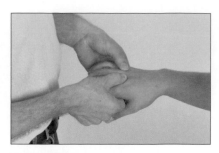

Fig. 14.172

Physiological end-feel:
firm and elastic

d) **Flexion** and **extension** of carpometacarpal joints II–V:

The therapist fixates one of the carpal bones (trapezoid, capitate, or hamate), moves the corresponding metacarpal passively in palmar direction, first in flexion and then dorsally in

extension, and tests the end-feel each time. This is accompanied by a gliding movement in the intermetacarpal joints.

Physiological end-feel:
firm and elastic

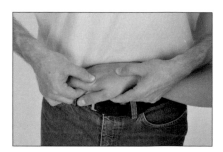

Fig. 14.173

14.11.3 Translatoric movement tests

Traction application to carpometacarpal joints II–V:

The therapist fixates the respective carpal bone (trapezoid, capitate, or hamate) with the thumb and index finger of his proximal hand. Using the thumb and index finger of his distal hand he holds the correspond-

ing metacarpal head, which he pulls at a right angle away from the treatment plane. The thumb of the proximal hand may be used to palpate the movement in the joint space.

Physiological end-feel:
firm and elastic

Compression of carpometacarpal

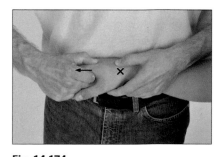

Fig. 14.174

joints II–V:

The therapist fixates the respective carpal bones (trapezoid, capitate, or hamate) with the thumb and index finger of his proximal hand. The thumb and index finger of the distal

hand hold the corresponding metacarpal bone, which he presses at a right angle toward the treatment plane.

Physiological end-feel: hard

Compression of the intermetacarpal

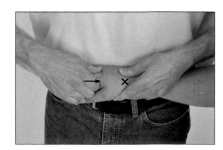

Fig. 14.175

joints II–V:

The therapist uses both hands to grasp the metacarpus from radial and ulnar and presses the second through fifth metacarpal bones together at a right angle toward the treatment plane. The application of compression may focus more on the distal or proximal intermetacarpal joints. If this provokes pain, compression between the individual metacarpal bones may be used for more precise localization.

Gliding in the proximal intermetacarpal joints has already been tested with the individual movements of

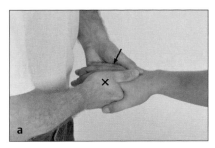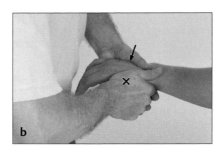

Fig. 14.176

the second through fifth metacarpal bones described above.

Physiological end-feel: hard

14.11.4   Treatment of Capsuloligamentous Hypomobility

Traction on the Carpometacarpal Joints II–V

The patient's forearm is resting with the hand face down on a wedge at the head of the treatment table. The carpal bone which will be fixated (trapezoid, capitate, or hamate) is lying on the wedge with the carpometacarpal joint space hanging over its edge. The therapist fixates the carpal bone against the wedge with the thenar

eminence. Next he grasps the corresponding metacarpal head with the thumb and index finger of his distal hand and pulls it at a right angle away from the treatment plane.

> **!** Pain-relieving traction may also be performed using the test version.

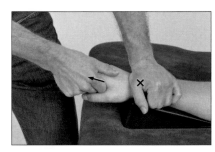

Fig. 14.177

▨ Mobilization of the Intermetacarpal Joints

The patient's forearm is resting on the head piece of the table with the palm of his or her hand on the wedge. The metacarpal bone (e.g., third) that is to be fixated is lying on the edge of the wedge with the metacarpal that is going to be mobilized (in the example, the second metacarpal) hanging over the edge. With the hand nearest the ulna, the therapist fixates the third metacarpal against the wedge with the thenar eminence. His radial hand grasps the second metacarpal and moves it toward the palm with pressure from the thenar eminence.

> **!** For mobilization dorsally, the back of the hand is held firmly against the wedge and the corresponding metacarpal bone is mobilized dorsally.

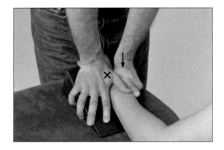

Fig. 14.178

For the proximal joint, both thenar eminences are at the height of the base of the metacarpal bone, and for the distal joint they are at the height of the head. Alternatively, for the proximal joint, the hypothenar of one hand pushes on the thumb of the other hand which is placed on the base of the metacarpal bone. If there is uncertainty, the proximal joint should be mobilized first.

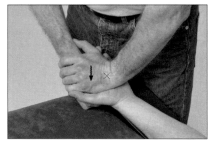

Fig. 14.179

> **!** For pain relief, specific movement within the slack of the joint capsule may also be performed with the test version.

Documentation template: Practice Scheme

Metacarpal joints II–V						
Symptoms						
Symptom-altering direction						
Contraindications?	Nervous system: Other:					
Symptom-altering joint						
General evaluation of adjacent joints						
Active movements, comparing sides						

Specific rotatory tests	Active	Continues passively?	Passive	End-feel	Symptoms/pain	Comments
Increasing the concavity of the palm						
Flattening the palm						
Individual movements of the intermetacarpal joints						
Flexion of the carpometacarpal joint						
Extension of the carpometacarpal joint						

Translatoric movement tests	Quantity	Quality	End-feel	Symptoms/pain	Comments
Carpometacarpal joint traction					
Carpometacarpal joint compression					
Intermetacarpal joint compression					

Summary Formulation aid: ■ Symptoms (often painful) ■ Direction ■ Contraindications ■ Site (joint) ■ Restricted mobility, hypermobility, or physiological mobility ■ Structure: muscle, joint, etc.	*Text:*
Trial treatment	
Physical therapy diagnosis	

Continued ▶

Documentation template: Practice Scheme (Continued)

Metacarpal joints II–V	
Treatment plan with treatment goal and prognosis	
Treatment progress	
Final examination	

Documentation: Practice Example

Metacarpal joints II–V (Movement limitation 3 weeks after cast immobilization due to scaphoid fracture in right hand)	
Symptoms	*Limited movement of the right hand*
Symptom-altering direction	*Hand opening and closing with different palmar grips*
Contraindications?	Nervous system: *no findings* Other: *no findings*
Symptom-altering joint	*Carpometacarpal joints II–V*
General evaluation of adjacent joints	*The entire right hand, especially the metacarpus, seems "stiff"; there is also stiffness of the metacarpophalangeal joints and the wrist.*
Active movements, comparing sides	*Restriction when trying to flatten the palm of the right hand or increase the hollow.*

Specific rotatory tests	Actively	Continues passively?	Passive	End-feel	Symptoms/ pain	Comments
Increasing the concavity of the palm	*Limited*	*< 5°*	*Increased resistance to movement*	*Very firm and elastic*		
Flattening the palm	*Limited*	*< 5°*	*Increased resistance to movement*	*Very firm and elastic*		
Individual movements of the intermetacarpal joints	*Limited*	*< 5°*	*Increased resistance to movement*	*Very firm and elastic*		
Flexion of the carpometacarpal joint	*Limited*	*< 5°*	*Increased resistance to movement*	*Very firm and elastic*		
Extension of the carpometacarpal joint	*Limited*	*< 5°*	*Increased resistance to movement*	*Very firm and elastic*		

Translatoric movement tests	Quantity	Quality	End-feel	Symptoms/pain	Comments
▪ Carpometacarpal joint traction	*Hypo 2*	*Increased resistance to movement*	*Very firm and elastic*	*No findings*	

Continued ▶

Documentation: Practice Example *(Continued)*

Metacarpal joints II–V (Movement limitation 3 weeks after cast immobilization due to scaphoid fracture in right hand)					
■ Carpometacarpal joint compression	*No findings*	*No findings*	*Hard*	*No findings*	
■ Intermetacarpal joint compression	*No findings*	*No findings*	*Hard*	*No findings*	

Summary Formulation aid: ■ Symptoms ■ Direction ■ Contraindications ■ Site (joint) ■ Restricted mobility, hypermobility, or physiological mobility ■ Structure: muscle, joint, etc.	*Text:* ■ *Restricted movement with different palmar grips.* ■ *The symptoms occur when increasing the hollow of the palm or flattening it.* ■ *There are no contraindications today for further movement testing.* ■ *The symptoms are in correlation with the carpometacarpal joints II–V,* ■ *in which flexion and extension are limited.* ■ *due to capsuloligamentous restriction.*
Trial treatment	*Grade III traction mobilization for 3 minutes each for carpometacarpal joints II–V, after which the patient says that movement is easier, and the therapist also notes less resistance.*
Physical therapy diagnosis	*See above*
Treatment plan with treatment goal and prognosis	■ *Continue grade III traction mobilization of the carpometacarpal joints II–V.* ■ *Treatment goal: pain-free physiological mobility.* **(Further information on examination and treatment techniques may be obtained through further education.)**
Treatment progress	
Final examination	

14.12 Carpometacarpal Joint of the Thumb

(Articulatio carpometacarpalis I)

14.12.1 Anatomy

Joint type:	saddle joint, unmodified sellar joint
Distal joint surface:	concave for flexion and extension, convex for abduction and adduction
Resting position:	intermediate position between flexion and extension, abduction and adduction
Close packed position:	maximum opposition
Capsular sign:	abduction > extension

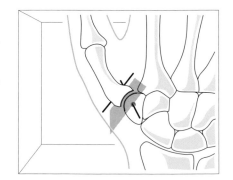

Fig. 14.180

14.12.2 Rotatory Tests

■ Active Movements, Comparing Sides

The patient moves the thumbs on both hands simultaneously, performing the four basic types of movement: flexion and extension, and abduction and adduction. The therapist may demonstrate the movements if necessary. In addition, all forms of opposition of the thumb to the fingers (= opposition) as well as returning from this position (= reposition) may be tested (not shown here).

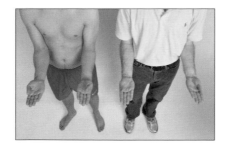

Fig. 14.181

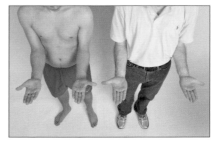

Fig. 14.182

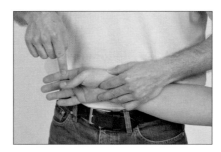

Fig. 14.183

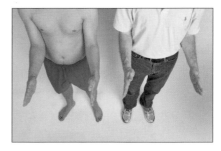

Fig. 14.184

■ Specific Active and Passive Movement Testing (Quantity and Quality)

a) **Flexion** from the zero position:

- The therapist fixates the trapezium and asks the patient, to actively flex the thumb.
- Then the therapist takes first metacarpal and tests whether the movement continues passively.
- Finally, the therapist moves the first metacarpal passively from the zero position through the en-

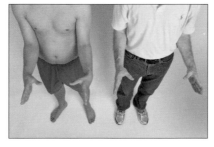

Fig. 14.185

tire range of motion and tests the end-feel.

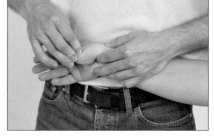

Fig. 14.186

Physiological end-feel: firm and elastic

b) **Extension** from the zero position:

- The therapist fixates the trapezium and asks the patient to actively extend the thumb.
- Then the therapist takes the first metacarpal and tests whether the movement continues passively.
- Finally, the therapist moves the first metacarpal passively from the zero position through the entire range of motion and tests the end-feel.

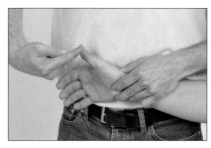

Fig. 14.187

Physiological end-feel: firm and elastic

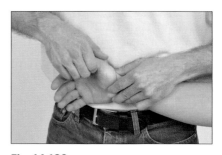

Fig. 14.188

c) **Abduction** from the zero position:

- The therapist fixates the trapezium and asks the patient to <u>actively</u> abduct the thumb.
- Then the therapist takes the first metacarpal and tests whether the movement <u>continues passively</u>.
- Finally, the therapist moves the first metacarpal <u>passively</u> from the zero position through the entire range of motion and tests the <u>end-feel</u>.

Physiological end-feel:
firm and elastic

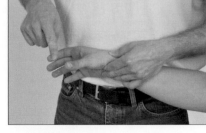

Fig. 14.189

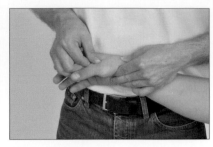

Fig. 14.190

d) **Adduction** from the zero position:

- The therapist fixates the trapezium and asks the patient to <u>actively</u> adduct the thumb.
- Then the therapist takes the first metacarpal and tests whether the movement <u>continues passively</u>.
- Finally, the therapist moves the first metacarpal <u>passively</u> from the zero position through the entire range of motion and tests the <u>end-feel</u>.

Physiological end-feel:
firm and elastic

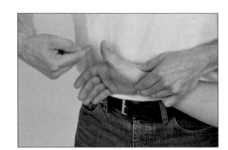

Fig. 14.191

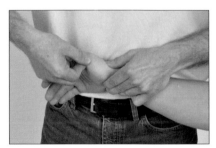

Fig. 14.192

14.12.3 Translatoric movement tests

Traction in the resting position:

The therapist fixates the trapezium and grasps the head of the first metacarpal, which he pulls <u>at a right angle away from the treatment plane</u>.

His proximal thumb may be used to palpate the movement dorsally in the joint space.

Physiological end-feel:
firm and elastic

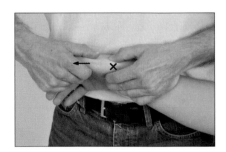

Fig. 14.193

Compression in the resting position:

The therapist fixates the trapezium and grasps the first metacarpal, which he presses <u>at a right angle to</u>ward the treatment plane.

Physiological end-feel: hard

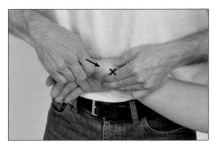

Fig. 14.194

14.12.4 Treatment of Capsuloligamentous Hypomobility

The ulnar border of the patient's forearm and hand are resting on the head piece of the treatment table with the thumb pointing toward the ceiling. The therapist supports himself against the bench with the lateral border of his forearm, and with his middle finger he stabilizes the trapezium from palmar. The thumb and index/middle finger of his medial hand grasp the first metacarpal head and pull it <u>at a right angle away from the treatment plane</u>. For sustained traction, the therapist may support himself with his medial elbow.

! To prevent slippage to due sweating fingers, a single layer of paper tissue may be placed between the thumband the therapist's hand.

! Pain-relieving traction may also be performed using the test version.

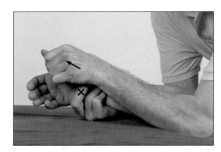

Fig. 14.195

Carpometacarpal joint of the thumb					
Symptoms					
Symptom-altering direction					
Contraindications?	Nervous system: Other:				
Symptom-altering joint					
General assessment of adjacent joints					
Active movements, comparing sides					

Specific rotatory tests	Active	Continues passively?	Passive	End-feel	Symptoms/ pain	Comments
▪ Flexion						
▪ Extension						
▪ Abduction						
▪ Adduction						

Translatoric movement tests	Quantity	Quality	End-feel	Symptoms/pain	Comments
▪ Traction					
▪ Compression					

Summary Formulation aid: ▪ Symptoms (often painful) ▪ Direction ▪ Contraindications ▪ Site (joint) ▪ Restricted mobility, hypermobility, or physiological mobility ▪ Structure: muscle, joint, etc.	*Text:*
Trial treatment	
Physical therapy diagnosis	
Treatment plan with treatment goal and prognosis	
Treatment progress	
Final examination	

Documentation: Practice Example

<table>
<tr><td colspan="2">Carpometacarpal joint of the thumb
(Pain in the right thumb when massaging and grasping)</td></tr>
<tr><td>Symptoms</td><td>Physical therapist with pain in the right thumb when massaging and grasping</td></tr>
<tr><td>Symptom-altering direction</td><td>Abduction and extension; flexion against resistance is also painful</td></tr>
<tr><td>Contraindications?</td><td>Nervous system: No findings
Other: No findings</td></tr>
<tr><td>Symptom-altering joint</td><td>Right carpometacarpal joint</td></tr>
<tr><td>General assessment of adjacent joints</td><td>The joints are otherwise generally very mobile.</td></tr>
<tr><td>Active movements, comparing sides</td><td>Abduction and extension of the thumb are significantly more limited on the right side than on the left, although there are mild symptoms there as well. Slightly restricted flexion on both sides.</td></tr>
</table>

Specific rotatory tests	Active	Continues passively?	Passive	End-feel	Symptoms/ pain	Comments
▪ Flexion	*Nearly 50°*	*< 5°*	*Increased resistance to movement*	*Firm and elastic*	*Somewhat painful at end range*	
▪ Extension	*40°*	*< 5°*	*Increased resistance to movement*	*Very firm and elastic*	*Somewhat painful at end range*	
▪ Abduction	*Nearly 30°*	*< 5°*	*Increased resistance to movement*	*Very firm and elastic*	*Somewhat painful at end range*	
▪ Adduction	*40°*	*< 5°*	*Increased resistance to movement*	*Firm and elastic*	*Somewhat painful at end range*	

Translatoric movement tests	Quantity	Quality	End-feel	Symptoms/pain	Comments
▪ Traction	*Hypo 2*	*Increased resistance to movement*	*Very firm and elastic*	*Somewhat painful at end range*	
▪ Compression	*No findings*	*No findings*	*Hard*		

Summary	
Formulation aid: ▪ Symptoms (often painful) ▪ Direction ▪ Contraindications ▪ Site (joint) ▪ Restricted mobility, hypermobility, or physiological mobility ▪ Structure: muscle, joint, etc.	*Text:* ▪ *The physical therapist has pain in the right thumb during massaging and grasping movements, which occurs especially* ▪ *with abduction and extension but also with flexion and less with adduction.* ▪ *There are no contraindications today to further movement testing.* ▪ *The pain is in correlation with the first carpometacarpal joint,* ▪ *which has restricted mobility* ▪ *due to restriction of the entire capsuloligamentous unit (capsular sign / osteoarthrosis?).*

Continued ▶

Carpometacarpal joint of the thumb (Pain in the right thumb when massaging and grasping)	
Trial treatment	▪ *5-minute pain-relieving grade I–II traction, after which the patient reports a reduction in end-range pain and the therapist feels less resistance to movement.* ▪ *This is followed by 5-minute traction mobilization (beginning of grade III), after which the patient reports that movement is easier. The end-feel seems to be rather less firm.*
Physical therapy diagnosis	*See above*
Treatment plan with treatment goal and prognosis	▪ *Continue preliminary pain-relieving traction followed by traction mobilization in grade III.* ▪ *Treatment goal: pain-free physiological mobility* **(Further information on examination and treatment techniques may be obtained through further education.)**
Treatment progress	
Final examination	

14.13   Wrist Joint

(Articulatio manus, consisting of the articulatio mediocarpalis, articulatio radiocarpalis, and articulatio ossis pisiformis)

14.13.1   Anatomy

Joint type:

▪ Midcarpal joint: ovoid joint, modified ovoid
  Distal joint surfaces: trapezium and trapezoid are concave, capitate and hamate are convex
▪ Radiocarpal joint: ovoid joint, modified oval shape
  Distal joint surfaces: scaphoid, lunate, and triquetrum are convex
▪ Pisiform joint: plane joint of a sesamoid bone
  Distal joint surface: irregular small curvature that is not significant for manual therapy

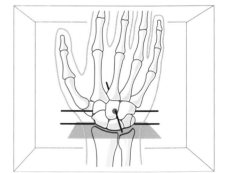

Fig. 14.196

Resting position: wrist joint = zero position with slight ulnar abduction

Close packed position: wrist joint = maximum dorsiflexion

Capsular sign: uniform restriction in all directions

! The pisiform joint is not a weight-bearing joint, but rather the pisiform is a sesamoid bone of the flexor carpi ulnaris muscle. Active and passive rotatory movements of the hand always occur simultaneously in the midcarpal and radiocarpal joints and thus allow initial global testing of the wrist joint.

14.13.2 Rotatory Tests

Active Movements, Comparing Sides

The therapist asks the patient to perform active palmar flexion and dorsiflexion of both hands as well as ulnar adduction and radial abduction.

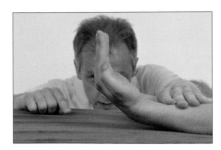

Fig. 14.197

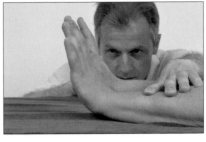

Fig. 14.198

> **Note**
>
> The patient's forearms should be resting parallel to one another on the treatment table for the evaluation of third metacarpal movements in relation to them. During abduction and adduction, the therapist can track the position of the third metacarpal with his index finger.

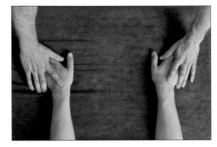

Fig. 14.199

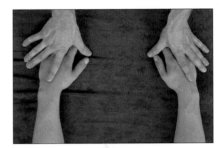

Fig. 14.200

Specific Active and Passive Movement Testing (Quantity and Quality)

a) **Palmar Flexion**:

- The therapist fixates the patient's forearm against his abdomen and asks him or her to actively perform palmar flexion of the hand.
- Then the therapist grasps the metacarpus from dorsal and tests whether the movement continues passively.
- Finally, the therapist moves the hand passively from the zero position through the entire range of motion and tests the end-feel.

Physiological end-feel:
firm and elastic

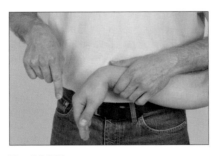

Fig. 14.201

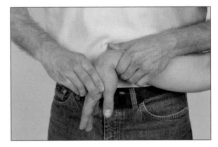

Fig. 14.202

b) **Dorsiflexion**:

- Still fixating the patient's forearm against his abdomen, the therapist asks the patient to <u>actively</u> dorsiflex the hand.
- Then the therapist grasps the metacarpus from palmar and tests whether the movement <u>continues passively</u>.
- Finally, the therapist moves the hand passively from the zero position through the entire range of motion and tests <u>the end-feel</u>.

Physiological end-feel:
firm and elastic

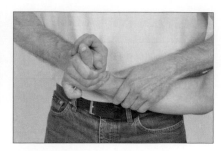

Fig. 14.203

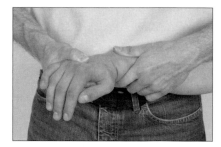

Fig. 14.204

> **Note**
> With wrist dorsiflexion (= extension), the rotatory range of motion is often slightly limited with movement quality and traction suggesting hypermobility; on rotatory extension the end-feel is loose and at the end it is rather hard and non-elastic in this case; and during translatoric movements the joint feels "like a worn out rubber band." These findings indicate a hypermobile wrist joint. The looseness of the capsuloligamentous unit allows the wrist bones or bases of the metacarpals, especially the third ray, to hit the distal border of the radius prematurely.

c) **Radial Abduction**:

- Still fixating the patient's forearm against his abdomen, the therapist asks the patient to <u>actively</u> move the hand toward the radius (radial abduction).
- Next the therapist grasps the metacarpus from the ulnar and tests whether the movement <u>continues passively</u>.
- Finally, the therapist moves the hand <u>passively</u> from the zero position through the entire range of motion and tests the <u>end-feel</u>.

Physiological end-feel:
firm and elastic

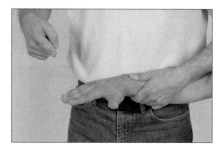

Fig. 14.205

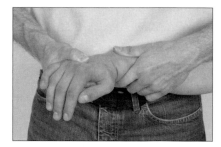

Fig. 14.206

d) **Ulnar Adduction**:

- As before, the therapist fixates the forearm against his abdomen and asks the patient to <u>actively</u> move the hand toward the ulna (ulnar adduction).
- Next the therapist grasps the metacarpus from the radial side and tests whether the movement <u>continues passively</u>.
- Finally, the therapist moves the hand <u>passively</u> from the zero position through the entire range of motion and tests the <u>end-feel</u>.

Physiological end-feel:
firm and elastic

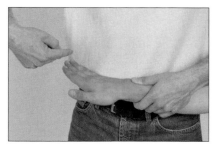

Fig. 14.207

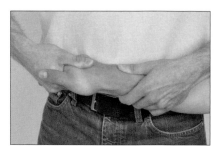

Fig. 14.208

> **Note**
> The end-feel during radial abduction and ulnar adduction is primarily ligamentous and thus firmer than during flexion or extension.

14.13.3 Translatoric movement tests

Traction:

Still fixating the patient's forearm against his abdomen, the therapist places the thumb and index finger of his proximal, stabilizing hand around the ulnar/radial styloid process. His distal hand fixates the bases of the metacarpals. The index finger and thumb of one hand are directly across from the index finger and thumb of the other. With his distal hand he pulls the metacarpus away at a right angle to the treatment plane.

Physiological end-feel:
firm and elastic

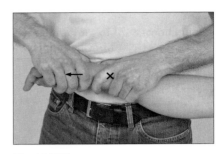

Fig. 14.209

Compression:

Continuing to hold the patient's forearm against his abdomen, the therapist places the thumb and index finger of his proximal stabilizing hand around the ulnar/radial styloid process. His distal hand grips the metacarpals, which he presses at a right angle toward the treatment plane.

Physiological end-feel: hard

Note
Pain felt in the wrist may also be related to the distal forearm joint.

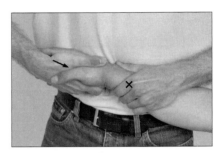

Fig. 14.210

14.13.4 Translatoric testing of the Intercarpal Joints

Wrist pain is often related to hypermobility if none of these three typical causes of joint stiffness is present in the patient's history: immobilization for a longer period of time, lacking use of the full range of motion for a longer period of time, and/or a specific disease such as complex regional pain syndrome (CRPS). If the patient's history contains any of these clues, and if general rotatory testing shows restricted movement, there nevertheless might often be hypermobility of individual intercarpal joints. Such a hypermobility might compensate stiffness in adjacent intercarpal joints. A hypermobile joint between the capitate and lunate, for example, can compensate for lacking mobility between the lunate and radius. Yet often there is hypermobility of certain intercarpal joints without any limitation of adjacent joints. Such hypermobility may be caused by rotatory mobilization attempts (also by the patient) or (minor) sprain injuries. Stabilization, especially passive stabilization with a wrist bandage, for example, is an important (trial) treatment. Because intercarpal hypermobility is a contraindication for grade III general traction, the specific examination of the intercarpal joints is shown in the following tests. Their specific mobilization is based on similar principles. The reader is referred to further education.

a) **Gliding between the capitate and trapezoid in the resting position** (Test 1)

The therapist stands distal to the patient's hand. The thumb of his ulnar hand fixates the capitate on the dorsal aspect and his index finger fixates on the palmar aspect. The thumb of his radial hand grasps the dorsal surface of the trapezoid and his index finger grasps the palmar aspect. The trapezoid is moved dorsally and palmarly, parallel to the treatment plane, which is approximately at a right angle to the back of the hand.

Physiological end-feel:
firm and elastic

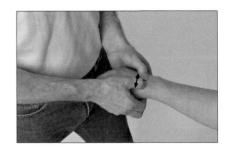

Fig. 14.211

b) **Gliding between the capitate and scaphoid in the resting position** (Test 2)

The therapist is still standing distal to the patient's hand. Again, his ulnar hand fixates the capitate. With the thumb of his radial hand, he grasps the dorsal aspect of the scaphoid and with his index finger he grasps its palmar aspect and moves it dorsally and palmarly, parallel to the treatment plane.

Physiological end-feel: firm and elastic

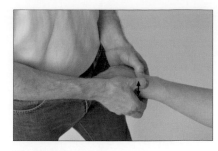

Fig. 14.212

c) **Gliding between the capitate and lunate in the resting position** (Test 3)

The therapist is still standing distal to the patient's hand, with his ulnar hand still fixating the capitate. His radial hand grasps the lunate and moves it dorsally and palmarly, parallel to the treatment plane.

Physiological end-feel: firm and elastic

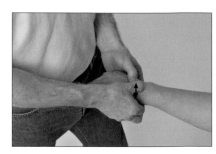

Fig. 14.213

d) **Gliding between the capitate and hamate in the resting position** (Test 4)

The therapist is still standing distal to the patient's hand. Now his radial hand fixates the capitate. The thumb of his ulnar hand grasps the dorsal aspect of the hamate and his index finger the palmar aspect, moving it dorsally and palmarly, parallel to the treatment plane.

Physiological end-feel: firm and elastic

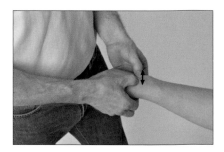

Fig. 14.214

e) **Gliding between the scaphoid and the trapezoid and trapezium in the resting position** (Test 5)

The therapist stands laterally to the patient's hand and places its ulnar side against his abdomen. The thumb of his proximal hand fixates the scaphoid on its dorsal aspect and his index finger on its palmar aspect. The thumb of his distal hand grasps the trapezoid and trapezium on their dorsal aspects and his index finger grasps them on their palmar aspects, moving them dorsally and palmarly, parallel to the treatment plane.

Physiological end-feel: firm and elastic

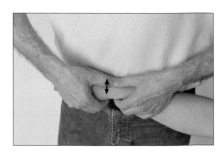

Fig. 14.215

f) **Gliding between the radius and scaphoid in the resting position** (Test 6)

As before, the therapist stands laterally to the patient's hand and fixates it against his abdomen. The two-handed grip is similar to the previous one, but is somewhat further proximal; thus the proximal hand fixates the radius while the distal one moves the scaphoid dorsally and palmarly, parallel to the treatment plane.

Physiological end-feel:
firm and elastic

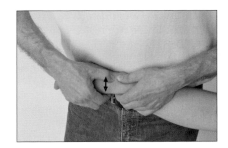

Fig. 14.216

g) **Gliding between the radius and lunate in the resting position** (Test 7)

The therapist stands as before and moves both hands toward the middle of the wrist joint so that the proximal hand continues to fixate the radius and the distal one moves the lunate dorsally and palmarly, parallel to the treatment plane.

Physiological end-feel:
firm and elastic

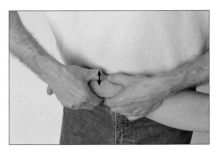

Fig. 14.217

h) **Gliding between the radius and triquetrum in the resting position** (Test 8)

The therapist now stands on the other side of the patient's hand, placing its radial side against his abdomen. The thumb of his proximal hand fixates the radius on its dorsal aspect and his index finger on its palmar aspect. With the thumb of his distal hand on the dorsal surface of the triquetrum and his index finger on its palmar aspect, he moves it dorsally and palmarly, parallel to the treatment plane.

Physiological end-feel:
firm and elastic

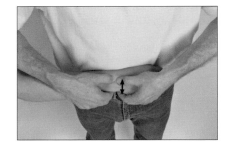

Fig. 14.218

i) **Gliding between the triquetrum and hamate in the resting position** (Test 9)

As before, the therapist stands laterally to the patient's hand and holds it against his abdomen. The grip with both hands is similar to previously, but somewhat further distal so that the proximal hand fixates the triquetrum and the distal one moves the hamate dorsally and palmarly, parallel to the treatment plane.

Physiological end-feel:
firm and elastic

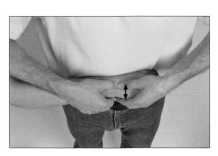

Fig. 14.219

j) **Gliding between the triquetrum and pisiform in the resting position** (Test 10)

The therapist again stands distal to the patient's hand, which he fixates with his radial hand. The thumb and index finger of his lateral hand wrap around the pisiform from the palmar side and move it toward the radius and ulna, parallel to the treatment plane.

Physiological end-feel: firm and elastic

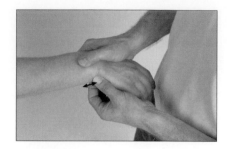

Fig. 14.220

> **Note**
>
> Certain intercarpal joints were not tested in the above. These are the joints between the trapezium and trapezoid, between the scaphoid and lunate, and between the lunate and triquetrum. These joints are seldom affected by dysfunction—perhaps because extreme or prolonged horizontal force is rare compared with vertical force which occurs, for instance, when carrying something or supporting oneself.

14.13.5 Treatment of Capsuloligamentous Hypomobility

The patient's distal forearm is lying on a wedge with the joint space hanging over its edge. With his ulnar hand, the therapist fixates the patient's forearm and with his radial hand he grasps the metacarpals, which he pulls at a right angle away from the treatment plane.

> **!** Pain-relieving traction may also be performed using the test version.

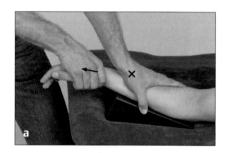

> **!** Alternatively, a belt may be placed around the wrist and around the pelvis of the therapist. By leaning backward, the therapist can increase the force of traction. Fixation of the patient's forearm may also be done using a belt.

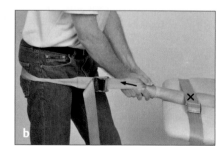

Fig. 14.221 a, b

Documentation template: Practice Scheme

Wrist joint						
Symptoms						
Symptom-altering direction						
Contraindications?	Nervous system: Other:					
Symptom-altering joint						
General assessment of adjacent joints						
Active movements, comparing sides						

Specific rotatory tests	Active	Continues passively?	Passive	End-feel	Symptoms/ pain	Comments
▪ Palmar flexion						
▪ Dorsiflexion						
▪ Radial abduction						
▪ Ulnar adduction						

Translatoric movement tests	Quantity	Quality	End-feel	Symptoms/pain	Comments
▪ Traction					
▪ Compression					

Summary Formulation aid: ▪ Symptoms ▪ Direction ▪ Contraindications ▪ Site (joint) ▪ Restricted mobility, hypermobility, or physiological mobility ▪ Structure: muscle, joint, etc.	*Text:*
Trial treatment	
Physical therapy diagnosis	
Treatment plan with treatment goal and prognosis	
Treatment progress	
Final examination	

Documentation: Practice Example

<table>
<tr><td colspan="7" align="center">Wrist joint
(Impaired movement of the right hand two months after conservative treatment of a "classic" distal radius fracture)</td></tr>
<tr><td>Symptoms</td><td colspan="6">Impaired mobility of the right hand during grasping movements</td></tr>
<tr><td>Symptom-altering direction</td><td colspan="6">Dorsiflexion and radial abduction</td></tr>
<tr><td>Contraindications?</td><td colspan="6">Nervous system: No findings
Other: No findings</td></tr>
<tr><td>Symptom-altering joint</td><td colspan="6">Wrist</td></tr>
<tr><td>General assessment of adjacent joints</td><td colspan="6">The entire right metacarpus appears somewhat "stiff."</td></tr>
<tr><td>Active movements, comparing sides</td><td colspan="6">Limited dorsiflexion and radial abduction of the right wrist</td></tr>
</table>

Specific rotatory tests	Active	Continues passively?	Passive	End-feel	Symptoms/ pain	Comments
Palmar flexion	60°	ca. 20°	No findings	Firm and elastic		
Dorsiflexion	50°	< 5°	Increased resistance to movement	Very firm and elastic		
Radial abduction	10°	< 5°	Increased resistance to movement	Very firm and elastic		
Ulnar adduction	30°	< 5°	No findings	Firm and elastic		

Translatoric movement tests	Quantity	Quality	End-feel	Symptoms/pain	Comments
Traction	Hypo 2	Increased resistance to movement	Very firm and elastic		
Compression	No findings	No findings	Hard		

<table>
<tr><td>Summary
Formulation aid:
■ Symptoms

■ Direction
■ Contraindications
■ Site (joint)
■ Restricted mobility, hypermobility, or physiological mobility
■ Structure: muscle, joint, etc.</td><td>Text:
■ Patient has impaired movement of the right hand after complete healing of a classic radius fracture.
■ There is limited dorsiflexion and radial abduction
■ There are no contraindications today to larger movements.
■ The symptoms are in correlation with the wrist joint,
■ which has restricted mobility

■ due to capsuloligamentous shrinkage.</td></tr>
<tr><td>Trial treatment</td><td>10-minute grade III traction, after which the patient reported that movement felt easier and the therapist felt less resistance to movement.</td></tr>
<tr><td>Physical therapy diagnosis</td><td>See above</td></tr>
</table>

Continued ▶

Wrist joint	
(Impaired movement of the right hand two months after conservative treatment of a "classic" distal radius fracture)	
Treatment plan with treatment goal and prognosis	▪ *Continue grade III traction mobilization.* ▪ *Treatment goal: pain-free physiological mobility* ***(Further information on examination and treatment techniques may be obtained through further education.)***
Treatment progress	
Final examination	

14.14 Forearm Joints

(Articulationes radioulnaris distalis et proximalis)

14.14.1 Anatomy

- Distal radioulnar joint:
  Joint type: trochoid joint – pivot joint
  Joint surface: articular circumference of the radius: concave
  Resting position: ca. 10° supination
  Close packed position: maximum pronation and supination

- Proximal radioulnar joint:
  Joint type: trochoid joint – rotary joint
  Joint surface: head of radius: convex
  Resting position: ca. 35° supination with ca. 70° elbow flexion
  Close packed position: maximum pronation and supination
  Capsular sign: uniformly restricted pronation and supination if the elbow joint is very restricted during flexion and extension

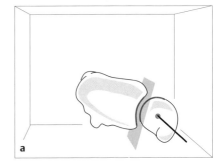

> **!** The distal and proximal radioulnar joints are necessarily coupled. During pronation and supination there is significant accompanying movement of the humeroradial joint and minimal movement of the humeroulnar joint.

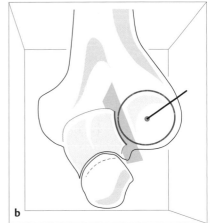

Fig. 14.222 a, b

14.14.2 Rotatory Tests

■ Active Movements, Comparing Sides

The patient flexes both elbows to 90° alongside the body with the thumbs pointing toward the ceiling (= zero position). Next he or she rotates the forearms to maximum supination and pronation.

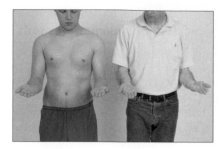

Fig. 14.223

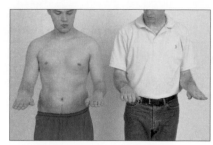

Fig. 14.224

■ Specific Active and Passive Movement Testing (Quantity and Quality)

a) **Supination** from the zero position:

- The therapist stands in front of the patient and asks them to <u>actively</u> supinate the forearm to its maximum.
- Then with his medial hand the therapist holds the ulna and tests with his lateral hand whether the movement of the radius around the ulna <u>continues passively</u>. There is acceptable minimal movement of the ulna.
- Finally, the therapist moves the ra-

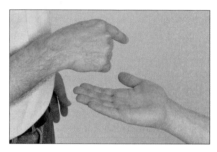

Fig. 14.225

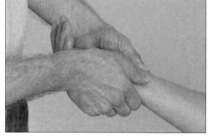

Fig. 14.226

dius <u>passively</u> from the zero position around the relatively still ulna through the entire range of motion and tests the <u>end-feel</u>.

Physiological end-feel:
firm and elastic

b) **Pronation** from the zero position:

- The therapist stands in front of the patient and asks him or her to <u>actively</u> pronate the forearm as far as possible.
- Then with his lateral hand he holds the patient's ulna and with his medial hand tests whether the radius <u>continues to move passively</u> around the ulna. The slight movement of the ulna is not prevented.
- Finally, the therapist moves the radius <u>passively</u> from the zero position around the relatively stable ulna through the entire range of motion and tests the <u>end-feel</u>.

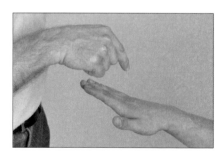

Fig. 14.227

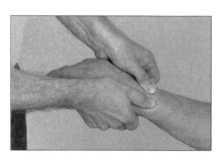

Fig. 14.228

Physiological end-feel:
initially firm and elastic, then with a significant overpressure, hard and elastic

14.14.3 Translatoric movement tests

▪ Distal Radioulnar Joint

Traction is not possible due to the poor grip possibilities.

a) **Compression** in the resting position:

The therapist grasps the ulna and the radius with both hands and presses the radius <u>perpendicularly toward the treatment plane</u>, which is on the radius.

Physiological end-feel: hard

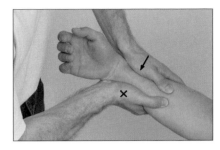

Fig. 14.229

b) **Gliding** from the resting position:

The therapist holds the distal ulna with the three radial fingers of his medial hand; the three radial fingers of his lateral hand grasp the distal radius, which he moves <u>posteriorly and anteriorly, parallel to the treatment plane</u>.

Physiological end-feel:
firm and elastic

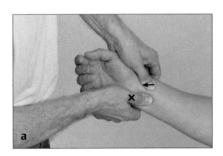

Fig. 14.230 a, b

▪ Proximal Radioulnar Joint

Traction is not possible due to the poor grip possibilities.

a) **Compression** in the resting position:

The therapist holds the ulna and the radius with both hands and presses the radius <u>perpendicularly toward the treatment plane</u>, which is on the ulna. The ulna is fixated mainly by the underlying surface.

Physiological end-feel: hard

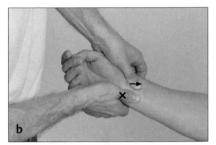

Fig. 14.231

b) **Gliding** from the resting position:

The patient's forearm is in the resting position on the bench, which is raised so that with abduction of the shoulder the treatment plane is nearly horizontal in space. The therapist's proximal hand fixates the proximal end of the ulna and his distal hand

holds the head of the radius which he moves <u>parallel to the treatment plane posteriorly and anteriorly</u>. With the thumb of the proximal hand he can feel the movement in the joint space.

Physiological end-feel:
firm and elastic

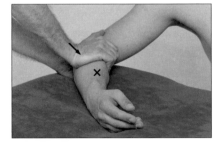
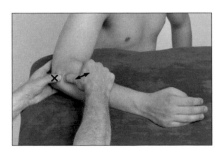

Fig. 14.232

14.14.4 Treatment of Capsuloligamentous Hypomobility

▪ Distal Radioulnar Joint

a) **Gliding posteriorly:**

The patient's forearm rests on the head piece of the bench and the therapist stands in front of it. The therapist fixates the ulna with the thenar eminence of his medial hand and his three radial fingers. The thenar eminence and the three radial fingers of his lateral hand hold the radius and push it posteriorly, parallel to the treatment plane. This improves restricted supination.

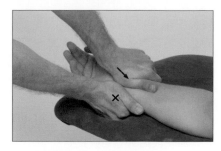

Fig. 14.233

b) **Gliding anteriorly:**

The patient's forearm is lying on the head piece of the bench, which is raised so that with abduction of the shoulder the treatment plane is nearly horizontal in space. The therapist stands posteriorly. He fixates the ulna with the thenar eminence of the lateral hand and the three radial fingers. The thenar eminence and the three radial fingers of the medial hand grip the radius and push it anteriorly, parallel to the treatment plane. This improves restricted pronation.

> **!** For pain-relief, intermittent grade I–II gliding may also be performed with the test version. Important: Hypomobility in the distal radioulnar joint occurs very uncommonly. Thus mobilization in grade III is hardly ever indicated.

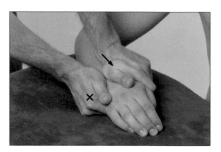

Fig. 14.234

▪ Proximal Radioulnar Joint

a) **Gliding posteriorly:**

The patient's forearm rests on the head piece of the bench and the therapist stands in front of it. His lateral hand holds the distal ulna, which is fixated against the bench. The medial hand lies with the pisiform on the anterior aspect of the head of the radius which it pushes posteriorly, parallel to the treatment plane. This improves restricted pronation.

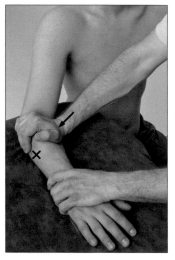

Fig. 14.235

b) **Gliding anteriorly:**

The patient's forearm rests on the head piece of the bench, which is raised so that with abduction of the shoulder the treatment plane is nearly horizontal in space. The therapist stands posteriorly. The distal hand holds the distal ulna, which is fixated against the bench. The proximal hand is resting with the pisiform on the posterior side of the head of the radius which it pushes anteriorly, parallel to the treatment plane. This improves restricted supination.

! For pain relief, intermittent grade I–II gliding may also be performed with the test version.

! Unlike the distal radioulnar joint, in the proximal joint there is minimal rolling of the radius on the circular joint surface of the ulna and the anular ligament. Hence gliding movements in the resting position place very little tension on the joint capsule. Thus early gliding mobilization should be done in a submaximal position as shown in **Figs. 14.235** and **14.236**.

Caution: Limited pronation and/or supination are often caused by restricted mobility of the proximal radioulnar joint.

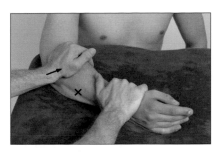

Fig. 14.236

Forearm joints						
Symptoms						
Symptom-altering direction						
Contraindications?	Nervous system: Other:					
Symptom-altering joint						
General assessment of adjacent joints						
Active movements, comparing sides						
Specific rotatory tests	**Active**	**Continues passively?**	**Passive**	**End-feel**	**Symptoms/ pain**	**Comments**
▪ Supination						
▪ Pronation						

Translatoric movement tests	**Quantity**	**Quality**	**End-feel**	**Symptoms/pain**	**Comments**
Distal radioulnar joint ▪ Compression					
▪ Posterior gliding					
▪ Anterior gliding					
Proximal radioulnar joint ▪ Compression					
▪ Posterior gliding					
▪ Anterior gliding					

Summary Formulation aid: ▪ Symptoms ▪ Direction ▪ Contraindications ▪ Site (joint) ▪ Restricted mobility, hypermobility, or physiological mobility ▪ Structure: muscle, joint, etc.	*Text:*
Trial treatment	
Physical therapy diagnosis	
Treatment plan with treatment goal and prognosis	
Treatment progress	
Final examination	

Documentation: Practice Example

<table>
<tr><td colspan="7">Forearm joints
(Handyman who complained of pain in the right forearm when inserting screws)</td></tr>
<tr><td>Symptoms</td><td colspan="6">Pain in the right forearm when inserting screws</td></tr>
<tr><td>Symptom-altering direction</td><td colspan="6">Supination</td></tr>
<tr><td>Contraindications?</td><td colspan="6">Nervous system: No findings
Other: No findings</td></tr>
<tr><td>Symptom-altering joint</td><td colspan="6">Proximal radioulnar joint</td></tr>
<tr><td>General assessment of adjacent joints</td><td colspan="6">No findings</td></tr>
<tr><td>Active movements, comparing sides</td><td colspan="6">End-range limitation of supination on the right side.</td></tr>
</table>

Specific rotatory tests	Active	Continues passively?	Passive	End-feel	Symptoms/ pain	Comments
▪ Supination	70°	< 5°	Increased resistance to movement	Very firm and elastic	Pain at end range	Triggers reported pain
▪ Pronation	80°	< 5°	No findings	Firm and elastic at the end		

Translatoric movement tests	Quantity	Quality	End-feel	Symptoms/pain	Comments
Distal radioulnar joint ▪ Compression	No findings	No findings	Hard	No findings	
▪ Posterior gliding	Hyper 4	Reduced resistance	Loose	No findings	
▪ Anterior gliding	Hyper 4	Reduced resistance	Loose	No findings	
Proximal radioulnar joint ▪ Compression	No findings	No findings	Hard	No findings	
▪ Posterior gliding	Slightly hypo	Mildly increased resistance to movement	Firm and elastic	No findings	
▪ Anterior gliding	Hypo 2	Increased resistance to movement	Very firm and elastic	Pain at end range	Triggers reported pain

Summary Formulation aid: ▪ Symptoms ▪ Direction ▪ Contraindications ▪ Site (joint) ▪ Restricted mobility, hypermobility, or physiological mobility ▪ Structure: muscle, joint, etc.	Text: ▪ Forearm pain ▪ during supination. ▪ There are no contraindications today for further movement testing. ▪ The symptoms are localized in the proximal radioulnar joint ▪ and in correlation with restricted mobility ▪ of the capsuloligamentous unit.

Continued ▶

Forearm joints **(Handyman who complained of pain in the right forearm when inserting screws)**	
Trial treatment	▪ *5-minute grade I–II intermittent gliding anteriorly in the proximal radioulnar joint. The patient felt that movement was easier afterward and there was less end-range pain.* ▪ *This was followed by 5-minute grade III anterior gliding in the proximal radioulnar joint. The patient felt afterward that movement was easier and there was less resistance to movement at the end range.*
Physical therapy diagnosis	*See above*
Treatment plan with treatment goal and prognosis	▪ *Continue with anterior gliding movements in the proximal radioulnar joint, first for pain relief and later grade III mobilization.* ▪ *Treatment goal: pain-free physiological mobility* **(Further information on examination and treatment techniques may be obtained through further education.)**
Treatment progress	
Final examination	

14.15   Elbow Joint

(Articulatio cubiti, consisting of the articulatio humeroradialis and articulatio humeroulnaris)

14.15.1   Anatomy

▪ Humeroradial joint
  Joint type: ball-and-socket joint
  Distal joint surfaces: concave
  Resting position: maximum extension and supination
  Close packed position: 90° flexion and 5° forearm supination

▪ Humeroulnar joint
  Joint type: saddle joint (often simplified in anatomy texts as a hinge joint)
  Distal joint surface: concave for flexion and extension, convex for abduction of the ulna with pronation as well as adduction of the ulna with supination
  Resting position: 70° flexion and 10° forearm supination
  Close packed position: maximum extension and supination
  Capsular sign: flexion > extension (with a limitation of ca. 90° flexion, there is only ca. 10° restriction of extension)

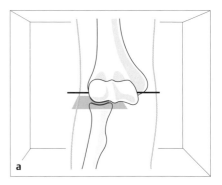
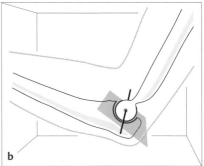

> ❗ Active flexion and extension occur in both joints simultaneously. Forearm supination and pronation are accompanied by rotation in the humeroradial joint and small lateral movements in the humeroulnar joint—abduction during pronation and adduction during supination.

Fig. 14.237 a, b

14.15.2 Rotatory Tests

■ Active Movements, Comparing Sides

The therapist asks the patient to flex and extend both elbows as far as possible. The amount of flexion may also be palpated and assessed by the distance between the acromion and the distal forearm.

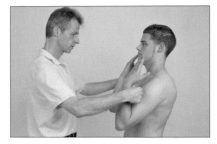

Fig. 14.238

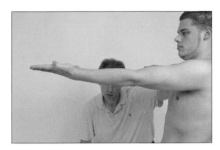

Fig. 14.239

■ Specific Active and Passive Movement Testing (Quantity and Quality)

a) **Flexion:**

- The therapist fixates the humerus and asks the patient to actively flex the elbow.
- Next the therapist grasps the distal forearm and tests whether the movement continues passively.
- Finally, the therapist moves the forearm passively from the zero position through the entire range of motion and tests the end-feel.

Physiological end-feel:
hard and elastic

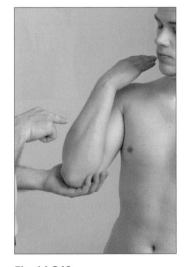

Fig. 14.240

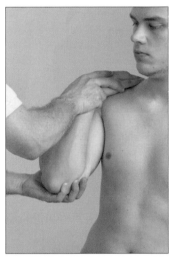

Fig. 14.241

! The application of overpressure to the distal ulna may be used to place emphasis on the humeroulnar joint; overpressure may be applied to the distal radius to emphasize the humeroradial joint.

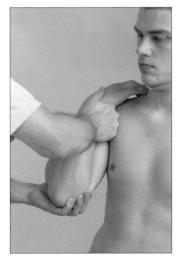

Fig. 14.242

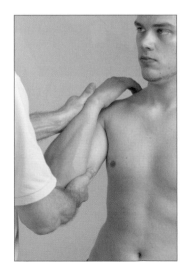

Fig. 14.243

b) Extension:

- The therapist fixates the humerus and asks the patient to <u>actively</u> extend the elbow.
- Next the therapist grasps the distal forearm and tests whether the movement <u>continues passively</u>.
- Finally, the therapist moves the forearm <u>passively</u> from the zero position through the entire range of motion and tests the <u>end-feel</u>.

Physiological end-feel:
hard and elastic

> **!** The application of overpressure to the distal ulna may be used to place emphasis on the humeroulnar joint; overpressure may be applied to the distal radius to emphasize the humeroradial joint.

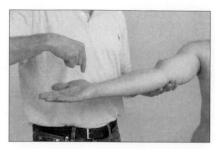

Fig. 14.244

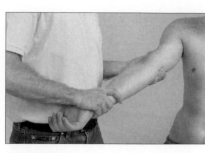

Fig. 14.245

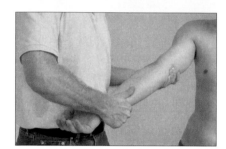

Fig. 14.246

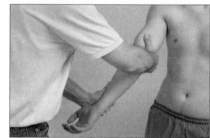

Fig. 14.247

c) Medial stability:

The therapist stands laterally and with the distal hand grasps the distal ulna from medial. The proximal hand holds the lateral epicondyle of the humerus from lateral. This holds the elbow joint in the neutral position. Next the therapist twists his torso causing the medial joint surfaces to separate. He should note the quantity (range of motion) and the quality (end-feel) of movement as well as any pain. This test primarily evaluates the humeroulnar joint, although there is accompanying movement of the humeroradial joint as well.

Physiological end-feel:
very firm and elastic

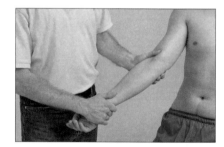

Fig. 14.248

d) Lateral stability:

The therapist stands medially and with the distal hand grasps the distal ulna from lateral. The proximal hand holds the medial epicondyle of the humerus from medial. This holds the elbow joint in the neutral position. Next the therapist twists his torso causing the lateral joint surfaces to separate. The therapist notes the quantity (range of motion) and the quality (end-feel) of movement as well as any pain. This test primarily evaluates the humeroulnar joint, although there is accompanying movement of the humeroradial joint as well.

Physiological end-feel:
very firm and elastic

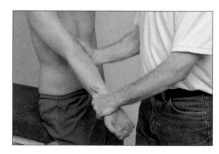

Fig. 14.249

14.15.3 Translatoric movement tests

■ Humeroulnar Joint

a) **Traction:**

The therapist fixates the humerus from posterior with his lateral hand. He should stabilize his arm against his body to keep his hand still. Next, using the ball of the little finger, he grasps the proximal ulna from medial and supports the distal forearm of the patient against his medial shoulder. Then he pulls the ulna at a right angle away from the treatment plane.

Physiological end-feel:
firm and elastic

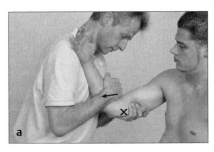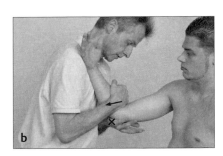

Fig. 14.250 a, b

> **!** During traction the range of motion is minimal. Thus the therapist "calibrates" his ability to sense joint movements by fixating the olecranon and then pulling on the ulna (**Fig. 14.250 b**). There will be no palpable joint movement, only soft tissue deformation. Afterward, he again fixates the humerus and performs traction on the ulna. What he senses more strongly now than before comes from the movement of the joint.

b) **Compression:**

The therapist fixates the humerus with his lateral hand. His medial hand presses the proximal ulna against the humerus at a right angle to the treatment plane. In a stronger compression test, the patient supports himself or herself on the forearm and presses the humerus against the ulna.

Physiological end-feel: hard

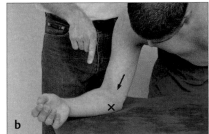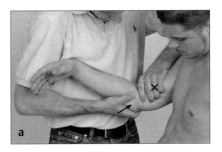

Fig. 14.251 a, b

■ Humeroradial Joint

a) **Traction:**

The patient is lying supine or sitting with his or her upper arm lying on the bench. With the ulnar border of his proximal hand, the therapist fixates the distal humerus so that his index finger can easily palpate the humeroradial joint space. His distal hand holds the thicker end of the distal radius. Next he rotates his body and pulls the radius at a right angle away from the treatment plane.

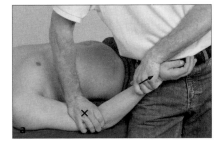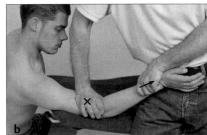

Fig. 14.252 a, b

b) **Compression:**

The patient is lying supine or seated at the head of the bench. With the ulnar border of his proximal hand, the therapist fixates the distal humerus and with his distal hand he grasps the thicker end of the distal radius. Next he pushes the radius at a right angle toward the treatment plane, using the weight of his own body to aid the application of pressure.

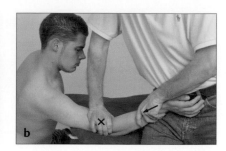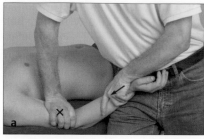

Fig. 14.253 a, b

> ❗ Unlike the other joints, the humeroradial joint is not in the anatomical resting position for traction and compression, but instead is slightly flexed. This is because, in a position of extension and maximum supination, it is difficult to fixate the humerus during application of longitudinal traction or compression to the radius.

14.15.4   Treatment of Capsuloligamentous Hypomobility

■ Humeroulnar Joint

Traction in the resting position:

The patient lies on his or her side. The patient's proximal humerus is held against the bench by his or her upper body with epicondyles resting on a sandbag placed near the edge of the bench. The olecranon is hanging over the edge of the bench. The therapist stands laterally and grasps the distal ulna with his lateral hand. The heel of his medial hand is on the proximal ulna which he presses at a right angle away from the treatment plane.

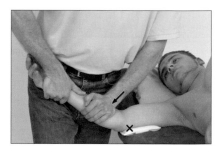

Fig. 14.254

■ Humeroradial Joint

Traction in the resting position:

The patient is lying in the supine position. The therapist stands medial to the patient's forearm. The therapist fixates the humerus with the ulnar part of his proximal hand or with a belt. His distal hand grasps the thick end of the distal radius. Then he rotates his body and pulls the radius at a right angle away from the treatment plane. If using a belt, the medial hand may assist the lateral one.

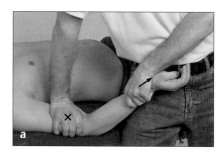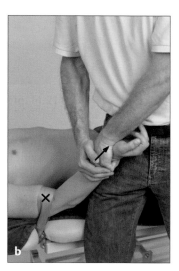

Fig. 14.255 a, b

> ❗ As explained above in the section on examination techniques, the humeroradial joint is not in the anatomical resting position. Soon after a trial treatment the joint should be prepositioned in submaximal flexion or extension in order to put tension on that part of the joint capsule which limits the movement, and less on the ligaments.

> ❗ Pain-relieving traction may also be performed with the examination techniques.

Documentation Template: Practice Scheme

Elbow joint	
Symptoms	
Symptom-altering direction	
Contraindications?	Nervous system: Other:
Symptom-altering joint	
General assessment of adjacent joints	

Active movements, comparing sides						
Specific rotatory tests	**Active**	**Continues passively?**	**Passive**	**End-feel**	**Symptoms/pain**	**Comments**
Humeroulnar joint: ▪ Flexion						
▪ Extension						
Humeroradial joint: ▪ Flexion						
▪ Extension						

Stability tests	**Quantity**	**Quality**	**End-feel**	**Symptoms/pain**	**Comments**
▪ Radial gaping					
▪ Ulnar gaping					
Translatoric movement tests	**Quantity**	**Quality**	**End-feel**	**Symptoms/pain**	**Comments**
Humeroulnar joint: ▪ Traction					
▪ Compression					
Humeroradial joint: ▪ Traction					
▪ Compression					

Summary Formulation aid: ▪ Symptoms ▪ Direction ▪ Contraindications ▪ Site (joint) ▪ Restricted mobility, hypermobility, or physiological mobility ▪ Structure: muscle, joint, etc.	*Text:*
Trial treatment	
Physical therapy diagnosis	

Continued ▶

Documentation Template: Practice Scheme *(Continued)*

Elbow joint	
Treatment plan with treatment goal and prognosis	
Treatment progress	
Final examination	

Documentation: Practice Example

Elbow joint	
(Painfully limited motion 7 weeks after conservative treatment of a fractured humeral trochlea)	
Symptoms	*Painfully limited elbow joint flexion and extension*
Symptom-altering direction	*Flexion and extension*
Contraindications?	Nervous system: *No findings* Other: *No findings*
Symptom-altering joint	*Elbow joint*
General assessment of adjacent joints	*Movements of right wrist joint are slightly restricted.*
Active movements, comparing sides	*Right elbow is painful with significantly limited movement (flexion/extension: 0–50° to nearly 90°).*

Specific rotatory tests	Active	Continues passively?	Passive	End-feel	Symptoms/pain	Com-ments
Humeroulnar: ■ Flexion	*Nearly 90°*	*< 5°*	*Increased resistance to movement*	*Empty or very slightly firm and elastic*	*End-range pain as reported by the patient*	
■ Extension	*Nearly −50°*	*< 5°*	*Increased muscular resistance to movement*	*Empty or very slightly firm and elastic*	*End-range pain, medial*	
Humeroradial: ■ Flexion	*Nearly 90°*	*Barely more than humeroulnar joint*	*Increased muscular resistance to movement*	*Empty or very slightly firm and elastic*	*End-range pain, lateral*	
■ Extension	*Nearly −50°*	*Somewhat more than humeroulnar joint*	*Increased muscular resistance to movement*	*Empty or very slightly firm and elastic*	*End-range pain, anterior*	

Stability tests	Quantity	Quality	End-feel	Symptoms/pain	Comments
■ Radial gaping	*?*	*?*	*?*	*?*	*Not yet tested due to pain and lacking signs*
■ Ulnar gaping	*?*	*?*	*?*	*?*	*ditto*

Continued ▶

Elbow joint (Painfully limited motion 7 weeks after conservative treatment of a fractured humeral trochlea)					
Translatoric movement tests	**Quantity**	**Quality**	**End-feel**	**Symptoms/ pain**	**Comments**
Humeroulnar joint: ■ Traction	*Hypo 1–2*	*Increased resistance to movement*	*Very firm and elastic*	Not painful	*In early grade III traction strong stretching feeling provoked*
■ Compression	*No findings*	*No findings*	*Hard and elastic*	*Supracondylar pain*	*Pain relief with soft-tissue massage*
Humeroradial joint: ■ Traction	*Hypo 2*	*Increased resistance to movement*	*Very firm and elastic*	Not painful	*In early grade III traction strong stretching feeling provoked*
■ Compression	*No findings*	*No findings*	*Hard and elastic*		

Summary Formulation aid: ■ Symptoms ■ Direction ■ Contraindications ■ Site (joint) ■ Restricted mobility, hypermobility, or physiological mobility ■ Structure: muscle, joint, etc.	*Text:* ■ *Painfully limited movement in the right elbow* ■ *with flexion (nearly 90°) and extension (50°).* ■ *There are no contraindications today to further movement testing.* ■ *The symptoms are in correlation with the elbow joint; both the humeroulnar and humeroradial joints* ■ *which have limited movement,* ■ *due to capsuloligamentous shrinkage following immobilization and pain provocation with humeroradial flexion (lateral) and with humeroulnar extension (medial).*
Trial treatment	■ *5-minute grade I–II pain-relieving traction each for the humeroradial and humeroulnar joints, after which the patient reports decreased pain and there is less resistance to movement.*
Physical therapy diagnosis	*This is followed by 5-minute traction mobilization (beginning grade III) of the humeroradial and humeroulnar joints, after which the patient reports a further decrease in pain and the end of movement is achieved with less resistance.*
Treatment plan with treatment goal and prognosis	*See above*
Treatment progress	
Final examination	

14.16   Shoulder and Shoulder Girdle Region

Active movements of the humerus occur in what is colloquially referred to as "the shoulder," although anatomically speaking the movements involve five joints: the glenohumeral joint, the acromioclavicular joint, the sternoclavicular joint, the subacromial gliding space, and the scapuloserrato-thoracic gliding space. Thus, if a patient complains of "shoulder" symptoms, the therapist must first determine in which of the five joints the problem is localized before conducting the actual specific examination.

Until now we have assumed that the location of the problem is identified by the examination and pain/hypomobility treatment. This didactic simplification for the purpose of learning specific examination techniques assumes conditions which the therapist first must ensure are present. There are various possibilities for **symptom localization**. In this discussion of the fundamentals, we use the basic principle of taking each joint involved in symptom provocation and moving that joint specifically to its end-range. The therapist should carefully note which joint changes the symptoms.

In patients with "shoulder pain" it is important to ask about the type of symptoms: is the problem one of pain or dysfunction, and is there hypomobility, hypermobility, or poor control of movements? Next, the therapist should determine which movement direction produces these symptoms. This should be possible based on the patient's history, an inspection of everyday movements, and a demonstration of active movements.

The therapist should also note whether there is simultaneous movement of the cervical or thoracic spine during painful arm movements and whether the symptoms intensify if the patient continues to move that spinal segment in the symptom-producing direction. If so, this should raise suspicion of cervical or thoracic spine involvement. The appropriate examination, as detailed in Chapter 15 on the spinal column, should be included in the "shoulder pain" examination.

Only if active movements fail to point out any symptom-altering direction does the therapist check all movement directions with passive tests as usual, which are described in the following sections. Once the symptom-altering direction has been identified, each joint involved should be moved as specifically as possible in the symptom-changing direction to determine which joint actually changes the symptoms. The joint whose movement correlates with the symptoms is tested as usual for hypomobility, hypermobility, and physiological mobility. Again, preliminary clues indicating the structure which alters the mobility are obtained from the quality of movement (end-feel) and Translatoric movement tests.

The following section describes a general examination for locating the symptom-altering direction and performing a general assessment of mobility of the entire shoulder girdle. The subsequent specific examination of the glenohumeral joint and the actual shoulder girdle, including the acromioclavicular and the sternoclavicular joints, enables symptom localization in one of these joints as well as an assessment of specific mobility and the movement-altering structure. This is followed by the treatment of capsuloligamentous pain and hypomobility as usual.

For specific examination techniques related to the subacromial space, which is always involved in glenohumeral joint movements, the reader is referred to further education. The same applies to symptom localization tests.

Note

General procedure for symptom localization

1. What is the pain or dysfunction reported by the patient (= **symptoms**)?
2. Which **direction of movement** causes pain to occur?
3. Which **joint** changes the symptoms during specific movement tests?
4. Does the responsible joint exhibit **restricted mobility, hypermobility, or physiological mobility**?
5. Which movement-altering **structure** is suggested by the quality of movement and the end-feel?

This simplified procedure may now be applied to the joints already discussed. If, for example, the patient has pain (= symptoms) with knee joint flexion (= movement direction) we try to influence the symptoms with end-range movements of the knee and hip joint. If knee movement is painful, Translatoric movement tests of end-range movements of the patella or tibia may be used to determine whether the pain is related more to the femoropatellar or femorotibial joint. One should also think of specific movements of the proximal tibiofibular joint whose dysfunction is often perceived as "knee pain" (= joint). Next the mobility of the corresponding joint is evaluated (restricted mobility, hypermobility, or physiological mobility?). Based on the rotatory movement quality and the Translatoric movement tests, one can then determine which structure probably changes the mobility (= structure).

14.17 | Should Girdle Region

(Articulatio humeri, articulatio acromioclavicularis, articulatio sternoclavicularis, articulatio subacromiales and scapulo-serrato-thoracic gliding space)

14.17.1 | Anatomy

A complex consisting of five joints, of which three are true joints and two are gliding spaces.

True joints:
- Glenohumeral joint
- Acromioclavicular joint
- Sternoclavicular joint

Gliding spaces:
- Subacromial and subdeltoid gliding space
- Scapulothoracic gliding space

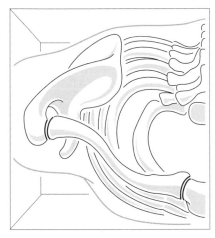

Fig. 14.256

14.17.2 | Rotatory Tests

■ Active Movements, Comparing Sides

The patient is seated on a stool and moves both arms simultaneously to maximum

- flexion/elevation and extension

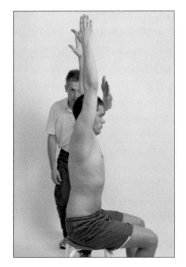

Fig. 14.257

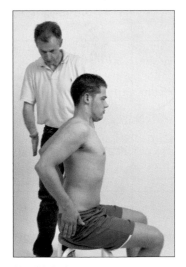

Fig. 14.258

In the same manner, bilateral active tests are done with

- abduction/elevation and adduction
- external and internal rotation

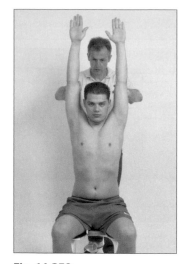

Fig. 14.259

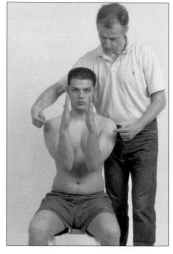

Fig. 14.260

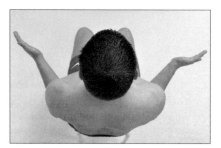

Fig. 14.261

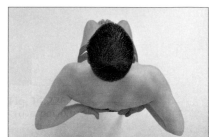

Fig. 14.262

■ Specific Active and Passive Movement Testing (Quantity and Quality)

a) **Flexion/elevation** from the zero position:

- The therapist stands behind the patient and asks him or her to actively flex the arm to its maximum height above the horizontal plane.
- Next the therapist stabilizes the thoracic spine by fixating the contralateral upper ribs from above, and placing his thumb on the spinous process of T1. He can also use his body to support the patient's back. Next he takes the patient's arm and tests whether the movement continues passively.
- Finally, the therapist moves the arm passively from the zero position through the entire range of motion and tests the end-feel.

Physiological end-feel:
soft and elastic, because several joints are involved in the movement

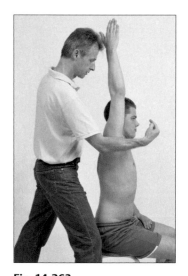

Fig. 14.263

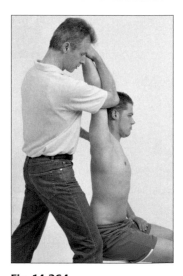

Fig. 14.264

b) **Extension** from the zero position:

- The therapist stands behind the patient and asks him or her to <u>actively</u> extend the arm, which is bent at the elbow, as far as possible.
- Next the therapist stabilizes the thoracic spine with his medial hand as described above, takes the patient's arm, and tests whether the movement <u>continues passively</u>.
- Finally, the therapist moves the arm <u>passively</u> from the zero position through the entire range of motion and tests the <u>end-feel</u>.

Physiological end-feel:
soft and elastic, because several joints are involved in the movement

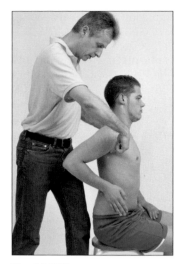

Fig. 14.265

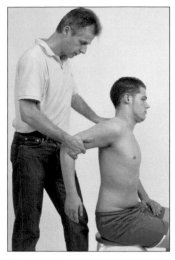

Fig. 14.266

c) **Abduction/elevation** from the zero position:

- The therapist stands behind the patient and asks him or her to <u>actively</u> abduct the arm as far as possible above the horizontal plane.
- Then the therapist stabilizes the cervical spine with his medial hand by fixating the contralateral upper ribs from above, and placing his thumb on the spinous process of T1. He can also use his body to support the patient's back. Then he takes the patient's arm and tests whether the movement <u>continues passively</u>.
- Finally, the therapist moves the arm <u>passively</u> from the zero position through the entire range of motion and tests the <u>end-feel</u>.

Physiological end-feel:
soft and elastic because several joints are involved in the movement

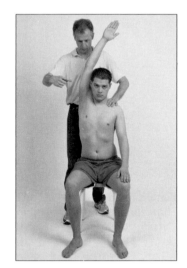

Fig. 14.267

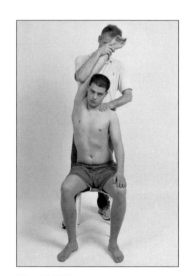

Fig. 14.268

d) **Adduction** from the zero position:

- The therapist stands behind the patient and asks him or her to <u>actively</u> adduct the arm with ca. 90° elbow flexion as far as possible in front of the abdomen.
- Next the therapist stabilizes the patient's sternum with the fingers of his medial hand and fixates the upper ribs with his thumb. He can also use his body to support the

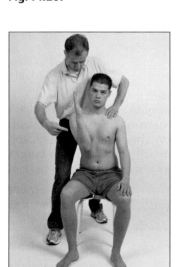

Fig. 14.269

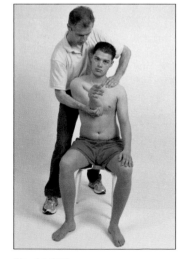

Fig. 14.270

patient's back. Then he takes the patient's arm and tests whether the movement continues passively.

- Finally, the therapist moves the patient's arm passively from the zero position through the entire range of motion and tests the end-feel.

Physiological end-feel:
soft and elastic, because several joints are involved in the movement

! The same grip may be used to examine horizontal abduction and adduction.

e) **External rotation** from the zero position:

- The therapist stands behind the patient and asks him or her to perform active maximum external rotation of the arm which is bent ca. 90°at the elbow.
- Next the therapist stabilizes the patient's body as described above, takes the arm and tests whether the movement continues passively.
- Finally, the therapist moves the arm passively from the zero position through the entire range of motion and tests the end-feel.

Physiological end-feel:
soft and elastic, because several joints are involved in the movement

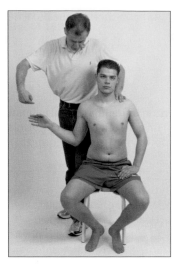

Fig. 14.271

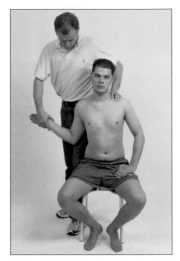

Fig. 14.272

f) **Internal rotation** from the zero position:

- The therapist stands behind the patient and palpates the humeral epicondyles (in the neutral joint position) with his thumb and fingers. Then the therapist asks the patient to actively perform maximum internal rotation of the arm, which is extended at the elbow. The thumb and fingers on the epicondyles follow the movement and enable an assessment of the end range of movement.
- Next the therapist stabilizes the patient's body as described above, grasps the epicondyles, and tests whether the movement continues passively.
- Finally, the therapist moves the arm passively from the zero position through the entire range of motion and tests the end-feel.

Physiological end-feel:
soft and elastic, because several joints are involved in the movement

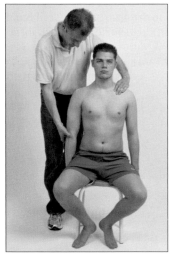

Fig. 14.273

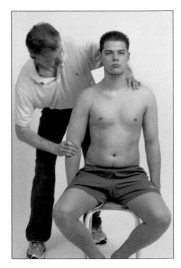

Fig. 14.274

Documentation Template: Practice Scheme

Shoulder girdle region						
Symptoms						
Symptom-altering direction						
Contraindications?	Nervous system: Other:					
Symptom-altering joint region						
General assessment of adjacent joints						
Active movements, comparing sides						
Specific rotatory tests	**Active**	**Continues passively?**	**Passive**	**End-feel**	**Symptoms/ pain**	**Comments**
▪ Flexion/elevation						
▪ Overall extension						
▪ Abduction/elevation						
▪ Overall adduction						
▪ Overall external rotation						
▪ Overall internal rotation						
Summary Formulation aid: ▪ Symptoms ▪ Direction ▪ Contraindications ▪ Restricted mobility, hypermobility, or physiological mobility	*Text:*					
Further joints to be examined						

Documentation: Practice Example

Shoulder girdle region						
(Painful abduction/elevation in right shoulder region)						
Symptoms	*Pain in the right shoulder when lifting the arm to the side*					
Symptom-altering direction	*Abduction/elevation*					
Contraindications?	Nervous system: *No findings* Other: *No findings*					
Symptom-altering joint region	*Shoulder girdle, right side*					
General assessment of adjacent joints	*No findings*					
Active movements, comparing sides	*Abduction/elevation on the right is limited and there is end-range pain.*					
Specific rotatory tests	**Active**	**Continues passively?**	**Passive**	**End-feel**	**Symptoms/ pain**	**Comments**
▪ Flexion/elevation	*ca. 160°*	*ca. 10°*	*Slightly increased resistance to movement*	*Somewhat more firm than extension*		
▪ Overall extension	*ca. 50°*	*ca. 30°*	*No findings*	*Soft or firm and elastic*		
▪ Abduction/elevation	*ca. 150°*	*< 5° and painful*	*Increased resistance to movement*	*Firm and elastic*	*Pain at end range*	*Deviation during external rotation*
▪ Overall adduction	*ca. 30°*	*ca. 15°*	*No findings*	*Soft or firm and elastic*		
▪ Overall external rotation	*ca. 50°*	*ca. 10°*	*Increased resistance to movement*	*Firm and elastic*	*Pain at end range*	
▪ Overall internal rotation	*ca. 100°*	*ca. 20°*	*Slightly increased resistance to movement*	*Soft or firm and elastic*		

Summary Formulation aid: ▪ Symptoms ▪ Direction ▪ Contraindications ▪ Restricted mobility, hypermobility, or physiological mobility	*Text:* ▪ *Pain in the right shoulder* ▪ *when lifting the arm to the side.* ▪ *There are no contraindications today to further movement testing.* ▪ *Abduction/elevation is restricted (ca. 150° with active movement) and there is pain with end-range movement; limited general external rotation (ca. 50° with active movement) with slight end-range pain. Active internal rotation is ca. 100° and thus only slightly restricted.*
Further joints to be examined	*Glenohumeral joint, acromioclavicular joint, sternoclavicular joint, scapulo-serrato-thoracic gliding space*

14.18 Shoulder Joint

(Articulatio humeri)

14.18.1 Anatomy

Joint type:	ball-and-socket joint, unmodified ovoid shape
Distal joint surface:	head of humerus is convex
Resting position:	55° abduction, 30° horizontal adduction (so that the humerus continues the line of the spine of the scapula), and ca. 90° elbow flexion with the forearm in the horizontal plane
Close packed position:	maximum abduction and external rotation
Capsular sign:	external rotation → abduction → internal rotation

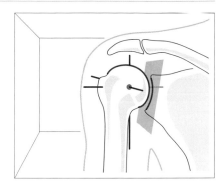

Fig. 14.275

14.18.2 Rotatory Tests

■ Active Movements, Comparing Sides

The movements of the glenohumeral joint cannot be isolated during active upper arm motions. We thus advise active movement testing on the shoulder girdle region with a comparison of sides. Certain movements, however, may be performed which emphasize the glenohumeral joint. For instance, in abduction, the external rotation that automatically occurs with abduction/elevation might be prevented if the elbows are bent and the forearm remains pointing forward, thus emphasizing the movement in the glenohumeral joint. During external rotation, the patient may be asked to hold the elbow against the torso and not to move the shoulders backward. During internal rotation the shoulders should not be moved forward. The remaining movements are difficult to actively emphasize in the glenohumeral joint. Hence in actual clinical practice, the therapist must usually be content with this comparison of sides.

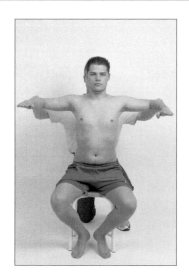

Fig. 14.276

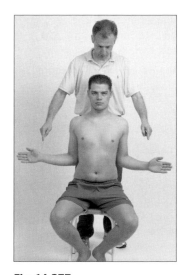

Fig. 14.277

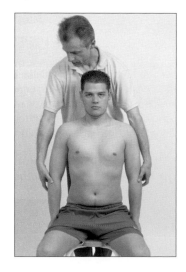

Fig. 14.278

■ Specific Active and Passive Movement Testing (Quantity and Quality)

a) **Flexion** from the zero position:

- The therapist stands behind the seated patient and with his medial hand, aided by the lateral one, fixates the scapula from above. His fingers fixate the coracoid process firmly. The patient is then asked to actively raise his or her arm in front of them until either the arm can go no further, or the pressure of the fingers on the coracoid process becomes too uncomfortable, or the therapist says "stop" because he feels that the stabilization can no longer be held against the strength of the patient.
- Next the therapist removes his lateral hand and takes the patient's forearm to test whether the movement continues passively.
- Finally, the therapist moves the arm passively from the zero position to maximum flexion and tests the end-feel.

Physiological end-feel: firm and elastic

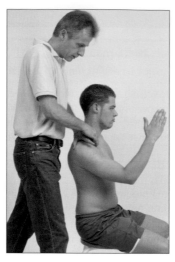

Fig. 14.279

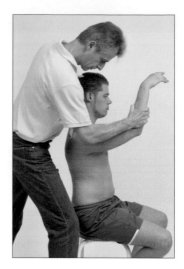

Fig. 14.280

b) **Extension** from the zero position:

- The therapist continues to fixate the scapula with the medial hand, increasing the stabilizing pressure dorsally with his lateral hand if needed. The patient is asked to actively extend the bent arm (relaxation of the biceps brachii muscle) posteriorly until it can either go no further, or the therapist says "stop" because he senses that he cannot fixate the scapula against the strength of the patient.
- Then the therapist removes the lateral hand from its position, takes the distal upper arm and tests whether the movement continues passively.
- Finally, the therapist moves the arm passively from the zero position to maximum extension and tests the end-feel.

Physiological end-feel: firm and elastic

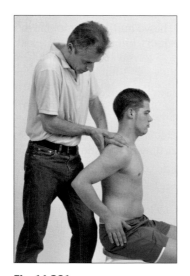

Fig. 14.281

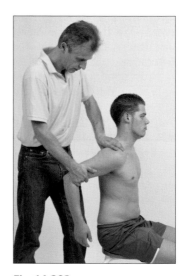

Fig. 14.282

c) **Abduction** from the zero position:

- The therapist fixates the scapula with the medial hand, increasing the stabilizing pressure with the lateral hand if needed. The patient is asked to <u>actively</u> lift the arm sideways, which is bent at the elbow, until either it can go no further, the pressure of the stabilizing hand becomes too uncomfortable, or the therapist says "stop" because he senses that he cannot fixate the scapula any longer against the strength of the patient.
- Then the therapist removes his lateral hand from its position, takes the proximal forearm and tests whether the movement <u>continues passively</u>.
- Finally, the therapist moves the arm <u>passively</u> from the zero position to maximum abduction and tests the <u>end-feel</u>.

Physiological end-feel:
firm and elastic

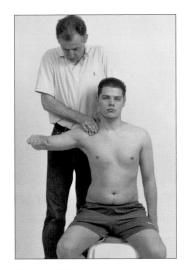

Fig. 14.283

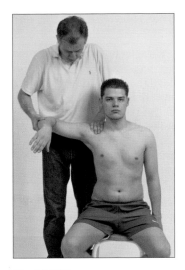

Fig. 14.284

> **!** During abduction the end-feel is often pathologically firm or hard and elastic due to subacromial impingement; the joint may be loose and hypermobile or "stiff" with restricted mobility.

d) **Adduction** from the zero position:

- The therapist stands behind the seated patient and fixates the scapula with the medial hand, increasing the stabilizing pressure with the lateral hand if needed. His fingers fixate the coracoid process. The patient is asked to <u>actively</u> adduct the arm, which is bent approximately 90° at the elbow, in front of the abdomen. This should continue until either the arm can go no further, the pressure of the therapist's fingers on the coracoid process becomes too uncomfortable, or the therapist says "stop" because he senses that he cannot hold the scapula still against the strength of the patient. The patient's forearm should be in the sagittal plane.
- Then the therapist releases the lateral hand, takes the patient's proximal forearm and elbow, and tests whether the movement <u>continues passively</u>.
- Finally, the therapist moves the patient's arm <u>passively</u> from the zero position to maximum flexion and tests the <u>end-feel</u>.

Physiological end-feel:
firm and elastic

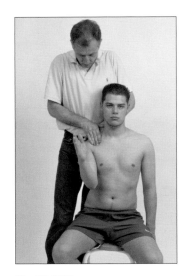

Fig. 14.285

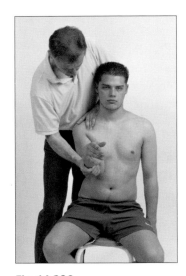

Fig. 14.286

e) **External rotation** from the zero position:

- The therapist continues to hold the scapula from above with his medial hand and uses his thigh to support the patient's upper arm, while the patient actively fixates his or her elbow against their side. The patient should then <u>actively</u> externally rotate the arm, which is bent about 90° at the elbow, which should continue until either the arm can go no further, the pressure of the stabilizing hand becomes too uncomfortable, or the therapist says "stop" because he senses that he cannot fixate the scapula against the strength of the patient.
- Then the therapist takes the patient's distal forearm with his lateral hand and tests whether the movement <u>continues passively</u>.
- Finally, the therapist moves the arm <u>passively</u> from the zero position to maximum external rotation and tests the <u>end-feel</u>.

Physiological end-feel:
firm and elastic

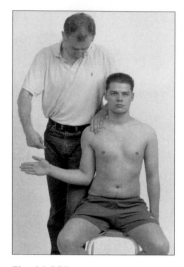

Fig. 14.287

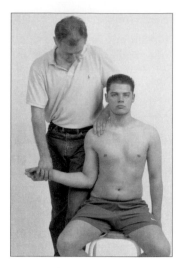

Fig. 14.288

f) **Internal rotation** from the zero position:

- The therapist continues to hold the scapula from above with his medial hand. The patient's elbow is extended. The patient is asked to <u>actively</u> rotate the extended arm internally until it can go no further, the pressure from the stabilizing hand becomes uncomfortable, or the therapist says "stop" because he senses that he can no longer fixate the scapula against the strength of the patient.
- Next the therapist grasps the patient's arm at the humeral epicondyles with his lateral hand and tests whether the movement <u>continues passively</u>.
- Finally, the therapist moves the arm <u>passively</u> from the zero position to maximum internal rotation and tests the <u>end-feel</u>.

Physiological end-feel:
firm and elastic

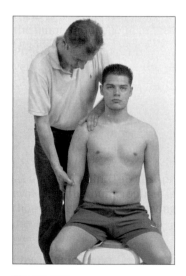

Fig. 14.289

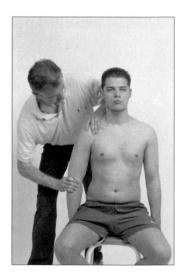

Fig. 14.290

For measuring the angle, the already-mentioned starting positions are used according to the neutral zero method. Horizontal abduction and adduction (not shown here) as well as external and internal rotation may also be tested in this way in 90° abduction. The therapist should note the position in which the movement was tested. On the one hand, movement tests should determine reproducible ranges of motion, which is possible with the neutral zero method. On the other hand, movement tests should tell the examiner about the symptom-altering joint and symptom-altering mechanism, for which the most useful starting position is the one in which the patient usually experiences the symptoms.

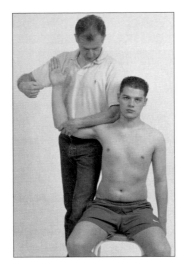

Fig. 14.291

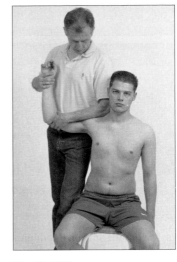

Fig. 14.292

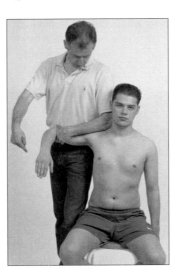

Fig. 14.293

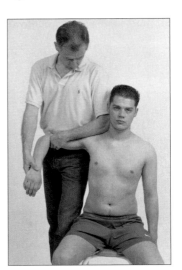

Fig. 14.294

14.18.3 Translatoric movement tests

Traction in the resting position:

The patient should be seated on the edge of the bench. The therapist's dorsal hand fixates the scapula from above; his ventral hand is placed deep in the axilla and around the head of the humerus. Next he pulls the head of the humerus at a right angle away from the treatment plane. His dorsal thumb is placed between the posterior aspect of the acromial angle and the head of the humerus to palpate the range of motion.

Physiological end-feel:

firm and elastic

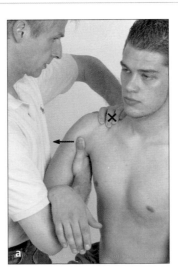

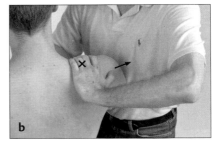

Fig. 14.295 a, b

Compression:

The therapist stands dorsolaterally to the patient and fixates the medial margin of the scapula with the ulnar border of his medial hand. His lateral hand presses the head of the humerus <u>at a right angle toward the treatment plane</u>.

> **!** Compression may also be performed in the resting position. The joint is in the zero position because the resistance tests of the shoulder joint muscles are performed here. Prior to each resistance test, the therapist should check that compression of the joint will be pain free.

Physiological end-feel: hard

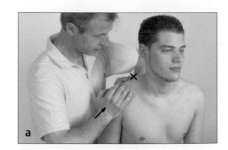

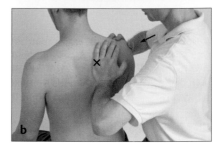

Fig. 14.296 a, b

14.18.4 Treatment of Capsuloligamentous Hypomobility

The patient lies in the supine position with a belt placed around his or her thorax to fixate the scapula firmly against it. The other end of the belt is tied to the contralateral side of the bench. The therapist stands laterally, places the joint in the actual resting position, and puts both hands on the head of the humerus. The patient's elbow is resting against the therapist's torso. The therapist leans back to move the head of the humerus <u>at a right angle away from the treatment plane</u>.

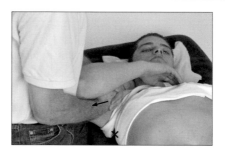

Fig. 14.297

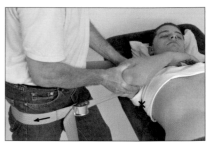

Fig. 14.298

Alternatively, the therapist may grasp the patient's elbow with his distal hand to hold the arm in the resting position of the glenohumeral joint. The patient's hand rests lightly on their chest. The therapist's proximal hand is as close as possible to the head of the humerus. A belt is placed across the dorsum of his hand and looped around the therapist's pelvis. By displacing his pelvis backward, the therapist can perform mobilizing traction. Use of a belt technique allows the therapist to maintain grade III traction for a longer period of time and with less effort.

> **!** For pain-relief, intermittent traction may also be performed with the test version.

Documentation Template: Practice Scheme

Shoulder joint						
Symptoms						
Symptom-altering direction						
Contraindications?	Nervous system: Other:					
Symptom-altering joint						
General assessment of adjacent joints						

Active movements, comparing sides						
Specific rotatory tests	**Active**	**Continues passively?**	**Passive**	**End-feel**	**Symptoms/ pain**	**Comments**
▪ Flexion						
▪ Extension						
▪ Abduction						
▪ Adduction						
▪ Horizontal abduction						
▪ Horizontal adduction						
▪ External rotation						
▪ Internal rotation						
▪ External rotation with 90° abduction						
▪ Internal rotation with 90° abduction						

Translatoric movement tests	**Quantity**	**Quality**	**End-feel**	**Symptoms/pain**	**Comments**
▪ Traction					
▪ Compression					

Summary Formulation aid: ▪ Symptoms ▪ Direction ▪ Contraindications ▪ Site (joint) ▪ Restricted mobility, hypermobility, or physiological mobility ▪ Structure: muscle, joint, etc.	*Text:*
Trial treatment	
Physical therapy diagnosis	

Continued ▶

Documentation Template: Practice Scheme *(Continued)*

Shoulder joint	
Treatment plan with treatment goal and prognosis	
Treatment progress	
Final examination	

Documentation: Practice Example

Shoulder joint (Painful restriction at the end-range of abduction 12 weeks after subcapital fracture of the humerus on the right side)	
Symptoms	*End-range pain when lifting the right arm to the side*
Symptom-altering direction	*Abduction*
Contraindications?	Nervous system: *No findings* Other: *No findings*
Symptom-altering joint	*Right glenohumeral joint*
General assessment of adjacent joints	*The right acromioclavicular joint appears slightly hypermobile.*
Active movements, comparing sides	*Abduction on the right side is slightly limited.*

Specific rotatory tests	Active	Continues passively?	Passive	End-feel	Symptoms/pain	Comments
▪ Flexion	*ca. 65°*	*ca. 30°*	*No findings*	*Firm and elastic*		
▪ Extension	*ca. 35°*	*ca. 15°*	*No findings*	*Firm and elastic*		
▪ Abduction	*ca. 70°*	*ca. 10°*	*Increased resistance to movement*	*Very firm and elastic, almost hard at the end*	*Pain at end range*	
▪ Adduction	*ca. 10°*	*ca. 10°*	*No findings*	*Firm and elastic*		
▪ Horizontal abduction	*Not tested*	*Not tested*	*Not tested*			
▪ Horizontal adduction	*Not tested*	*Not tested*	*Not tested*			
▪ External rotation	*ca. 40°*	*< 5°*	*Increased resistance to movement*	*Very firm and elastic*		
▪ Internal rotation	*ca. 80°*	*< 5°*	*Slightly increased resistance to movement*	*Firm and elastic*		

Continued ▶

Documentation: Practice Example *(Continued)*

Shoulder joint (Painful restriction at the end-range of abduction 12 weeks after subcapital fracture of the humerus on the right side)						
External rotation with 90° abduction	*Not tested*	*Not tested*	*Not tested*			
Internal rotation with 90° abduction	*Not tested*	*Not tested*	*Not tested*			

Translatoric movement tests	Quantity	Quality	End-feel	Symptoms/pain	Comments
Traction	*Hypo 2*	*Increased resistance to movement*	*Very firm and elastic*	*Not painful*	
Compression	*No findings*	*No findings*	*Hard*	*No findings*	

Summary Formulation aid:	Text:
• Symptoms • Direction • Contraindications • Site (joint) • Restricted mobility, hypermobility, or physiological mobility • Structure: muscle, joint, etc.	• *Pain with* • *end-range abduction of the right arm.* • *There are no contraindications today to further movement testing.* • *The pain correlates with the glenohumeral joint,* • *which is hypomobile* • *due to shrinkage of the capsuloligamentous unit (capsular pattern). The slightly hard end-feel with abduction is suggestive of subacromial impingement syndrome.*
Trial treatment	• *5-minute intermittent grade I–II traction after which the joint feels lighter with less pain and less resistance to movement.* • *This is followed by 5-minute long grade III traction, after which there is less end-range resistance to movement and the patient reports that the movement feels easier.*
Physical therapy diagnosis	*See above*
Treatment plan with treatment goal and prognosis	• *Continue brief preliminary pain-relieving traction followed by mobilizing traction in grade III.* • *Treatment goal: pain-free physiological mobility* **(Further information on examination and treatment techniques may be obtained through further education.)**
Treatment progress	
Final examination	

14.19 Joints of the Shoulder Girdle

(Articulatio acromioclavicularis, articulatio sternoclavicularis, scapulo-serrato-thoracic gliding space)

14.19.1 Anatomy

■ Acromioclavicular Joint

Joint type:	plane joint, unmodified ovoid
Distal joint surface:	acromion concave
Resting position:	physiological position of the shoulder girdle
Close packed position:	arm in 90° abduction in glenohumeral joint
Capsular sign:	not described

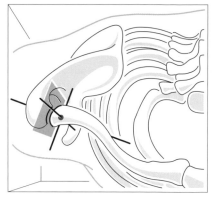

Fig. 14.299

■ Sternoclavicular Joint

Joint type:	saddle joint, unmodified sellar joint
Distal joint surface:	medial end of clavicle convex for elevation and depression, concave for protraction and retraction
Resting position:	physiological shoulder girdle position
Close packed position:	arm in full elevation
Capsular sign:	not described

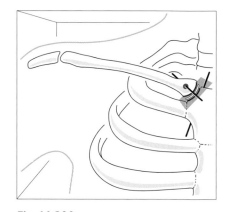

Fig. 14.300

■ Scapulo-serrato-thoracic Gliding Space

Joint type:	"gliding joint" between the thoracic wall and the serratus anterior muscle on the one side, and between the serratus anterior and the scapular surface, covered by the subscapularis muscle, on the other side
Distal joint surface:	scapula concave
Resting position:	physiological shoulder girdle position
Close packed position:	not described
Capsular sign:	not described

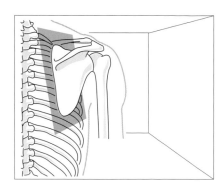

Fig. 14.301

14.19.2 Rotatory Tests

■ Active Movements, Comparing Sides

The patient sits and moves both shoulders up to the ears and then down toward the floor. Then he or she moves them forward and backward. During the up-and-down movements, the therapist observes from anterior or posterior, and for the forward–backward movements he should preferably look from above.

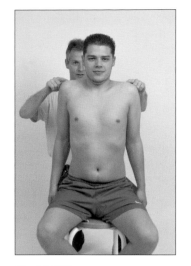

Fig. 14.302

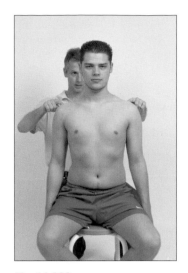

Fig. 14.303

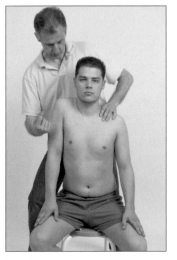

Fig. 14.304

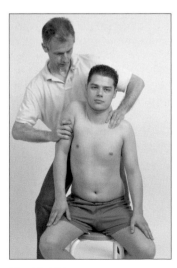

Fig. 14.305

■ Specific Active and Passive Movement Testing (Quantity and Quality)

a) **Elevation** from the zero position:

■ The therapist stands behind the sitting patient and stabilizes the thorax from above with his contralateral hand. His thumb is held against the spinous process at about T1. The patient is asked to actively elevate the shoulder.

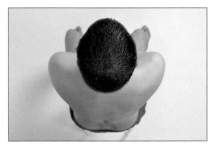

Fig. 14.306

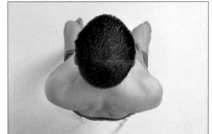

Fig. 14.307

- Next the therapist fixates the shoulder girdle, either by grasping the lateral proximal upper arm or by grasping the scapula in the axilla. He then checks whether the movement continues passively.

- Then the therapist moves the joint from the zero position passively through the entire range of motion to maximum elevation and tests the end-feel.

Physiological end-feel:
firm to soft and elastic

b) **Depression** from the zero position:

- Using the same fixating grip the therapist asks the patient to actively depress the shoulder.
- Then the therapist places his hand on the patient's shoulder and tests whether the movement continues passively.
- Finally, he moves the joint from the zero position passively through the entire range of motion to maximum depression and tests the end-feel.

Physiological end-feel:
firm to soft and elastic

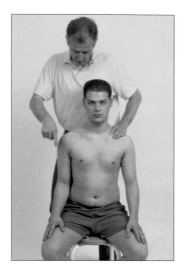

Fig. 14.308

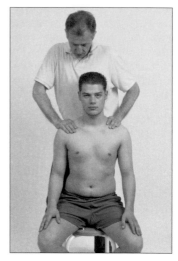

Fig. 14.309

c) **Protraction** in the zero position:

- The therapist is still standing behind the seated patient. He fixates the sternum from ventral with his fingers so that his thumb is lying on the patient's upper ribs. Then the patient is asked to actively press the shoulders forward.
- The therapist takes the shoulder girdle from dorsal along the scapular spine and acromion and tests whether the movement continues passively.
- Then he moves the joint from the zero position passively through the entire range of motion to maximum protraction and tests the end-feel.

Physiological end-feel:
firm to soft and elastic

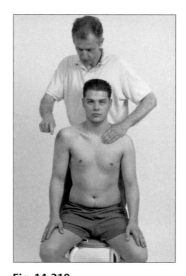

Fig. 14.310

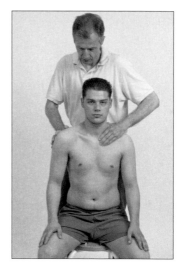

Fig. 14.311

d) **Retraction** in the zero position:

- The therapist's contralateral hand fixates the patient's thorax from above and his thumb holds the spinous process at about T1. The patient is then asked to <u>actively</u> press his shoulder backward.
- The therapist takes the shoulder girdle from anterior at the acromion and coracoid process and tests whether the movement <u>continues passively</u>.
- Then he moves the joint from the zero position <u>passively</u> through the entire range of motion to maximum retraction and tests the <u>end-feel</u>.

Physiological end-feel:
firm to soft and elastic

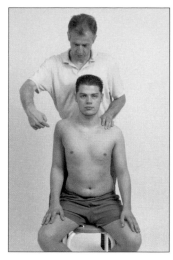

Fig. 14.312

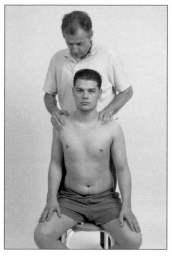

Fig. 14.313

e) **External rotation** of the scapula:

The patient lies on their side and the therapist stands in front of him or her at the height of the thorax. The patient's arm is resting on the lower forearm of the therapist whose hand grasps the inferior angle of the scapula with the fingers or ulnar border. The cranial hand wraps around the acromion from ventral and cranial.

Given that this specific movement cannot be performed actively, the therapist can only <u>passively</u> test external rotation of the scapula. Fixating the clavicle causes maximum stress on the acromioclavicular joint. If the clavicle is allowed to move with the motion, then the sternoclavicular joint is also under stress.

Physiological end-feel:
firm to soft and elastic

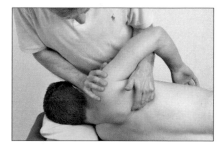

Fig. 14.314

f) **Internal rotation** of the scapula:

The patient lies on their side. The therapist uses the same grip to grasp the scapula, which he rotates <u>passively</u> to produce internal rotation.

This specific movement is also impossible to perform actively. If the therapist fixates the scapula during the movement, this produces maximum stress on the acromioclavicular joint. If he allows the clavicle to move with it, the sternoclavicular joint is also placed under stress.

Physiological end-feel:
firm to soft and elastic

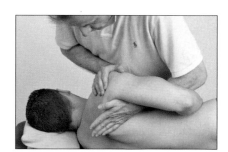

Fig. 14.315

14.19.3   Translatoric movement tests

■ Acromioclavicular Joint

Traction in the resting position:

The therapist stands behind the seated patient and grasps the acromion with the thumb and middle finger of his lateral hand from dorsal and ventral, and with his index finger he palpates the acromioclavicular joint space. The middle and ring finger and thumb of his medial hand hold the lateral end of the clavicle still. The therapist's abdomen or pelvis, with the ASIS, presses against the medial border of the scapula and pushes it laterally. His lateral hand guides the movement of the acromion so that it moves at a right angle away from the treatment plane.

Physiological end-feel:
firm and elastic

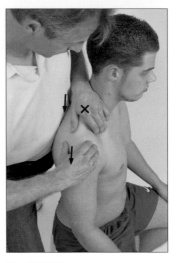

Fig. 14.316

Compression in the resting position:

The therapist is still standing behind the seated patient, using his body to support the patient's back. His medial hand fixates the sternum from ventral. The lateral hand presses the lateral border of the acromion to move the acromion at a right angle toward the treatment plane. This movement also compresses the sternoclavicular joint.

Physiological end-feel: hard

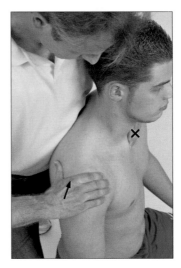

Fig. 14.317

■ Sternoclavicular Joint

Traction in the resting position:

The therapist stands behind the seated patient and supports the patient's back with his body. His medial hand fixates the sternum; the index finger of the medial hand is loosely placed in the sternoclavicular joint space from ventral. The lateral hand is lying with the thenar eminence on the forward-facing hollow of the lateral clavicle, which it pulls laterally and dorsally. This moves the clavicle at a right angle away from the treatment plane.

Physiological end-feel:
firm and elastic

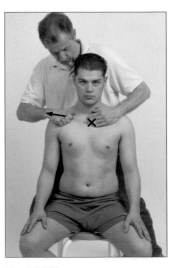

Fig. 14.318

Compression in the resting position:

The technique is identical to compression of the acromioclavicular joint because both joints are compressed simultaneously.

Physiological end-feel: hard

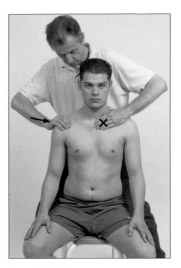

Fig. 14.319

■ Scapulo-serrato-thoracic Gliding Space

Lifting the scapula off the thorax:

The patient lies on their side and the therapist stands in front of him or her at the level of the thorax. The patient's arm is resting on the lower forearm of the therapist, who grasps the inferior angle of the scapula and its medial border with his fingers or the ulnar border of his caudal hand. His cranial hand is wrapped from ventral and cranial around the acromion. With this grip the therapist lifts the scapula perpendicularly off the thorax.

> **!** The test may also be done with the patient in the prone position.

Physiological end-feel:
soft and elastic

> **!** The grip for lifting the scapula may also be used for all passive rotatory movements of the scapula.

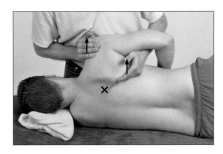

Fig. 14.320

Pressure of the scapula against the thorax:

The patient is lying on their side. The therapist stands in front of him or her at the level of the thorax. The patient's arm is resting on the lower forearm of the therapist, whose hand is on the inferior dorsal surface of the scapula. His cranial hand grasps the acromion from cranial. With this grip the therapist presses the scapula perpendicularly against the thorax.

> **!** The test may also be done with the patient in the prone position.

Physiological end-feel:
hard and elastic

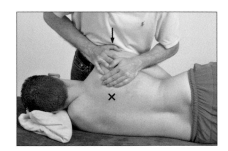

Fig. 14.321

14.19.4 Treatment of Capsuloligamentous Hypomobility

▪ Acromioclavicular Joint

The same technique may be used for treatment as for the test. The applica-

tion may be longer as needed for mobilization therapy.

> **Note**
> Pain relief can often be more easily obtained by gliding the clavicle ventrally and dorsally in grade I–II using the same position of both hands as for traction but without pushing with the abdomen.

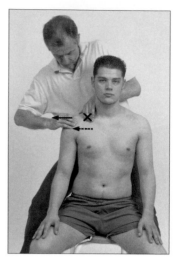

Fig. 14.322

▪ Sternoclavicular Joint

The therapist stands behind the seated patient and supports the back with his body; with his medial hand he fixates the sternum. The lateral hand is lying with the ulnar border and the ulnar fingers in the forward-facing concavity of the lateral clavicle. The patient's arm is resting in the crook of the therapist's elbow which is supported on the treatment table. The acromioclavicular joint is locked in this position of 90° abduction,

allowing the therapist's lateral hand to also be on the acromion. Next the therapist pulls the clavicle at a right angle away from the treatment plane. The therapist can support himself with the elbow of the mobilizing arm on the table in order to hold the traction for a longer period of time.

> ❗ Pain-relieving traction may also be performed with the test version.

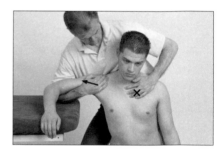

Fig. 14.323

▪ Scapulo-serrato-thoracic Gliding Joint

The same technique may be used for treatment as for the test. The applica-

tion may be longer as needed for mobilization therapy.

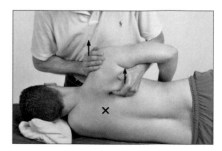

Fig. 14.324

Documentation Template: Practice Scheme

Shoulder girdle joints	
Symptoms	
Symptom-altering direction	
Contraindications?	Nervous system: Other:
Symptom-altering joint	
General assessment of adjacent joints	
Active movements, comparing sides	

Specific rotatory tests	Active	Continues passively?	Passive	End-feel	Symptoms/ pain	Comments
▪ Elevation						
▪ Depression						
▪ Protraction						
▪ Retraction						
▪ External rotation of the scapula						
▪ Internal rotation of the scapula						

Translatoric movement tests	Quantity	Quality	End-feel	Symptoms/pain	Comments
Acromioclavicular ▪ Traction					
▪ Compression					
Sternoclavicular ▪ Traction					
▪ Compression					
Scapulo-serrato-thoracic ▪ Lifting					
▪ Compression					

Summary Formulation aid: ▪ Symptoms ▪ Direction ▪ Contraindications ▪ Site (joint) ▪ Restricted mobility, hypermobility, or physiological mobility ▪ Structure: muscle, joint, etc.	*Text:*
Trial treatment	
Physical therapy diagnosis	

Continued ▶

Documentation Template: Practice Scheme (Continued)

Shoulder girdle joints	
Treatment plan with treatment goal and prognosis	
Treatment progress	
Final examination	

Documentation: Practice Example 1

Shoulder girdle joints (Pain in the right shoulder when playing handball)	
Symptoms	End-range pain in the right arm when winding up to throw during handball
Symptom-altering direction	Abduction and external rotation
Contraindications?	Nervous system: No findings Other: No findings
Symptom-altering joint	Shoulder girdle joints; the glenohumeral joint is not involved
General assessment of adjacent joints	No findings
Active movements, comparing sides	More abduction and horizontal external rotation on the right compared to the left; these movements provoke the reported pain at the end-range.

Specific rotatory tests	Active	Continues passively?	Passive	End-feel	Symptoms/ pain	Comments
▪ Elevation	Right > left	> 10°	Slight resistance to movement	Soft to firm and elastic		
▪ Depression	No findings	< 5°	No findings	Firm and elastic		
▪ Protraction	No findings	< 5°	No findings	Firm and elastic		
▪ Retraction	No findings	< 5°	No findings	Soft to firm and elastic		
▪ External rotation of the scapula	Not possible	Not possible	Right > left, slight resistance to movement	Soft to firm and elastic	End-range pain	Provokes the reported pain
▪ Internal rotation of the scapula	Not possible	Not possible	No findings	Firm and elastic		

Translatoric movement tests	Quantity	Quality	End-feel	Symptoms/pain	Comments
Acromioclavicular joint ▪ Traction	Hyper 4	Slight resistance to movement	Soft or firm and elastic	Provokes reported end-range pain	
▪ Compression	No findings	No findings	Hard		

Continued ▶

Documentation: Practice Example 1 *(Continued)*

Shoulder girdle joints (Pain in the right shoulder when playing handball)					
Sternoclavicular ▪ Traktion	*No findings*	*No findings*	*Firm and elastic*	*No findings*	
▪ Compression	*No findings*	*No findings*	*Hard and elastic*	*No findings*	
Scapulo-serrato-thoracic ▪ Lifting	*No findings*	*No findings*	*Soft to firm and elastic*	*No findings*	
▪ Compression	*No findings*	*No findings*	*Hard and elastic*	*No findings*	

Summary Formulation aid: ▪ Symptoms ▪ Direction ▪ Contraindications ▪ Site (joint) ▪ Restricted mobility, hypermobility, or physiological mobility ▪ Structure: muscle, joint, etc.	*Text:* ▪ *Pain in the right shoulder* ▪ *with end-range abduction and external rotation of the right arm.* ▪ *There are no contraindications today to further movement testing.* ▪ *The pain is in correlation with the right acromioclavicular joint,* ▪ *which is hypermobile* ▪ *due to a loose capsuloligamentous unit.*
Trial treatment	*5-minute long grade I–II pain-relieving traction after which the patient reports less end-range pain with movement*
Physical therapy diagnosis	*See above*
Treatment plan with treatment goal and prognosis	▪ *Continue pain-relieving traction. Grade III traction mobilization is contraindicated.* ▪ *Treatment goal: pain relief* **(Further information on examination and treatment techniques may be obtained through further education.)**
Treatment progress	
Final examination	

Documentation: Practice Example 2

Shoulder joints (End-range pain in the right clavicle 8 weeks after conservative management of a fractured clavicle)	
Symptoms	*Pain with end-range arm elevation as well as end-range shoulder movements*
Symptom-altering direction	*All directions of the arm and shoulder girdle movements are painful*
Contraindications?	Nervous system: *No findings* Other: *No findings*
Symptom-altering joint	*Shoulder girdle joints; the glenohumeral joint is not involved*
General assessment of adjacent joints	*No findings*

Continued ▶

Documentation: Practice Example 2 *(Continued)*

Shoulder joints
(End-range pain in the right clavicle 8 weeks after conservative management of a fractured clavicle)

Active movements, comparing sides	*All general arm movements as well as shoulder movements are slightly limited on the right compared to the left.*					
Specific rotatory tests	**Active**	**Continues passively?**	**Passive**	**End-feel**	**Symptoms/ pain**	**Comments**
▪ Elevation	*Right < left*	*< 5°*	*Increased resistance to movement*	*More firm and elastic*	*Slight pulling pain at end range*	
▪ Depression	*Right slight < left*	*< 5°*	*No findings*	*Firm and elastic*		
▪ Protraction	*Right slight < left*	*< 5°*	*Increased resistance to movement*	*More firm and elastic*	*Slight pulling pain at end range*	
▪ Retraction	*Right < left*	*< 5°*	*Increased resistance to movement*	*More firm and elastic*	*Slight pulling pain at end range*	
▪ External rotation of the scapula	*Right < left*	*< 5°*	*No findings*	*Firm and elastic*		
▪ Internal rotation of the scapula	*Right < left*	*< 5°*	*No findings*	*Firm and elastic*		

Translatoric movement tests	Quantity	Quality	End-feel	Symptoms/pain	Comments
Acromioclavicular ▪ Traction	*Slightly hypo*	*Slightly increased resistance to movement*	*Firm and elastic*		
▪ Compression	*No findings*	*No findings*	*Hard*		
Sternoclavicular ▪ Traction	*Hypo 2*	*Increased resistance to movement*	*Very firm and elastic*	*Provokes reported end-range pain*	
▪ Compression	*No findings*	*No findings*	*Hard*	*No findings*	
Scapulo-serrato-thoracic ▪ Lifting	*Slightly limited*	*Slightly increased resistance to movement*	*Soft to firm and elastic*	*No findings*	
▪ Compression	*No findings*	*No findings*	*Hard*	*No findings*	

Summary Formulation aid:	Text:
▪ Symptoms ▪ Direction ▪ Contraindications ▪ Site (joint) ▪ Restricted mobility, hypermobility, or physiological mobility ▪ Structure: muscle, joint, etc.	▪ *Pain with end-range arm and shoulder movements* ▪ *in all directions.* ▪ *There are no contraindications today to further movement testing.* ▪ *The pain primarily correlates with the sternoclavicular joint,* ▪ *which is hypomobile* ▪ *due to shrinkage of the capsuloligamentous unit.*

Continued ▶

Shoulder joints	
(End-range pain in the right clavicle 8 weeks after conservative management of a fractured clavicle)	
Trial treatment	▪ *5-minute long grade I–II pain-relieving traction, after which the patient reported less end-range pain.* ▪ *This was followed by mobilizing grade III traction for 5 minutes, after which the patient felt movement was easier and end-range resistance was less.*
Physical therapy diagnosis	*See above*
Treatment plan with treatment goal and prognosis	▪ *Continue initial pain-relieving traction, followed by grade III traction mobilization.* ▪ *Treatment goal: pain-free, physiological mobility* **(Further information on examination and treatment techniques may be obtained through further education.)**
Treatment progress	
Final examination	

15.1   Introduction

From the occiput to the coccyx, the spine contains 76 joints. Due to their close functional relationship, the spine is discussed along with the two sacroiliac joints and with the pubic symphysis, the ribs, and the temporomandibular joints.

For manual therapy (MT), the main difference between the extremity joints and those in the spine is the presence of the nervous system. Because of this, extra caution is warranted when examining and treating the patient, as injury can cause serious and sometimes irreparable damage. The physical therapist must therefore be able to identify the most important **contraindications** for comprehensive movement testing and intensive treatment.

Again, the first goal of movement testing is to ascertain the **symptom-altering direction** of movement. Tests are generally performed in the position in which the alteration of symptoms can be identified easily and with the fewest associated risks. Given that spinal symptoms are generally more intense when standing or sitting than when lying down, the following tests are described in these positions.

As with the extremities, the patient is first asked to perform all movements **actively**. If active movement elicits symptoms, and if there is severe pain, further passive movement should be avoided for the present. Immediate consideration of potential **contraindications** to further movement tests is warranted.

Given that such contraindications affect the nervous system, before testing actual movement, the physiological function of impulse conduction should be examined, at least roughly. The reader is referred to the relevant literature and coursework for more information. An early indication of compression of neural structures is limited mechanical mobility. Related tests are described in detail. As reported in 1864 by Ernest-Charles Lasègue in Paris, the movement of the sciatic nerve is limited if the nerve, its root, or the dura mater become compressed and/or irritated in the spinal canal (Kügelgen 1991). Based on this principle, the great nerves of the lower and upper extremities and the mobility the dura mater are examined.

Symptoms of neural structure compression (e.g., herniated disk) often decrease with traction and increase with compression. Hence these two test procedures may be used. The compression test may also positively detect fractures, extensive inflammation, or instability.

Testing of the cervical spine is more challenging. The upper end of the spinal canal in the cervical region contains the medulla oblongata and thus holds vital neural centers. It is imperative to perform **"safety tests"** prior to initiating larger passive movements. The stability of the most important ligaments in this area (transverse ligament of the atlas and alar ligament) as well as the stability of the bony structures must be checked before performing larger passive movements with the head. Given that a significant portion of the blood is carried to the brain by the vertebral arteries in the spinal column, circulation to the central nervous system (CNS) must also be tested before performing end-range movements.

Only after active movements fail to demonstrate a symptom-altering direction, and after ruling out contraindications to further movement tests, can one proceed with passive movements of the trunk with overpressure. Movements in the sagittal and frontal planes tend to push the weight of the spine further in the direction of motion, while the antagonistic muscles work eccentrically to control the movement. Any passive continuation of movement thus is often associated with worsening of symptoms and warrants extra caution.

Performing **passive movements** through the entire range of motion is extremely difficult on the standing or sitting patient due to the weight of the trunk around the lumbar and thoracic spine. Depending on the difference in size between the patient and therapist, it may even be impossible. Only movements in the horizontal plane and movements of the thoracic spine may be performed passively through the entire range of motion. The quality of movement, resistance to movement, and the end-feel are useful for assessing the severity of symptoms and mobility-limiting structures.

Once a **symptom-altering direction** has been identified, accentuated movements of individual sections of the spine can help to localize the symptom-altering region. Further education and training can provide information on refining techniques that enable a more specific localization of the symptom-altering spinal segment.

Finally, the therapist assesses whether the affected site demonstrates **restricted mobility, hypermobility,** or **physiological mobility**.

Because it is impossible to actively move isolated segments of the spinal column, but rather, the segments move together in chain-like fashion, the focus is on an **evaluation of consecutive segments or regions in the spinal column and the "root joints"** (= the roots of the extremities: hip and shoulder girdle joints). Diminished mobility in one region often leads to hypermobility in the next. Thus, for instance, limited hip joint extension is often associated with lumbar spine hypermobility. Similarly, restricted thoracic spine mobility often causes mechanical stress on the lower lumbar spine and the lower cervical spine which may become hypermobile.

When evaluating movement **quantity**, not only do physiologically normal ranges and a comparison of sides (lateral bending and right/left rotation) serve as a guide, but so too does the harmonious distribution of individual spinal curves.

Ventral and dorsal flexion is normally greater in the lumbar and cervical spine than in the thoracic spine. Lateral bending as well as rotation occurs mainly in the cervical spine and lower thoracic spine. It is also important to note whether the transitions between more mobile spinal segments and less mobile ones are gradual or abrupt. Junctions between highly mobile spinal segments and those with much less mobility represent zones of increased mechanical stress. These transitional zones are often symptom-triggering: the lumbosacral, thoracolumbar, cervicothoracic, and craniovertebral junctions.

Another aspect is the **quality** of movement: whether the patient performs it carefully or carelessly, slowly or quickly, "elegantly" or jerkily, according to the instructed movement or with deviations. This also serves as an indication of symptom severity and of the patient's coordination.

According to Junghans, a spinal motion segment consists of two adjacent vertebral bodies and the structures between them. When attempting to mobilize a single motion segment, one can almost achieve a segmental **end-feel**. This can yield information about the mobility-limiting **structure**. Such techniques are extremely difficult, however, and the information in this book is limited to movements of the main sections of the spine. Thus, as mentioned above, we primarily test the end-feel such as in rotation and cervical spine movements. The increased pressure during movements of the lumbar spine and thoracic spine in the sagittal and frontal planes gives an idea of how the movement stops and thus about the mobility-limiting structure.

Since we are dealing with a chain of joints—that is, several joints moving simultaneously—it is very difficult to precisely determine a structure-specific end-feel. Still, protective muscle contraction, inability of the patient to relax the muscle, and "firm" movement limitations are readily detectable. Passively increasing pressure or performing passive movements with the patient standing or sitting are to be avoided if these methods (potentially) exacerbate symptoms. This is often the case in everyday practice. Nevertheless, the physical therapist should be able to perform these techniques if they are indicated. Further education can provide experience in passive movement tests with the patient lying down.

The examination of the spinal column is as complex as its structure and function. A complete discussion would be beyond the scope of this book. The principles of MT described here should enable the physical therapist to:

- identify contraindications to movement testing and treatment of the spine;
- treat acute compression of the neural system with traction, immobilization, and protective and analgesic measures;
- determine the symptom-altering movement direction and roughly identify the symptom-altering spinal section;
- evaluate the overall mobility of individual spinal segments;
- treat painful spinal segments, especially the zygapophyseal joints and the sacroiliac joints, ribs, and temporomandibular joints using pain-relieving traction or pain-relieving gliding techniques (sacroiliac joints); and
- mobilize areas of the spine with limited mobility using traction.

Note

Symptoms

↓

Direction

Primarily active, continue passive movement only if necessary

↓

Contraindications for large movements?

Compression of the nervous system, fractures, instability (especially transverse ligament of the atlas, alar ligaments), blood circulation (especially vertebral arteries)

↓

Spinal segment or segment region?

Identify as precisely as possible

↓

Restricted mobility, hypermobility, or normal physiological mobility?

Also assess adjacent joints or spinal segments

↓

Structure?

Painfully limited mobility with suspected nervous system involvement due to protective muscle contraction or limited joint mobility

15.2   Pubic Symphysis and Sacroiliac Joints

(Symphysis pubica and articulatio sacroiliaca)

15.2.1   Anatomy

■ Pubic Symphysis

Joint type:	symphysis (cartilaginous joint (= synchondrosis), connected by a fibrocartilaginous junction; both pubic bones are covered with hyaline cartilage)
Distal joint surface:	the two pubic bones are convex; and the interpubic disk is concave
Close packed position:	not described
Capsular pattern:	not described

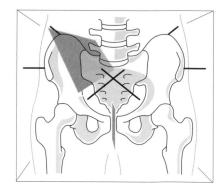

■ Sacroiliac Joint

Fig. 15.1

Joint type:	amphiarthrosis
Distal joint surface:	Although the propeller like shape of the sacral articular surface is concave and the corresponding ilium convex (Vleeming et al. 2012), the movement of sacrum between the ilia is according to the convex rule.
Resting position:	not described
Close packed position:	not described
Capsular pattern:	not described

■ Pain Management in the Sacroiliac Joint

The reported prevalence of sacroiliac joint pain ranges from 10 to 80% (Zelle et al 2005). This reflects the difficulty of identifying the condition and making an accurate clinical diagnosis. It has long been recommended that a group of tests be used (Laslett et al. 2005a, b; Laslett 2009). According to one study, where the examination was based on such a clinical test group (e.g., a positive result for three out of five sacroiliac joint provocation tests), the sacroiliac joint was the cause of the low back pain in 90% of 34 inlineskaters (Ruhe et al 2012). Yet if one takes into account only studies which diagnose sacroiliac joint pain using a local anesthetic (still considered the current gold standard, despite limita-

tions), the prevalence would be 15% in patients with low back pain (Bogduk 2000).

The sacroiliac joint transfers loads from the trunk to the pelvis as well as in the reverse direction, thereby lessening load spikes (Bussey et al 2009). In the prone patient (= no weight-bearing), movements of the leg in the hip joint into external rotation or abduction, or combination of the two, lead to movements of the ipsilateral and contralateral ilium and thus influence the sacroiliac joint (Bussey et al 2009). The ilium moves in the same direction as the femur and thus increases the range of hip joint movement, albeit by only 1 to 2° (Bussey et al 2009). The joint therefore acts as a shock absorber and should, above all, be stable (Calvillo et al 2000; Schomacher 2003).

Medical treatment includes intra-articular injection of local anesthetic, prolotherapy (injection of sclerosing agents into the ligaments), surgical denervation, and arthrodesis; administration of a local anesthesia is also commonly used to confirm the diagnosis before proceeding with larger interventions (Zelle et al 2005).

Nonsurgical treatments include mobilization/manipulation, stabilizing measures such as the sacroiliac belt, and exercises for the deep muscles such as the transversus abdominis, and superficial muscles such as the gluteus maximus and latissimus dorsi (Zelle et al 2005). Current scientific evidence tends to advise stabilizing, active training programs (Vleeming et al 2006) and does not recommend mobilization (Vleeming et al. 2008).

Use of the following mobilizations is thus primarily recommended at pain-relieving dosages. In joints with little mobility, however, this may also require movement beyond the first resistance to stimulate the mechano-receptors which transmit the pain-relieving sensory input (Schmid et al 2008; Nijs and Van Houdenhove 2009). The minimal amount of movement which perhaps could be achieved with grade III mobilization hardly improves the movement functions of the trunk or the lower extremities. Comparative studies on the different nonsurgical treatment options for managing sacroiliac joint pain are unfortunately still lacking (Zelle et al 2005).

15.2.2 Rotational Tests

■ Active Movements, Comparing Sides

The sacroiliac joint does not allow for conscious, active movements. Instead, slightly "springy" movements occur when there is movement of the lumbar spine above or the legs in the hip joints below. Given the limited mobility that is characteristic of amphiarthroses, visual inspection is inadequate for comparing sides. Gait analysis may reveal deviations from the physiological gait, such as pain during the stance phase. Such disturbances may be an indication of abnormal sacroiliac mobility. The sacroiliac joint should be stable. The reader is referred to the literature for more information on the underlying concepts of form closure and force closure.

Targeted active movements in the pubic symphysis are also impossible. Here, too, a slight movement occurs when weight is shifted from the supporting leg to the free leg, along with movement of the sacroiliac joint. Toward the end of pregnancy, there is increased mobility of the symphysis and the sacroiliac joint in preparation for birth.

Trainees in manual therapy should try for themselves to feel these tiny movements when walking. For the symphysis, the middle finger of one hand is placed on the gap in the symphysis from cranial. For identifying movement in the sacroiliac joint, the middle fingers of both hands are placed on the median sacral crest and the index fingers on the posterior superior iliac spine in order to feel their movement against the sacrum. Contact with the muscle should be avoided as contraction of the muscle interferes with palpation of the bony reference points.

■ Pubic Symphysis

The supine patient pushes one heel and then the other distalward. The therapist may help guide the movement by placing one hand on the patient's thigh. Performing this action causes alternating slight abduction and adduction in the hip joints. The movement is transmitted to the symphysis because the pubic bone on the side where the leg moves distally, also moves caudally. The therapist can palpate the movement by placing the fingers on the gap in the pubic symphysis from cranial.

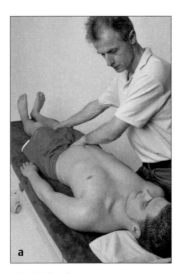
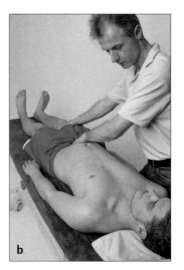

Fig. 15.2 a, b

Note

This palpation test may also be done while standing, while the patient shifts his or her weight from one leg to the other.

! If palpation reveals little or no movement of the symphysis, the joint is considered stable. This is not an indication for grade III stretching mobilization. Rather, the aim of the test is to identify hypermobility.

Sacroiliac Joint

a) Shifting weight from supporting to free leg:

The therapist sits or kneels on one knee behind the patient who is standing with the legs hip-width apart. Next the therapist places his thumbs on the posterior superior iliac spines. The therapist uses his fingers to guide the pelvis to the right or left causing the patient to place more weight on the right and then the left leg. While doing so, the therapist notes any difference in the range of motion of the right and left posterior superior iliac spines. If there is any asymmetry, first the right thumb remains on the right posterior superior iliac spine while the left palpates the sacrum in order to assess mobility of the right sacroiliac joint. Then the same is done on the opposite side.

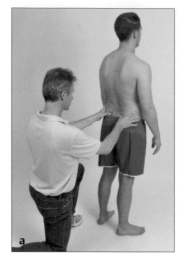
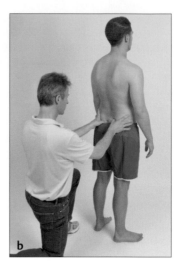

Fig. 15.3 a–c

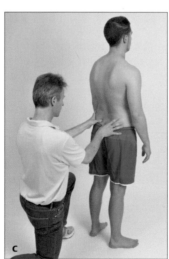

> **Note**
>
> A difference of 2.54 cm should be palpated between the posterior superior iliac spines on both sides during the movements in order to consider this and the following two tests (a–c) positive (Cibulka and Koldehoff 1999).

b) Forward bending test (standing):

The therapist remains positioned behind the patient and asks him or her to roll forward through the spine. The therapist again uses his thumbs to palpate both posterior superior iliac spines and observes whether both joints move forward simultaneously or consecutively. In physiological motion, first the lumbar spine bends forward and then the sacrum, which causes simultaneous nutation in both sacroiliac joints, and finally there is flexion of the hip joints. On the side with less sacroiliac joint mobility, the sacrum will pull the ipsilateral sacroiliac joint anteriorly with it sooner. The therapist will note that on that side the posterior superior iliac spine "goes forward" earlier.

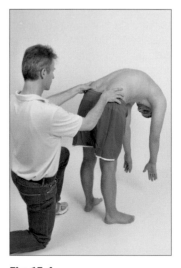

Fig. 15.4

c) **Standing hip flexion test:**

As before, the therapist stands behind the patient and palpates both posterior superior iliac spines. The patient holds onto the bench with one hand for balance and slowly lifts the right leg, flexing the hip joint. Then he or she lifts the left leg. In physiological motion, first the hip joint flexes and then the movement passes to the innominate bone so that the ilium moves dorsally. Then the ilium pulls the sacrum with its basis dorsally. Finally, there is ventral flexion of the lumbar spine. The therapist palpates and compares posterior superior iliac spine motion on both sides. If one side seems to move dorsally sooner than the other, there may be restricted mobility on that side in the hip joint. Then the right thumb remains on the right posterior superior iliac spine and the left one palpates the sacrum in order to feel movement in the right sacroiliac joint. The same is done on the left side. If there is restricted mo-

bility of the sacroiliac joint, the posterior superior iliac spine and sacrum move dorsally nearly simultaneously.

This gives an impression of which sacroiliac joint is less mobile than the other. The question remains, however, whether the less mobile side has restricted mobility and the contralateral side has physiological mobility, or whether the less mobile side has physiological mobility and the other side is hypermobile. Given the limited range of motion and the lack of precise measurement techniques, these tests cannot answer this question and their reliability on the standing patient is low. They are useful mainly for noting any major differences between the two sides, but do not warrant spending a great deal of time on them. Afterward, with the patient in the prone position, end-range mobilization of the sacroiliac joint is performed in order to ascertain in which sacroiliac joint the nutation or counternutation is painful and altered.

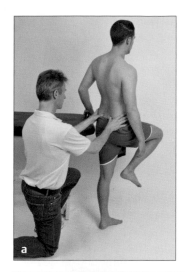

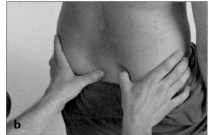

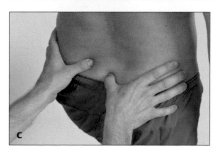

Fig. 15.5 a–c

■ **Specific Passive Movement Tests (Quantity and Quality)**

Passive movements of the pubic symphysis to assess movement quantity and quality are hardly technically feasible. Creating end-range movement stress is possible with the patient in the supine position and by pressing the two coxae apart and toward each other. This also causes stress on the sacroiliac joint. The following sections are restricted to passive movements of the sacroiliac joint in which there is also slight movement of the symphysis.

a) **Nutation as a symptom-provoking test:**

With the patient lying prone, a firm cushion is placed ventrally under the lumbar spine to reduce motion during the test. A sandbag or wedge is placed under the anterior superior iliac spine on the test side to prevent movement of the ilium ventrally. The therapist stands laterally and places the thumb of his caudal hand on the base of the sacrum on the test side, which is opposite to the therapist. The ulnar border of the cranial hand is placed over the thumbnail and pressure is applied ventrally and somewhat caudally so that nutation of the sacroiliac joint occurs. The

therapist observes the range of motion, the end-feel, and especially any pain associated with movement.

Physiological end-feel:
firm and elastic

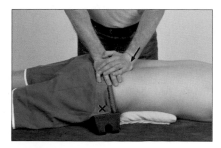

Fig. 15.6

b) Counternutation as a symptom-provoking test:

With the patient in the prone position, a stable cushion continues to support the lumbar spine. The sandbag or wedge is removed from underneath the anterior superior iliac spine, leaving it free. The therapist stands laterally and fixes the apex of the sacrum on the homolateral side with the ulnar side of the caudal hand. The ulnar side of the cranial hand rests on the iliac crest of the contralateral side and pushes the ilium ventrally. This produces stress in the direction of counternutation in the sacroiliac joint on the side op-posite to the therapist. The therapist again observes the range of motion, the quality of the end-feel, and especially any pain associated with movement.

Physiological end-feel:
firm and elastic

! Nutation and counternutation tests may be repeated without fixation. This causes more stress on the lumbar spine than on the sacroiliac joint. The localization of symptoms can be more precisely identified in the sacroiliac joint or lumbar spine.

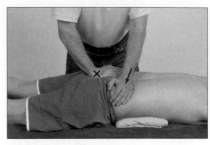

Fig. 15.7

c) Nutation as a mobility test ("lifting test"):

The patient is in the same position as for the counternutation test. The therapist places the caudal hand around the contralateral anterior superior iliac spine and, using minimal effort, lifts the ilium dorsally and slightly medially and then allows it to slide back into position. This movement can be performed slowly to the end-range position or quickly with a "rocking motion." The fingertips of the three middle fingers of the cranial hand rest on the posterior superior iliac spine so that the volar surface of the fingers is in contact with the median sacral crest. With these fingers, the therapist can palpate the movement of the posterior superior iliac spine against the sacrum in the sacroiliac joint. The therapist observes the range of motion as well as quality, that is, resistance to movement.

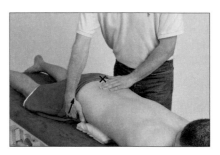

Fig. 15.8

d) Counternutation as a mobility test:

The patient remains in the prone position and the cranial hand of the therapist is placed, as before, between the median sacral crest and the posterior superior iliac spine on the opposite side. The hypothenar eminence of the caudal hand rests on the apex of the sacrum on the side closest to the therapist and pushes it ventrally and slightly cranially. The movement can be done slowly to the end-range position or quickly as a "rocking movement." The range of motion in counternutation is usually much smaller than that in nutation.

! Nutation and counternutation are movements around an axis of rotation. Although the end-feel may be tested with the mobility tests, it is better assessed with the techniques used in symptom-provoking nutation and counternutation tests.

! After standing tests have provided an initial impression of mobility and after passive movement tests have shown the symptom-altering direction and the responsible joint, the lifting test and counternutation test can further show whether the affected sacroiliac joint demonstrates restricted mobility, hypermobility, or whether there is physiological mobility. The reliability of mobility tests for the sacroiliac joint is low, however, and careful interpretation of results is warranted.

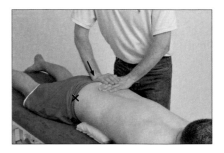

Fig. 15.9

15.2.3 Translatoric Tests

Linear translatoric movements cannot be performed passively in the sacroiliac joint. In nutation and counter nutation, the bones move nearly parallel to the treatment plane, but around axes of rotation. These movements, which are used for examination and treatment, are thus rotational.

15.2.4 Treatment of Capsuloligamentous Hypomobility

Although mobility testing of the sacroiliac joint is not conclusive (Pescioli and Kool 1997), it is necessary for determining treatment.

Treatment of a painful joint with normal physiological mobility consists of pain-relieving movements such as the lifting test. Pain is presumably related to inflammation of the capsuloligamentous apparatus—caused by mild distortion, for example.

In a hypermobile joint, pain-relieving treatment again consists of non–end-range movements, and causal trial treatment consists of placing a pelvic support belt for stabilization of the sacroiliac joint.

If there is apparent restricted mobility of the sacroiliac joint, pain-relieving measures include pain-relieving movements in the remaining range of motion and causal treatment consists of mobilization in grade III.

Clinical symptoms are not reported in conjunction with reduced mobility of the pubic symphysis. Only hypermobility seems to produce symptoms. A hypermobile pubic symphysis should be immobilized with a stable pelvic belt.

Mobilization in restricted nutation:

One may use the same technique as for testing. The initial position and placement of the hands are identical. The application pressure in grade III is longer, however.

An alternative is as follows: The patient lies in the supine position on the edge of the bench, with the sacrum resting on the edge of the bench on a sandbag and the ilium hanging laterally over it. The therapist stands caudally and holds the patient's leg, which is flexed at the hip and knee joints, against his trunk. The medial hand is placed from ventral on the anterior superior iliac spine and presses the ilium dorsally. This results in nutation of the sacrum due to the fixation of the sacrum to the sandbag. The lateral hand palpates the movement with the fingers between the posterior superior iliac spine and the sacrum. The median aspect of the therapist's thigh is placed against the patient's pelvis as a precaution.

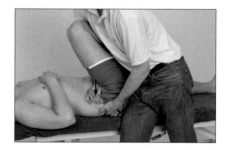

Fig. 15.10

Mobilization in restricted counter-nutation:

Here, too, the test version for mobilization is suitable. The initial position and technique are identical. In order to increase the intensity, the hand used for fixation on the apex of the sacrum can be supported by placing the leg closest to the therapist on the floor in maximum hip flexion. The force of the mobilizing hand can be increased by raising the part of the bench with the opposite leg on it. This causes maximum extension of the opposite hip joint, pulling the ilium ventrally.

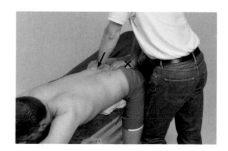

Fig. 15.11

Documentation Template: Practice Scheme

Pubic symphysis and sacroiliac joint						
Symptoms						
Symptom-altering direction						
Contraindications?	Nervous system: Other:					
Symptom-altering joint						
General assessment of adjacent joints						

Specific rotational tests	Active	Continues passively?	Passive	End-feel	Symptoms/ pain	Comments
Symphysis: (with hip abduction/adduction)						
Sacroiliac joint: ▪ Shifting between supporting and non-supporting leg						
▪ Standing forward bending test						
▪ Standing hip flexion test						
▪ Nutation as symptom-provoking test						
▪ Counternutation as symptom-provoking test						

Translatoric tests (in this case, specific rotatory tests):	Quantity	Quality	End-feel	Symptoms/pain	Comments
▪ Nutation as a mobility test					
▪ Counternutation as a mobility test					

Summary Formulation aid: ▪ Symptoms ▪ Direction ▪ Contraindications ▪ Site (joint) ▪ Restricted mobility, hypermobility, or physiological mobility ▪ Structure: muscle, joint, etc.	*Text:*
Trial treatment	
Physical therapy diagnosis	
Treatment plan with treatment goal and prognosis	
Treatment with periodic control tests	
Final examination	

Documentation: Practice Example

<table>
<tr><td colspan="7">Pubic symphysis and sacroiliac joint
(Pain in right sacroiliac joint after falling onto an outstretched leg 3 months previously)</td></tr>
<tr><td>Symptoms</td><td colspan="6">Pain in lower right back and buttock region when weight is on the supporting leg following a fall onto the outstretched leg (extended knee)</td></tr>
<tr><td>Symptom-altering direction</td><td colspan="6">Weight on supporting leg, right</td></tr>
<tr><td>Contraindications?</td><td colspan="6">Nervous system: No findings
Other: No findings</td></tr>
<tr><td>Symptom-altering joint</td><td colspan="6">Sacroiliac joint, right</td></tr>
<tr><td>General assessment of adjacent joints</td><td colspan="6">When walking, the patient shortens the amount of time on the (right) supporting leg due to pain, and there is avoiding movement of the trunk in the opposite direction.</td></tr>
<tr><td>Specific rotational tests</td><td>Active</td><td>Continues passively?</td><td>Passive</td><td>End-feel</td><td>Symptoms/ pain</td><td>Comments</td></tr>
<tr><td>Symphysis: (with hip abduction/adduction)</td><td>No findings</td><td></td><td></td><td>No findings</td><td></td><td></td></tr>
<tr><td>Sacroiliac joint:
■ Shifting between supporting and non-supporting leg</td><td>Less on right than left</td><td></td><td></td><td>Pain on right supporting leg</td><td></td><td></td></tr>
<tr><td>■ Standing forward bending test</td><td>Positive on right side (= less mobile) than left</td><td></td><td></td><td>None</td><td></td><td></td></tr>
<tr><td>■ Standing hip flexion test</td><td>Positive on right side (= less mobile) than left</td><td></td><td></td><td>None</td><td></td><td></td></tr>
<tr><td>■ Nutation as symptom-provoking test</td><td></td><td></td><td>Increased resistance to movement, right</td><td>Empty</td><td>Provokes symptoms on right</td><td></td></tr>
<tr><td>■ Counternutation as symptom-provoking test</td><td></td><td></td><td>Less on right than left</td><td>Very firm and elastic</td><td>No findings</td><td>More pain-relieving</td></tr>
<tr><td>Translatoric tests (in this case, specific rotatory tests):</td><td>Quantity</td><td colspan="2">Quality</td><td>End-feel</td><td>Symptoms/pain</td><td>Comments</td></tr>
<tr><td>■ Nutation as a mobility test</td><td>Less on right than left</td><td colspan="2">Increased resistance to movement</td><td>Ilium very firm and elastic dorsalward</td><td>None</td><td>Grade I–II tends to be pain-relieving if done rhythmically; moving ilium dorsally in grade III causes pain</td></tr>
<tr><td>■ Counternutation as a mobility test</td><td>No findings</td><td colspan="2">No findings</td><td>Firm and elastic</td><td>None</td><td></td></tr>
</table>

Continued ▶

Pubic symphysis and sacroiliac joint (Pain in right sacroiliac joint after falling onto an outstretched leg 3 months previously)	
Summary Formulation aid: ▪ Symptoms ▪ Direction ▪ Contraindications ▪ Site (joint) ▪ Restricted mobility, hypermobility, or physiological mobility ▪ Structure: muscle, joint, etc.	*Text:* ▪ *Pain in right side of back and buttock region when weight is on supporting leg* ▪ *with nutation.* ▪ *There are no contraindications today to further movement testing.* ▪ *Right sacroiliac joint involvement* ▪ *due to restricted joint mobility* ▪ *as a result of capsuloligamentous restriction. Pain with nutation may be explained by a sprain of the capsuloligamentous unit.*
Trial treatment	▪ *5-minute long pain-relieving movements (grade I–II) using the lifting test on the right sacroiliac joint, leading to less pain when walking.* ▪ *Then 5-minute grade III mobilization in the direction of counternutation, leading to a significant decrease in symptoms and diminished resistance during the lifting test.*
Physical therapy diagnosis	*See above*
Treatment plan with treatment goal and prognosis	▪ *After initial pain-relieving movements, further (grade III) mobilization in the direction of counternutation.* ▪ *Treatment goal: pain-free physiological mobility.* **(Further information on examination and treatment techniques may be obtained by attending further education.)**
Treatment with periodic control tests	
Final examination	

15.3   Sacrococcygeal Joint

(Articulatio sacrococcygea)

15.3.1   Anatomy

Joint type:	synchondrosis (thin intervertebral disk)
Distal joint surface:	The coccyx is considered in movement as a concave bone.
Resting position:	not described
Close packed position:	not described
Capsular pattern:	not described

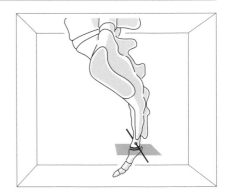

Fig. 15.12

15.3.2 Rotational Tests

It is impossible to actively move the sacrococcygeal joint, although a certain amount of movement might occur passively during birth. Thus this barely movable joint is very stable or even stiff and does not need to be mobilized. Owing to its attachment to the dorsal surface of the coccyx, the gluteus maximus muscle has the ability to pull the bone dorsally. The portions of the perineal muscle that attach to the lateral and ventral aspects of the coccyx (pubococcygeus muscle as part of the levator ani on the front and the coccygeus muscle on the side) can draw the coccyx ventrally.

The minimal mobility of the sacrococcygeal joint as well as its intimate location does not enable visual evaluation of movement of the joint.

During a fall onto the buttocks, or after prolonged sitting in a "slumped" position, unphysiologically large ventral movements of the coccyx can occur and cause a sprain. Application of pressure with a finger to move the coccyx ventrally reproduces the reported pain. Given the intimate site, one can first ask patients to try to do so themselves. Students of manual therapy are advised to practice first by palpating the mobility of their own sacrococcygeal joint. The therapist should perform the test movement after describing it to the patient and through a towel or the patient's underwear. The therapist then places the middle finger of the palpating hand on the coccyx, increasing the pressure with the middle finger of the other hand. If this specific move-

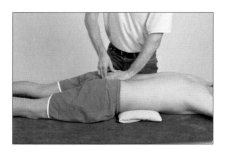

Fig. 15.13

ment causes the reported pain, then the symptoms are probably correlated with the sacrococcygeal joint.

Physiological end-feel:
very firm and elastic

15.3.3 Translatoric Tests

Due to the difficulty of the grip, although theoretically possible, translatoric movements are all but impossible to perform.

15.3.3 Treatment of Capsuloligamentous Hypomobility

Treatment may be attempted with isometric contraction of the gluteus maximus, which pulls the coccyx dorsally. The patient should press his or her buttocks together and not allow them to separate against the pressure from the therapist's hands.

If this technique is not sufficient, the coccyx should be manually mobilized dorsally. The patient should first try to do so alone at home after the therapist

has explained the technique. Only if this is inadequate should the therapist perform mobilization. The patient should be informed about what the procedure involves, and it should be carried out in the presence of another colleague in order to avoid any misunderstanding related to the intimate site and potential legal repercussions. The reader is referred to the appropriate further education courses.

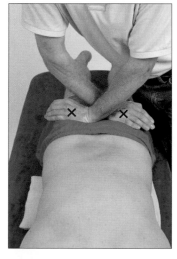

Fig. 15.14

Documentation Template: Practice Scheme

Sacrococcygeal joint						
Symptoms						
Symptom-altering direction						
Contraindications?	Nervous system: Other:					
Symptom-altering joint						
General assessment of adjacent joints						

Specific rotational tests	Active	Continues passively?	Passive	End-feel	Symptoms/ pain	Comments
▪ Movement of coccyx ventrally						

Translatoric tests	

Summary Formulation aid: ▪ Symptoms ▪ Direction ▪ Contraindications ▪ Site (joint) ▪ Restricted mobility, hypermobility, or physiological mobility ▪ Structure: muscle, joint, etc.	*Text:*
Trial treatment	
Physical therapy diagnosis	
Treatment plan with treatment goal and prognosis	
Treatment with periodic control tests	
Final examination	

Documentation: Practice Example

Sacrococcygeal joint	
Symptoms	*Pain in buttocks after a fall from standing height onto the buttocks*
Symptom-altering direction	*Sitting*
Contraindications?	Nervous system: *No findings* Other: *No findings*
Symptom-altering joint	*Sacrococcygeal joint*
General assessment of adjacent joints	*No findings*

Specific rotational tests	**Active**	**Continues passively?**	**Passive**	**End-feel**	**Symptoms/ pain**	**Comments**
Movement of coccyx ventrally			*Barely testable*	*Empty*	*Provokes reported pain*	

Translatoric tests	*Not tested*

Summary Formulation aid: • Symptoms • Direction • Contraindications • Site (joint) • Restricted mobility, hypermobility, or physiological mobility • Structure: muscle, joint, etc.	*Text:* • *Pain in lower buttock region* • *when sitting.* • *There are no contraindications today to further movement testing.* • *The sacrococcygeal joint correlates with the symptoms and triggers pain during ventral flexion,* • *which is why dorsiflexion is believed to be limited and also pain-alleviating.* • *The cause is presumably posttraumatic inflammatory irritation of the sacrococcygeal joint.*
Trial treatment	• *Repeated static tensing of the gluteus maximus to dorsiflex the coccyx, after which the patient reports a slight decrease in pain when sitting. When the therapist presses the coccyx ventrally, there is a more clearly palpable "stopping point" and less pain.*
Physical therapy diagnosis	*See above*
Treatment plan with treatment goal and prognosis	• *Continue the trial treatment measure and protect the sacrococcygeal joint to allow the inflammation to subside.* • *Treatment goal: pain relief.* **(Further information on examination and treatment techniques may be obtained by attending further education.)**
Treatment with periodic control tests	
Final examination	

15.4   Lumbar spine

(Columna lumbalis)

15.4.1   Anatomy

The functional unit of the spinal column is the motion segment based on Junghans. It consists of a complex made up of three connections: the intervertebral disk, which is between two vertebral bodies and the two zygapophyseal joints belonging to these, and all of the structures between the two vertebrae.

■ Intervertebral Disk Connection

Joint type: synchondrosis

Joint surface: the top and bottom vertebral end-plates move in the same direction as the vertebral body

■ Zygapophyseal Joint (Articulatio zygoapophysealis)

Joint type: plane joint (nearly flat joint; also known as an "arthrodial joint")

Joint surface: nearly flat; for manual therapy the inferior articular process is considered concave

> **!** The joint surfaces are at about a 90° angle to the upper vertebral end-plate and are tilted about 45° laterally to the median plane of the vertebral body, so that the inferior articular process "faces" ventrally and laterally.

Resting position: physiological lordosis

Close packed position: end-range, uncoupled movement

Capsular pattern: not described

> **!** The zygapophyseal joints are sometimes simply called "facetjoints."

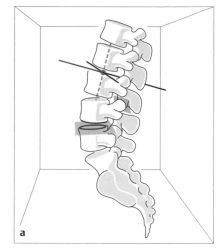

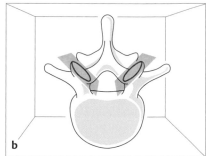

Abb. 15.15 a, b

15.4.2   Rotational Tests

■ Testing the Mobility of the Nerves

Sciatic nerve:

The patient should be in the position in which he or she normally feels the symptoms—often standing with one hand holding onto something for balance, or sitting. Alternatively, the patient may lie on his or her back or side. The therapist should help steady the patient with one hand on their back. In this position, he helps the patient to raise the leg, which is extended at the knee, using hip flexion. The patient should raise the leg until the symptoms just begin to be felt. Then the patient moves the leg slightly back until just before the symptom-altering point is reached. Next, the therapist should ask the patient to first dorsiflex the ankle joint and then to bend the cervical spine forward. This causes maximum elongation of the neural structures of the sciatic nerve and the dura mater.

The therapist should observe and note the degree of hip flexion at which the symptoms occur, the nature of the symptoms (tingling, stabbing pain, etc.), where they occur (radicular pain?), whether they correspond to those reported by the patient, and whether they worsen if the test is made more difficult with ankle or cervical spine movement.

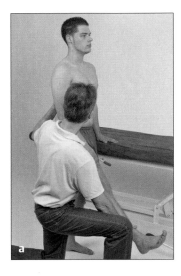
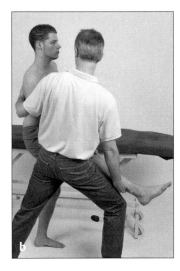
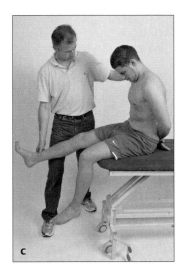

Fig. 15.16 a–c

Femoral nerve:

The patient should still be in the starting position in which the symptoms are most strongly felt—seated, or if standing, he or she should hold onto something to maintain their balance. Side-lying or prone positions are also possible. The therapist supports the patient's shoulder, grasps the distal lower leg with his dorsal hand, and bends the knee joint until the patient just begins to feel the symptoms. To prevent deviation occurring with hip joint flexion—often due to contraction or shortening of the rectus femo- ris muscle—the therapist should hold the patient's anterior thigh by placing his leg in front of it. Just before the symptom-altering point is reached, he asks the patient to first move the ankle joint in plantar flexion and then to bend the cervical spine forward. This changes the neural structures of the dura mater and the femoral nerve including its sensory terminal branch, the saphenous nerve. Occasionally, a few saphenous fibers also pass to behind the malleolus and thus the ankle joint should also be moved in dorsiflexion. As the saphenous nerve is relaxed when the knee is in flexion, tension in the neural structures of the femoral nerve is changed only slightly by ankle movements in this position. The important thing, however, is whether or not ankle motion produces a change in symptoms.

The same parameters as for the sciatic nerve are tested.

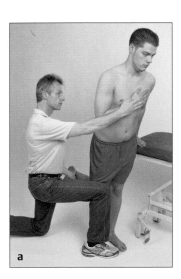
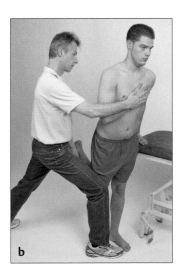
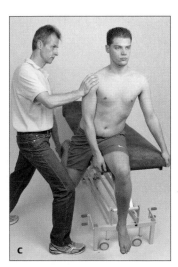

Fig. 15.17 a–c

■ Active Movements

The patient should still be in the starting position in which his or her symptoms are strongest. Due to the mechanics involved, stress on the lumbar spine is greatest during end-range movements when standing. The following section thus describes testing in the standing patient.

The patient should move actively in ventral flexion and dorsiflexion, right and left lateral flexion, and rotation to the right and left. For the majority of people it is exceedingly difficult to move only the lumbar spine, and thus there are often accompanying movements of the thoracic spine. During dorsiflexion the patient should place their hands on the opposite shoulders and lean back while lifting the sternum forward and upward. When rotating, the patient may also place their hands on the lower ribs of the opposite side and pull on them to increase the rotation of the lumbar spine. To limit rotation of the pelvis with the lumbar spine rotation, the patient should hold both thighs actively in contact with the treatment table in front of them.

One often observes the following:

- Ventral flexion:
  less in the (lower) lumbar spine and more in the thoracic spine (often too much)
- Dorsiflexion:
  more in the (lower) lumbar spine and less in the thoracic spine (often too little)
- Lateral flexion:
  more in the lower to mid thoracic spine (physiological if there is a harmonious transition to the adjacent regions)
- Rotation: more in the lower thoracic spine (physiological if there is a harmonious transition to the adjacent regions)

Patients with lumbar hypermobility often have an extreme curvature of the lower lumbar spine in dorsiflexion accompanied by a slight wiggling of the lower lumbar spine during lateral flexion and when returning from ventral flexion (= lacking control of movement).

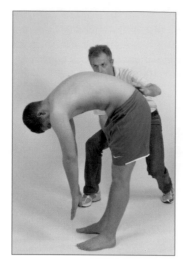

Fig. 15.18

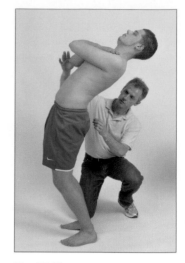

Fig. 15.19

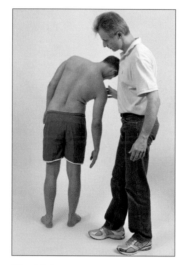

Fig. 15.20

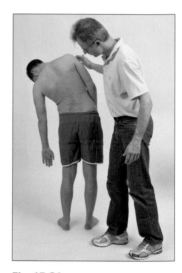

Fig. 15.21

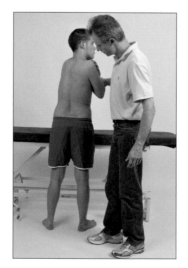

Fig. 15.22

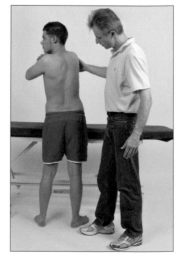

Fig. 15.23

Active movements with a comparison of sides are a part of the **orienting and specific examination**. They serve to localize the **symptoms** and for a **general assessment of the adjacent joints** as well as the **affected vertebral region**. The patient should perform the movements alone. If necessary, the therapist may indicate tactilely the desired direction of movement.

▆ Active and Passive Movement Testing (Quantity and Quality)

Generally speaking, passive flexion/extension as well as lateral bending movements cannot be performed in the standing patient. The application of passive overpressure after the patient has performed the active movement is only advisable if it does not cause pain and if the therapist wishes to know whether passive continuation of the movement elicits any pain or symptoms. In everyday practice, however, active movement is often already painful and hence the application of passive overpressure is avoided.

a) **Ventral flexion** from the zero position:

- The therapist should stand at the patient's side and ask him or her to actively bend the upper body as far forward as possible. The therapist should evaluate how the movement is performed and whether there is a harmonious curvature of the spine at the end of the movement.
- Next the therapist stabilizes the patient's pelvis by supporting it with his medial hand against his own side. His lateral hand is used to apply overpressure ventrally at about L1 to assess whether the movement continues passively and how the end of movement feels.
- Completely passive movement through the entire range of motion is not possible in the standing patient.

Physiological end of movement: firm and elastic

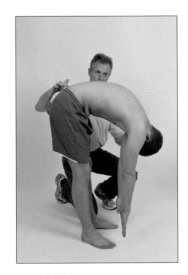

Fig. 15.24

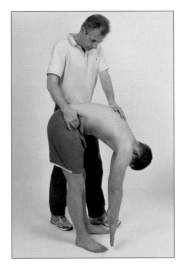

Fig. 15.25

b) **Dorsiflexion** from the zero position:

- The therapist stands at the patient's side and asks him or her to place their hands on the contralateral lower ribs. The patient then actively bends their whole back backward as far as possible. This displaces the pelvis anteriorly.
- Next, using his dorsal hand to support the patient's sacrum, the therapist grasps the patient's lower arms with his ventral arm and, using this grip, pushes the lumbar spine into dorsiflexion. He then tests whether the movement continues passively and how the end of movement feels.
- Completely passive movement through the entire range of motion is not possible in the standing patient.

Physiological end of movement: firm and elastic

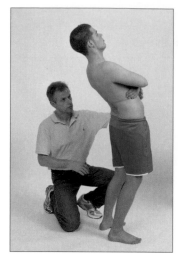

Fig. 15.26

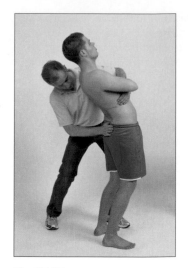

Fig. 15.27

c) **Lateral flexion** from the zero position:

- The therapist stands contralaterally and asks the patient to place each hand on the lower ribs on the opposite side. The patient then bends his or her rib cage laterally as far as possible to actively flex the lumbar spine laterally. There is some displacement of the pelvis to the opposite side.
- Next, with his dorsal hand the therapist stabilizes the patient's pelvis against his own body and then presses his ventral hand against the patient's hand on the lower costal arch. This increases the lateral flexion of the lumbar spine. Whether the movement continues passively and also the feel of the end of movement are also tested.
- Completely passive movement through the entire range of motion is not possible in the standing patient.

Lateral flexion should be performed to both sides.

Physiological end of movement: firm and elastic

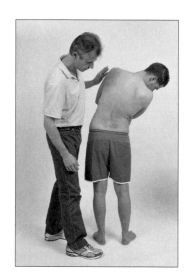

Fig. 15.28

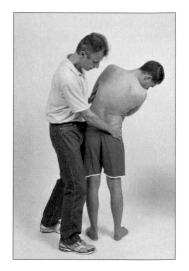

Fig. 15.29

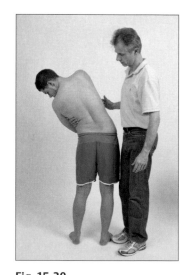

Fig. 15.30

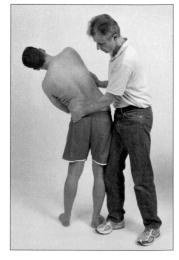

Fig. 15.31

d) **Rotation** from the zero position:

- The therapist stands on the side to which the patient will rotate. His dorsal hand stabilizes the patient's pelvis against his own. Next he asks the patient to grasp the lower ribs on the opposite side and to actively rotate his upper body as far as possible toward the therapist.
- Next the therapist takes hold of patient's upper body by placing his ventral hand over the patient's hand on the opposite lower ribs. He then can test whether the movement continues passively. The therapist's ventral shoulder leads the movement together with his ventral hand.
- Because he does not carry the weight of the upper body, the therapist can now passively rotate from the zero position and test the end-feel.

Rotation should be performed in both directions.

Physiological end-feel:
firm and elastic

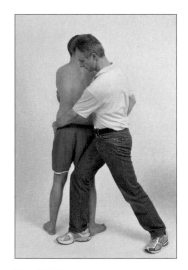

Fig. 15.32

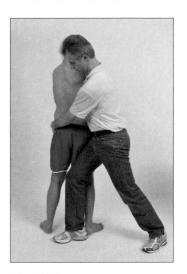

Fig. 15.33

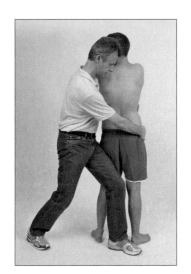

Fig. 15.34

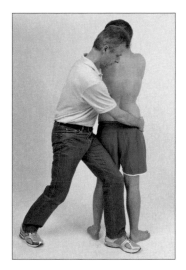

Fig. 15.35

15.4.3 Translatoric Tests

◾ Intervertebral Disk Connection

Traction:

The patient should be in the position in which he or she feels the symptoms, that is, just as they reach the pain threshold. If the symptoms are acute, the actual resting position may be used; or, for milder symptoms, three-dimensional prepositioning may be used. The patient should be standing with the feet hip-distance apart; the arms are crossed and grasping the lower ribs on the opposite side. The therapist stands behind the patient and grasps the forearms, pulling them dorsally so that the patient's upper body is firmly held between the therapist's hands and chest, which is in contact with the patient's lower thoracic spine. Next the therapist extends his knees, which were slightly bent at the beginning, in order to prevent his own clothing from slipping and to prevent movement of the patient's skin. The therapist shifts his weight onto his back leg without bending the knees.

This shifts the patient's body straight backward. Even a minimal range of movement is sufficient to feel the weight taken off as a type of traction. The therapist should not allow the patient to lean too far back because the fear of falling causes an increase in muscle contraction which counteracts the effects of traction.

The therapist should note any change in symptoms in particular.

Physiological end-feel:
firm and elastic (difficult to feel)

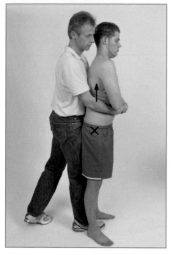

Fig. 15.36

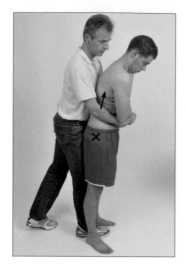

Fig. 15.37

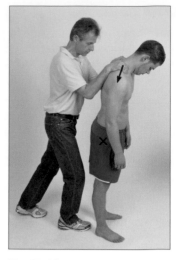

Fig. 15.38

If the patient only experiences symptoms with neural structure elongation, then traction should be done in the position in which this occurs. If the slump test causes symptoms, the patient may sit and extend the knee until he or she just begins to feel the symptoms. Staying in that position, the patient should plant the fists on either side of the pelvis and slightly extend the elbows to take the weight off the buttocks. This decreases the pressure on the lumbar spine, similar to traction maneuvers. The test result is considered positive if doing so alleviates the symptoms and the patient can extend the knee further. Similar to a positive compression result, once the patient relaxes the elbows, the symptoms should worsen and they should feel that they have to bend the knee. This form of self-traction should also be chosen if the therapist cannot or does not wish to perform passive traction.

Compression:

The patient should assume a position just before where the pain begins, which may require three-dimensional prepositioning. If the pain is constant, the test should be done with the patient in the actual resting position. The therapist should stand behind the patient, place both hands on the upper ribs, and press them caudally. The force of compression is transferred from the ribs and

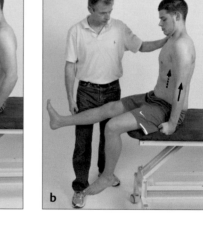

Fig. 15.39 a, b

thoracic spine to the lumbar spine. It should be noted that application of perpendicular downward pressure in patients with strong lumbar lordosis often causes dorsiflexion of the lumbar spine. In such instances, the patient should bend the upper body slightly forward so that the compression force occurs parallel to the longitudinal axis of the lumbar spine.

The therapist should pay special attention to any change in symptoms.

Physiological end-feel:
firm or hard and elastic

! General traction and compression methods applied to the intervertebral disk plane do not yield any information on the range of motion, but only tell whether the symptoms change—especially neurological ones. If neurological compression is suspected, it is advisable to perform traction and compression in the position in which the patient experiences the neurological symptoms. The therapist may instruct the patient, for instance, to sit with an extended knee to test symptoms correlating with sciatic nerve movement (**Fig. 15.39 a, b**).

▪ Zygapophyseal Joint

Traction on one joint and **compression** of the opposite joint:

The patient should be lying in the prone position. A firm cushion is placed beneath the abdomen to support the lumbar spine. The therapist stands caudally and laterally. His left thumb holds the spinous process of S1 from the left, and his right thumb pushes the right side of the spinous process of L5 leftward. This produces right rotation of L5 against S1. Then the therapist changes the position of the thumbs: the right thumb holds the spinous process of S1 and the left pushes the spinous process of L5 toward the right. This produces left rotation of L5 against S1. Then, in the same manner the therapist tests the L4–L5 segment and all lumbar segments above this level.

Physiological end-feel:
hard or firm and elastic

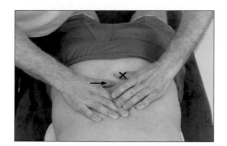

Fig. 15.40

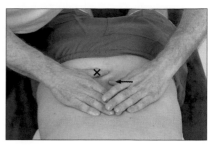

Fig. 15.41

! The therapist should note the quantity and quality of movement, the end-feel, and any change in symptoms. He should first perform the movement repeatedly with minimal force as far as the first stop, and then test the end-feel. Fixating S1 and rotating L5 to the right produces traction on the right zygapophyseal joint and compression on the left. Depending on the orientation of the zygapophyseal joint surfaces, these movements do not occur at a 100% right angle to the treatment plane but only approximately.

! The therapist should place his thumbs flat on the patient's back in splintlike fashion. He should always avoid overextension of his thumb joints with end-range stress to protect his own joints during application of the technique(s).

15.4.4 Treatment of Capsuloligamentous Hypomobility

▪ Traction in Relation to the Intervertebral Disk Plane

General traction in the supine position:

The patient should be lying in the supine position at the end of the bench with his or her hip and knee joints flexed so that the lumbar spine is in ventral flexion. Moving the legs allows one to establish the actual resting position of the lumbar spine in flexion, lateral bending, and rotation. The therapist stands caudally and places a long belt or two connected belts around the patient's proximal thigh. It is often useful to add padding to the belt, such as a towel. The other end of the belt is looped around the therapist's pelvis. The therapist then shifts his weight backward which produces traction at a right angle away from the treatment plane of the intervertebral disk.

Grade I–II traction technique is used in particular for relief of symptoms in patients with acute neural compression (e.g., physician diagnosis of disk herniation).

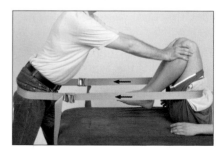

Fig. 15.42

General traction in the side-lying position

Patients should be lying on their side while the therapist stands ventrally. His cranial hand fixates L1 with the tips of his index and middle fingers which are on the articular process. The "soft" medial side of his caudal proximal forearm presses the patient's sacrum and thus the entire pelvis against his own body. By shifting the weight of his upper body caudally, he also moves the patient's pelvis caudally. This produces traction at a right angle away from the treatment plane of the intervertebral disk.

This technique (grade I–II traction) is also suitable for the treatment of acute neural compression symptoms.

> **!** General traction primarily serves to alleviate symptoms of neural compression. The therapist controls the treatment not only by asking about possible changes in symptoms, but also by testing neurological function, e.g., neurodynamics.

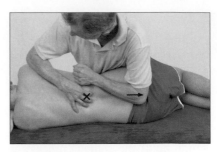

Fig. 15.43

Specific traction in the side-lying patient: L1–L2

The starting position and fixation are the same as described in the previous technique. The tips of the index and middle fingers of the caudal hand are in contact with the L2 articular processes. The patient's pelvis is still held firmly between the forearm and body of the therapist. When he shifts his body weight caudally, it pulls the patient's pelvis with it. The contact between the fingers and the articular processes of the caudal vertebra transfers the traction force specifically to this segment. The procedure is readily felt, but mechanically difficult to imagine, taking into account the complex anatomy of the surrounding soft tissues. Presumably, neurological factors such as tactile stimuli play a role in this phenomenon.

This technique may be used with grade I–II traction as well as grade III mobilization.

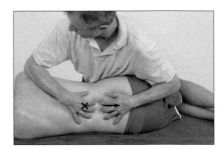

Fig. 15.44

Specific traction in the side-lying patient: L5–S1

The starting position and grip are similar as for the general side-lying techniques. The therapist's stabilizing hand is in contact with L5 instead of L1. Movement of the pelvis caudally, with fixation of the L5 vertebra, emphasizes the traction on the L5–S1 segment. Instead of using his caudal hand, the therapist may pull the patient's sacrum caudally with the part of his forearm near the elbow.

This technique may also be used with grade I–II traction as well as grade III mobilization.

> **!** Specific grade III traction is indicated in particular to increase the range of motion.

> **!** For all traction techniques in the supine and side-lying positions, the patient's pelvis and legs should be on a surface that allows them to move; or they may be on the foot-piece of the bench, which can be moved distally, or suspended in a sling table. This minimizes any friction between the patient and bench. Without such aids, it is very difficult to perform traction with sufficient force or for an adequate length of time.

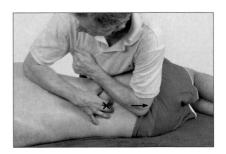

Fig. 15.45

Traction on the Zygapophyseal Joint

The starting position and grip are the same as for the translatoric test of the zygapophyseal joints. Pain-relieving traction may be performed with the examination technique. This technique may also be used for grade III mobilization by holding the thumb stable or by pushing against the spinous process with the pisi-form. The direction of movement is the one that produces maximum pain relief or in the direction of the greatest limitation.

> **!** Findings of quantity, quality of movement with end-feel, and any change in symptoms using traction in relation to the intervertebral disk plane in the supine or side-lying patient, or traction on the zygapophyseal joints in the prone patient can complete the assessment.

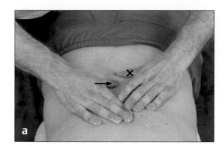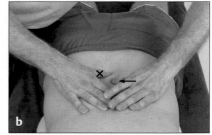

Fig. 15.46 a, b

Documentation Template: Practice Scheme

Lumbar spine	
Symptoms	
Symptom-altering direction	
Contraindications?	Nervous system: ▪ Mobility ▪ Impulse conduction Other:
Symptom-altering joint	
General assessment of adjacent joints and the affected vertebral region	

Rotational tests	Active	Continues passively?	Passive	End of movement / end-feel	Symptoms/ pain	Comments
▪ Ventral flexion						
▪ Dorsal flexion						
▪ Lateral flexion, right						
▪ Lateral flexion, left						
▪ Rotation, right						
▪ Rotation, left						
▪ Combined movements						

Translatoric tests	Quantity	Quality	End-feel	Symptoms/pain	Comments
▪ Traction, intervertebral disk plane					
▪ Compression, intervertebral disk plane					
▪ Traction (and compression) of the zygapophyseal joints					

Summary	
Summary Formulation aid: ▪ Symptoms ▪ Direction ▪ Contraindications ▪ Site (joint) ▪ Restricted mobility, hypermobility, or physiological mobility ▪ Structure: muscle, joint, etc.	*Text:*
Trial treatment	
Physical therapy diagnosis	

Continued ▶

Lumbar spine	
Treatment plan with treatment goal and prognosis	
Treatment with periodic control tests	
Final examination	

Documentation: Practice Example 1

Lumbar spine (Acute sciatic pain)		
Symptoms	Extreme pain in the lower back which radiates through the right buttocks, into the right thigh, the posterior lateral calf muscle, and the lateral border of the foot and to the small toe (S1 dermatome). Sudden onset of pain the previous day while lifting a heavy object with extended knees and torso bent forward.	
Symptom-altering direction	The patient is in a guarding position with ventral flexion and left lateral flexion. Any movement in the direction of the guarding position, as well as, and especially in, the opposite direction, severely exacerbates the symptoms.	
Contraindications?	Nervous system:	
	▪ Mobility	The sciatic nerve mobility test provokes the reported pain in the back and the right leg at 20° hip flexion on the right and 30° hip flexion on the left in the standing patient. Increasing the test difficulty with ankle and cervical spine movement leads to a clearly positive result.
	▪ Impulse conduction	The sensation at S1 dermatome, the ability to stand on tips of toes (triceps surae muscle test value of 4) and the Achilles tendon reflex are diminished.
	Other: *No findings*	
Symptom-altering joint	Not tested today.	
General assessment of adjacent joints the affected vertebral region	The patient moves the back very little and extremely carefully.	

Rotational tests	Active	Continues passively?	Passive	End of movement / end-feel	Symptoms/ pain	Comments
▪ Ventral flexion						
▪ Dorsiflexion						
▪ Lateral flexion, right						
▪ Lateral flexion, left			*Not tested today.*			
▪ Rotation, right						
▪ Rotation, left						
▪ Combined movements						

Translatoric tests	Quantity	Quality	End-feel	Symptoms/pain	Comments
Traction, intervertebral disk plane	Only grade I–II tested; quantity cannot be assessed	Muscular guarding	Not tested today.	Relieves reported symptoms	Tested in the actual resting position in standing patient
Compression, intervertebral disk plane	Only with minimal pressure application	Patient tenses muscles against pressure	Not tested today.	Provokes reported symptoms	Tested in the actual resting position in standing patient
Traction (and compression) of the zygapophyseal joints	Not tested today.				

Continued ▶

Documentation: First Practice Example 1 *(Continued)*

Lumbar spine (Acute sciatic pain)	
Summary Formulation aid: ■ Symptoms ■ Direction ■ Contraindications ■ Site (joint) ■ Restricted mobility, hypermobility, or physiological mobility ■ Structure: muscle, joint, etc.	*Text:* ■ *Acute lumbar pain which radiates radicularly into dermatome S1 of the right leg.* ■ *All movements performed from the guarding position of ventral flexion and left lateral flexion exacerbate the pain, especially movements in the opposite direction. Traction relieves and compression provokes the reported symptoms.* ■ *Movement is contraindicated today both for further examination and treatment. We thus stopped the examination today.* ■ *Presumably the symptoms are from the nerve root at S1, which might be related to mechanical compression.*
Trial treatment	*Relieving grade I–II traction, which alleviates symptoms*
Physical therapy diagnosis	*See above*
Treatment plan with treatment goal and prognosis	■ *Information to the treating physician. If further physiotherapy is prescribed for these symptoms, the following measures may be used:* 　■ *Traction:* 　*Static grade I–II traction in the actual resting position with the aim of relief and increasing space. If performed intermittently, traction also stimulates metabolism and inhibition of pain.* 　■ *Resting position:* 　*1–3 days bed rest in the actual resting position may be beneficial during this highly acute phase.* 　■ *Protection:* 　*If the patient must move about, he is advised to use a lumbar belt for stabilization of the actual resting position.* 　■ *Analgesia:* 　*Pain-relieving PT treatments such as application of heat and massage may be given.* 　■ *Information/Instruction:* 　*The patient is informed about his disorder and instructed about protective movements such as how to sit up from a supine position as well as self-help measures such as self-traction.* ■ *Treatment goal: relief of neural structures, pain relief.* *Neural structure mobility, impulse conduction, active movements of the patient, and symptoms are used as controls.* *Only after the highly acute symptoms have subsided can the examination of the first session be continued.* **(Further information on examination and treatment techniques may be obtained by attending further education.)**
Treatment with periodic control tests	
Final examination	

Documentation: Practice Example 2

Lumbar spine (Low back pain)	
Symptoms	*Patient has pain and stiffness with forward bending of the torso.*
Symptom-altering direction	*Ventral flexion*
Contraindications?	Nervous system: *No findings* ■ Mobility ■ Impulse conduction Other: *No findings*
Symptom-altering joint	*Lower lumbar spine*
General assessment of adjacent joints and the affected vertebral region	*The patient appears to have generally more "stiff" movements.*

Rotational tests	Active	Continues passively?	Passive	End of movement / end-feel	Symptoms/ pain	Comments
■ Ventral flexion	*Hypo 2*	*< 5°*	*Not tested*	*Rather more firm and elastic*	*Triggers end-range reported pain*	*Tested in the standing patient*
■ Dorsiflexion	*Rather hyper*	*> 10°*	*Not tested*	*Soft to firm and elastic*	*Unpleasant pulling sensation at end-range*	*Visible "fold" in the lower lumbar spine at maximum extension*
■ Lateral flexion, right	*No findings*	*No findings*	*Not tested*	*Firm and elastic*	*None*	*None*
■ Lateral flexion, left	*No findings*	*No findings*	*Not tested*	*Firm and elastic*	*None*	*None*
■ Rotation, right	*No findings*	*No findings*	*No findings*	*Firm and elastic*	*None*	
■ Rotation, left	*No findings*	*No findings*	*No findings*	*Firm and elastic*	*None*	
■ Combined movements	*Not tested today*					

Translatoric tests	Quantity	Quality	End-feel	Symptoms/pain	Comments
■ Traction, intervertebral disk plane	*General technique difficult to evaluate*	*Increased resistance to movement*	*Very firm and elastic*	*Relieves reported pain*	*Tested in the standing patient and specifically L5–S1 in the side-lying position*
■ Compression, intervertebral disk plane	*No findings*	*No findings*	*Very firm*	*None*	*Tested in the standing patient*
■ Traction (and compression) of the zygapophyseal joints	*L5–S1 hypo 2*	*Increased resistance to movement*	*Very firm and elastic*	*None*	

Continued ▶

Documentation: Practice Example 2 *(Continued)*

Lumbar spine (Low back pain)	
Summary Formulation aid: ■ Symptoms ■ Direction ■ Contraindications ■ Site (joint) ■ Restricted mobility, hypermobility, or physiological mobility ■ Structure: muscle, joint, etc. ■ Causal or influencing factors	*Text:* ■ *The patient reports low back pain and stiffness* ■ *during ventral flexion.* ■ *There are no contraindications today to further movement testing.* ■ *The symptom-altering region is the lower lumbar spine, especially the segment L5–S1,* ■ *which has restricted mobility during ventral flexion* ■ *due to capsuloligamentous shrinkage.* ■ *In addition there is hypermobility in dorsiflexion of the lower lumbar spine which provokes an unpleasant pulling sensation if the movement is continued passively.*
Trial treatment	■ *5-minute intermittent traction applied to L5–S1, after which the patient reports improved symptoms during ventral flexion.* ■ *This is followed by 5-minute specific grade III traction applied to L5–S1, after which the patient says he feels additional improvement during ventral flexion.* ■ *Finally, 5-minute traction applied to the zygapophyseal joints of L5–S1, after which the patient says he feels additional improvement during ventral flexion, although dorsiflexion is somewhat more painful.*
Physical therapy diagnosis	*Hypomobility of L5–S1 during ventral flexion*
Treatment plan with treatment goal and prognosis	■ *After initial pain-relieving traction on L5–S1, continue mobilization of this segment with grade III traction applied in relation to the intervertebral disk plane. To prevent stress on the intervertebral disk, which is unavoidable during traction on the zygapophyseal joints, first traction should be applied in relation to the intervertebral disk plane. To enhance the effectiveness of this technique, the segment may be placed in ventral flexion before performing traction.* ■ *Treatment goal: pain-free physiological mobility.* **(Further information on examination and treatment techniques may be obtained by attending further education.)**
Treatment with periodic control tests	
Final examination	

15.5   Thoracic Spine

(Columna dorsales)

15.5.1   Anatomy

■ Intervertebral Disk Connection

Joint type: synchondrosis

Joint surface: the top and bottom vertebral end-plates move in the same direction as the vertebral body

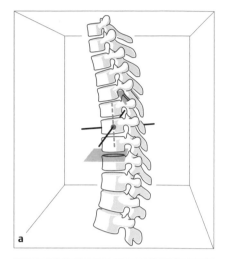

■ Zygapophyseal Joint (Articulatio zygoapophysealis)

Joint type: plane joint (nearly flat gliding joint; arthrodial joint)

Joint surface: nearly flat; in manual therapy the inferior articular process is considered concave

> **!** The joint surfaces are directed about 60° superiorly in relation to the upper vertebral end-plate; and they are directed 20° medially in relation to a frontal plane through the vertebral body so that the inferior articular process "faces" ventrally and slightly medially.

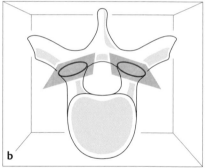

Resting position: physiological kyphosis

Close packed position: end-range, uncoupled movement

Capsular pattern: not described

Fig. 15.47 a, b

15.5.2   Rotational Tests

■ Testing Nerve Mobility

Mechanical compression of thoracic spinal nerves causes belt-like radicular symptoms around the trunk such as pain and paresthesia. Motor problems can affect the intercostal and abdominal muscles as well as the thoracic portion of the autochthonous back muscles.

The therapist should note any symptoms which may be caused by compression of the spinal cord or blood vessels. These are characterized by disruption in the conduction pathways affecting the lower extremity. Therapists must specifically search for and ask the patient about paresthesia, motor deficits, and autonomic nervous system symptoms in the legs. Bilateral—symmetrical or asymmetrical—appearance in particular raises the suspicion of a problem affecting the spinal cord. Autonomic nervous system symptoms caused by thoracic spine dysfunction are also very common. This may occur due to direct mechanical irritation of autonomic nerve fibers in the spinal nerve or directly in the sympathetic chain which runs near the costotransverse joints. Autonomic symptoms can also occur with spinal cord disorders, especially involving the sympathetic nuclei in the thoracic portion of the spinal cord (about C8/T1 to L2). Mechanical dysfunctions—especially involving the thoracic spine—may also disrupt autonomic nervous system equilibrium via afferent nociceptive fibers and are probably the most common cause in the thoracic spine of neurovegetative disorders.

Direct movement of the thoracic spinal nerves is possible only to a limited extent because they end in the trunk wall. Yet the nerves of the lower and upper extremities may be used to move the dura mater in the thoracic spine region. If irritation is present, the patient's symptoms will change with caudal tension on the dura via leg movements, or cranial tension via arm movements.

The mobility of neural structures is again tested in the position in which the symptoms are usually the strongest. If the patient has thoracic symptoms when standing, then the test is performed in a similar fashion as the lumbar spine test.

When sitting on the treatment table the patient should allow him or her self to "slump." Next the patient moves the cervical spine forward and then extends the knees (first one after the other and then possibly together). Finally, he or she raises the tips of the toes to maintain the dorsiflexion in the ankle joint. In order to further increase the tension in the neural structures, the upper extremity may also be positioned so as to lengthen its neural structures—in the example (**Fig. 15.48**), the median nerve.

❗ The movement components should be performed one after the other with caution. If symptoms are caused by neural structures, no additional components of the test should be performed.

The complex final position places the neural structures under a significant amount of tension. Every therapist should feel the test on themselves before performing it on a patient.

If the test results are positive, caution must be exercised. The therapist should perform a thorough clinical examination of the nervous system. If there are positive neurological symptoms and signs which are triggered by the thoracic spine region, the patient's physician should be informed.

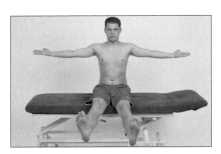

Fig. 15.48

■ Active Movements

For symptom provocation, the patient is again placed in the position in which he or she normally feels the symptoms most strongly. From a mechanical standpoint, it is best to have the patient sitting for the test. In this position the thoracic spine may be moved in a simple fashion to end-range positions without moving the upper body's center of gravity too far from the lumbar spine, which would place it under more stress. The patient is then asked to place each hand on the opposite shoulder. For ventral flexion, the patient then pulls both shoulders perpendicularly downward toward the hip joints. For dorsiflexion the patient raises his or her sternum anteriorly and superiorly. For lateral flexion, the patient moves

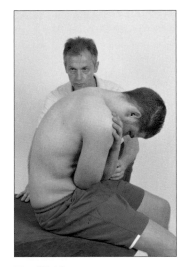

Fig. 15.49

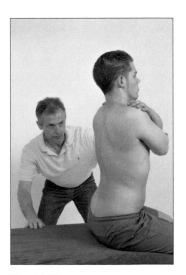

Fig. 15.50

one shoulder vertically down toward the ipsilateral hip. And for rotation, it is usually sufficient to ask patients to twist their upper body.

The following findings are commonly observed:

- Ventral flexion:
  readily possible, although different regions have more movement (often too much),
- Dorsal flexion:
  often significantly limited, especially in the upper and mid thoracic spine (often too little)
- Lateral flexion:
  occurs mainly in the lower to mid thoracic spine (physiological if there is a harmonious transition to the adjacent regions)
- Rotation:
  occurs mainly in the lower thoracic spine (physiological if there is a harmonious transition to the adjacent regions)

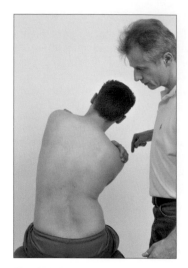

Fig. 15.51

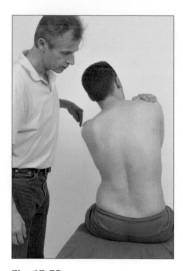

Fig. 15.52

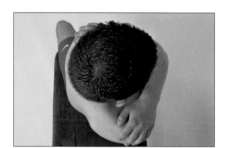

Fig. 15.53

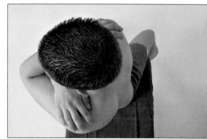

Fig. 15.54

■ Active and Passive Movement Testing (Quantity and Quality)

a) **Ventral flexion** from the zero position:

- The patient is seated on a wedge-shaped cushion or on the edge of the treatment table. This allows for easier pelvic anteversion, increasing the amount of lumbar lordosis which diminishes transmission of forward flexion of the thoracic spine to the lumbar spine. The therapist stands alongside the patient and asks him or her to pull their shoulders perpendicularly downward and <u>actively</u> bend the thoracic spine as far forward as possible.
- Next, with his dorsal hand the therapist stabilizes the patient's upper lumbar spine. His ventral hand grasps the contralateral shoulder. The therapist's ventral axilla or shoulder is placed against the patient's shoulder on the same

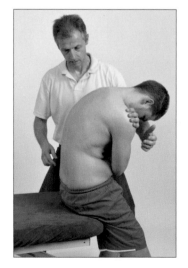

Fig. 15.55

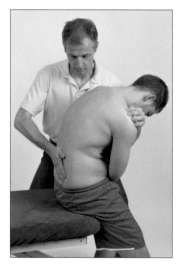

Fig. 15.56

side. With this grip, the therapist takes over the movement and presses both shoulders further straight down. This allows one to test whether the movement continues passively and how the end of movement feels.

- If there is a good relationship between the strength of the therapist and the patient's weight and size, the movement may also be performed passively through the entire range of movement and the end-feel may be tested.

Physiological end of movement or end-feel: firm and elastic

b) **Dorsiflexion** from the zero position:

- The patient is seated on the end of the treatment table with his or her feet on a stool. Maximum hip flexion enhances retroversion of the pelvis and thus ventral flexion of the lumbar spine. This reduces transmission of the dorsiflexion of the thoracic spine to the lumbar spine. The more the patient leans forward and is held there by the therapist, the greater the stability of the lumbar spine is for extension.
- The therapist stands alongside the patient and asks him or her to lift their sternum anteriorly and superiorly in order to <u>actively</u> bend the thoracic spine as far back as possible.
- Next, the therapist uses his dorsal hand to stabilize the upper lumbar spine. His ventral hand grasps the contralateral shoulder of the patient. The ventral shoulder of the therapist rests from anterior and inferior against the patient's shoulder on the same side. The patient's elbow closest to the body rests in the crook of the therapist's arm. With this grip, the therapist takes over the movement and, via the patient's elbow closest to the body, pushes dorsally and cranially, causing extension of the thoracic spine. The therapist uses the patient's shoulders to control the other movement components. In this manner he tests whether the movement of the thoracic spine <u>continues passively</u> and how the <u>end of movement</u> feels.
- If there is a good relationship between the strength of the therapist and the patient's weight and size, the movement may also be performed <u>passively</u> through the entire range of movement and the <u>end-feel</u> tested.

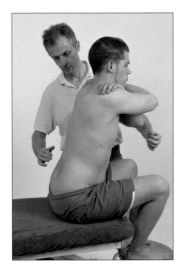

Fig. 15.57

Physiological end of movement or end-feel: firm and elastic, often very firm and less elastic

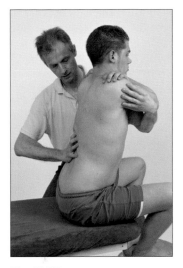

Fig. 15.58

! For maximum end-range movement and evaluation of the end of movement or end-feel, it may be necessary to place the stabilizing hand on the lower, middle, or upper portion of the thoracic spine. This can also allow for targeted movement in each region.

c) **Lateral flexion** from the zero position:

- The patient should be seated on a horizontal or anteriorly tilted surface, depending on which position allows the lumbar spine to best be held in its mid-position.
- The therapist stands on the side toward which the patient will bend laterally. The patient is asked to move the shoulder on that side perpendicularly down toward the hip joint to <u>actively</u> bend the thoracic spine sideways as far as possible.
- Next, the therapist places the thumb of his dorsal hand on the opposite side of the spinous process at L1. This grip enables him to control when the lateral flexion of the thoracic spine reaches the lumbar spine. The fingers rest on the lateral trunk to stabilize the hand. The ventral hand grasps the contralateral shoulder. The ventrally located axilla of the therapist is placed on the patient's shoulder on the same side. With this grip the therapist takes over the movement and presses the ipsilateral shoulder further downward. In this fashion he tests whether the movement <u>continues passively</u> and how the <u>end of movement</u> feels.
- If there is a good relationship between the strength of the therapist and the patient's weight and size, the movement may also be performed <u>passively</u> through the entire range of movement and the <u>end-feel</u> tested.

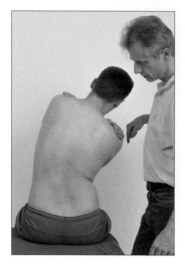

Fig. 15.59

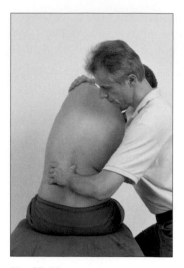

Fig. 15.60

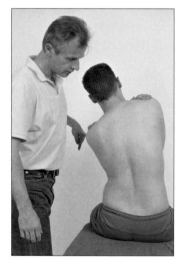

Fig. 15.61

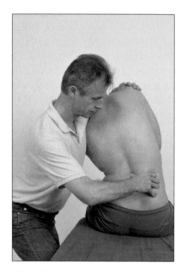

Fig. 15.62

Lateral flexion should be performed to both sides.

Physiological end of movement or end-feel: firm and elastic

d) **Rotation** from the zero position:

- The patient is still sitting on a horizontal or tilted surface, depending on which position allows the lumbar spine to best be held in its mid-position. The therapist stands on the side to which rotation will be performed. He asks the patient to place each hand on the opposite shoulder and <u>actively</u> rotate their torso as far as possible.
- Next, the therapist takes the patient's upper body with his ventral hand on the patient's opposite shoulder, and with his ventral shoulder he supports the patient's ipsilateral shoulder from anterior. The thumb of his dorsal hand is on the opposite side of the spinous process of L1 and his fingers rest on the sides of the trunk. Then he tests whether the movement <u>continues passively</u> and how the <u>end of movement</u> feels.
- If there is a good relationship between the strength of the therapist and the patient's weight and size, the movement may also be performed <u>passively</u> through the entire range of movement and the <u>end-feel</u> tested.

Rotation should be performed to both sides.

Physiological end of movement or end-feel: firm and elastic

❗ All movements might also be performed in a smaller region of the thoracic spine by placing the fixating hand more cranially, such as at the level of approximately T5, for example.

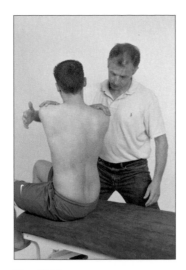

Fig. 15.63

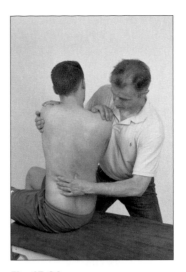

Fig. 15.64

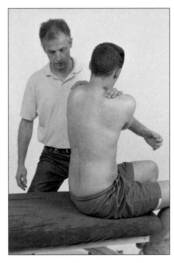

Fig. 15.65

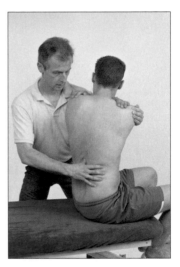

Fig. 15.66

15.5.3 Translatoric Tests

■ Intervertebral Disk Connection

Traction:

The patient is on a low seat in the position in which his or her symptoms just begin. The hands are resting on opposite shoulders. The therapist stands in a lunge behind the patient and with his hands folded, he grips the patient's elbow that is closest to the body (or both elbows simultaneously). The therapist's arms are lying on the lateral aspects of the patient's shoulders. Next, the therapist stretches his knees to perform end-range elevation of the patient's shoul-

der girdle. Now he shifts his weight onto his back leg without bending his knees. This pulls the patient's shoulder girdle backward in a straight line in space. The shoulder girdle pulls the uppermost thoracic vertebra along via the first rib, and the relief of weight has a traction effect. A minimal range of movement is sufficient for traction. The patient should not be moved too far backward, as the fear of falling increases muscle tension and prevents the effects of traction.

If symptoms only occur with elongation of the neural system, then traction should be performed in that position. For instance, in the slump-test position patients may support themselves on outstretched arms to relieve the weight of the thoracic spine (and lumbar spine) in the direction of traction. This method of self-traction is also the preferred technique if the therapist cannot or does not wish to perform passive traction. Adding lateral thoracic spinal flexion as well changes the length of the sympathetic chain: the contralateral side lengthens and the ipsilateral side relaxes.

The therapist should especially note any change in symptoms.

Physiological end-feel:
firm and elastic (difficult to feel)

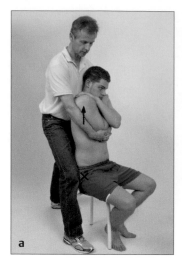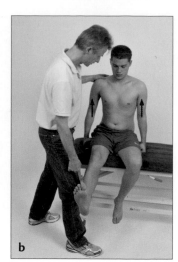

Fig. 15.67 a, b

Compression:

The patient is sitting in a position just before where he or she feels pain. The therapist stands behind the patient, places both hands on their upper ribs and presses them caudally. The force applied is transferred via the first rib to the uppermost thoracic vertebra and thus to the entire thoracic spine. In patients with extreme kyphosis, pressure applied perpendicularly downward often causes ventral flexion of the thoracic spine. In such patients, the therapist should support the thoracic spine with his own body and allow the compression pressure from anterior and superior to have an effect so that it arrives parallel to the longitudinal axis of the thoracic spine. Alternatively, the release after performing self-traction may be used as a compression test.

The therapist should especially note any change in symptoms.

Physiological end-feel:
firm or hard and elastic

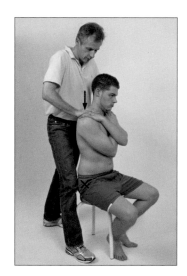

Fig. 15.68

> **!** If the test of neural mobility was positive, traction and compression should be performed in the position in which the patient just begins to feel symptoms, for example, sitting with knee extension and ankle joint dorsiflexion.

■ Zygapophyseal Joints

Traction and compression:

The patient should be lying in the prone position. A firm cushion is placed underneath the abdomen and chest to support the lumbar spine and thoracic spine and to hold them in the resting position. The head piece of the treatment table is tilted slightly downward. The therapist stands caudally and laterally and places the index and middle fingers of his medial hand at the level of the articular process or the origin of the transverse process of T12 on both sides. Skin tension should be prevented. The ulnar border of his lateral hand is resting on the fingernails of both fingers and he applies pressure ventrally and slightly caudally. The idea is that this causes the superior articular processes of T12 to move away at a right angle to the treatment plane from the inferior articular processes of T11, producing traction in both zygapophyseal joints. At the same time, the inferior articular processes of T12 are pressed against the superior articular processes of L1 causing compression in the caudal segment. This notion of what happens mechanically has not yet been tested. The important thing

for the therapist is what he senses during the test as well as the response of the patient.

In this manner the vertebrae are tested one by one, moving cranially to test traction in the cranial segment and compression in the caudal segment. In the direction of pressure, one must take into account the altered position of the joint surfaces in space due to thoracic spine kyphosis. As a rough guide, the cranial forearm, which determines the direction of the force application, should always be at a right angle to the thoracic spine (and directed slightly caudally). Depending on the orientation of the articular surfaces of the zygapophyseal joints, these movements may not always be 100% at a right angle to the treatment plane. It is also possible that extension might occur during this test as in the lumbar spine.

The therapist should again note the quantity of movement, its quality including end-feel, and any change in symptoms. The movement should be slightly springy (elastic) and should be repeated until the first stop and then performed slowly until the therapist senses the end-feel or if the patient's symptoms change.

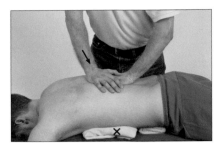

Fig. 15.69

This test is also known as the "springing test"—but not because the patient should spring off the bench with pain!

> **!** As regards the springing test, see also the note in the section on the costal joints on simultaneous compression of the costotransverse joint. When the patient is in the prone position, application of pressure on the thoracic spine or ribs from dorsal to ventral places stress on the ribs. In patients with predisposing factors, such as osteoporosis, excessive pressure carries a risk of fracture.

Physiological end-feel:
firm and elastic

15.5.4 Treatment of Capsuloligamentous Hypomobility

■ Traction in Relation to the Intervertebral Disk Plane: General Traction in the Supine Position

The patient should be in the supine position with his or her legs bent so that there is ventral flexion of the lumbar spine with hip joint flexion.

To apply traction on the lower and mid thoracic spine, the therapist places a long belt around the patient's thorax at the level at which traction should start. The other end of the belt is looped around the therapist's pelvis. The patient's arms are crossed over his or her chest, which enables the thoracic spine to be more easily preposi-

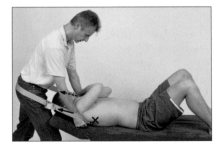

Fig. 15.70

tioned in flexion. The therapist stands in a lunge with his weight on his back leg which transfers the traction through the belt to the thoracic spine.

It is impossible to use a belt on the upper thoracic spine because the arms

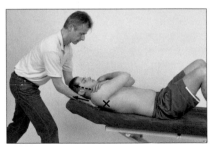

Fig. 15.71

are in the way. To perform traction there, the therapist places his fingertips on both sides of the spinous process at the level of the transverse process of the vertebra. Next he bends his fingers, which increases the contact between the fingers and the transverse process, and pulls the vertebra cranially causing traction caudally from this point.

This traction technique (grade I–II) relieves pressure and is thus especially useful for acute compression symptoms.

! Before performing this traction technique to treat neural compression symptoms affecting the thoracic spine, the therapist must ensure that the patient's physician is aware that the technique will be performed and has agreed to the procedure. Compression of the thoracic spine may be—or become—dangerous (even resulting in paraplegia). Clinical experience with this type of traction is very limited. The treatment of neural compression involving the thoracic spine should therefore be discussed within an expert team.

Application of Traction to the Zygapophyseal Joints

Pain-relieving traction may be performed using the test technique applied in the springing test. A mobilization wedge may be used for mobilization rather than the fingers. The middle finger is used to palpate in the groove in the wedge between the two spinous processes. For grade III mobilization, the patient is best placed in the supine position. The hand nearest the therapist is placed on the opposite shoulder so that his or her elbow is in the median plane. The other hand supports the neck and head. The therapist, who is standing laterally, turns the patient onto the side so that their back is off the table. Next, he identifies the segment that is to be mobilized. His medial hand is in contact with the articular or transverse process of the caudal vertebra. Its thenar eminence is tensed (= "hardened") and placed against the articular process or transverse process. Its index finger is extended and out of the way. The remaining three fingers are in maximum flexion, so that the other articular process or transverse process will come to rest on the second phalanges. To prevent end-range pain in the flexed fingers during mobilization, it is advisable to hold a firmly rolled tissue or similar padding between them.

Next, the therapist rolls the patient back into the supine position. He uses his sternum to press the patient's elbow down toward the abdomen to maintain the kyphotic position of the thoracic spine.

Next, the patient is instructed to exhale and relax. The mere weight of the upper body is often sufficient

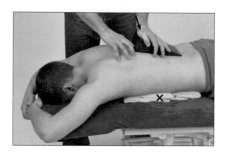

Fig. 15.72

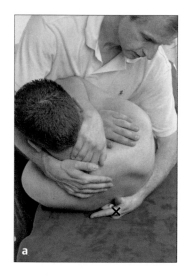

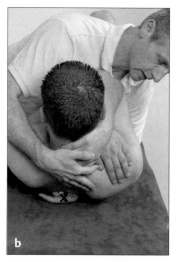

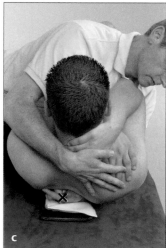

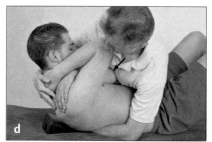

Fig. 15.73 a–d

for grade III mobilization. More intense mobilization may be achieved by applying a cranially and dorsally directed force to the elbow in the direction of the longitudinal axis of the patient's upper arm.

If the patient's upper body is too large or the therapist needs more distance, then the lateral hand on the therapist's side may be placed under the vertebrae and the movement guided by pressure of the medial hand on the elbow. Before the therapist increases the intensity of this mobilization with pressure from the sternum, he should place a sandbag or wedge underneath his fist. This gets his hand closer to the spinal column and the pressure is increased.

> **!** It is crucial to maintain the kyphosis of the thoracic spine. The technique may otherwise be painful if the patient lies on the therapist's fist in a position of extreme dorsiflexion. If the contact between the fist and the transverse process causes too much discomfort, a wider surface to lie on must be found or the soft tissues must be first massaged or otherwise treated to reduce the pain.

Alternative technique:

Instead of using the fist, a mobilization wedge may be placed in such a manner that both articular or transverse processes of the caudal vertebra are on the upper edge of the wedge. The spinous processes are in the groove of the wedge and not it contact with the underlying surface. Using the middle finger of his cranial hand, the therapist palpates the movement between the spinous processes of the target segment. The forearm of his cranial hand may also support the patient's head. His caudal hand controls the amount of kyphosis of the thoracic spine through the elbow. Especially in patients with more pronounced kyphosis, a second wedge must often be placed underneath the first to move it closer to the thoracic spine and increase the intensity of the treatment.

These techniques are especially indicated in patients with thoracic spine hypomobility.

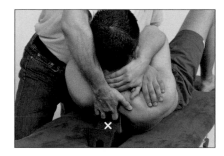

Fig. 15.74

Thoracic spine	
Symptoms	
Symptom-altering direction	
Contraindications?	Nervous system: ■ Mobility ■ Impulse conduction Other:
Symptom-altering segment region	
General assessment of adjacent joints and affected spinal region	

Active movements, comparing sides	

Rotational tests	Active	Continues passively?	Passive	End of movement / end-feel	Symptoms/ pain	Comments
■ Ventral flexion						
■ Dorsal flexion						
■ Lateral flexion, right						
■ Lateral flexion, left						
■ Rotation, right						
■ Rotation, left						
■ Combined movements						

Translatoric tests	Quantity	Quality	End-feel	Symptoms/pain	Comments
■ Traction, intervertebral disk plane					
■ Compression, intervertebral disk plane					
■ Traction (and compression) zygapophyseal joints					

Summary Formulation aid: ■ Symptoms ■ Direction ■ Contraindications ■ Site (joint) ■ Restricted mobility, hypermobility, or physiological mobility ■ Structure: muscle, joint, etc.	*Text:*

Continued ▸

Documentation Template: Practice Scheme (Continued)

Thoracic spine	
Trial treatment	
Physical therapy diagnosis	
Treatment plan with treatment goal and prognosis	
Treatment with periodic control tests	
Final examination	

Documentation: Practice Example

Pain in thoracic spine	
Symptoms	*Pain in mid thoracic spine when "sitting upright," which the patient has been trying to do since attending a course on back training exercises 7 weeks earlier.*
Symptom-altering direction	*Dorsiflexion*
Contraindications?	Nervous system: *No findings* ▪ Mobility ▪ Impulse conduction Other: *No findings*
Symptom-altering joint	*Thoracic spine*
General assessment of adjacent joints and affected spinal region	*The patient has a strongly rounded back with an increased curvature of the mid thoracic spine. The lower lumbar spine is markedly hypermobile during dorsiflexion.*

Active movements, comparing sides						
Rotational tests	**Active**	**Continues passively?**	**Passive**	**End of movement / end-feel**	**Symptoms/ pain**	**Comments**
▪ Ventral flexion	*No findings*	*ca. 10°*	*No findings*	*Firm and elastic*	*None*	*Tested with the patient sitting*
▪ Dorsal flexion	*Clearly hypo 1–2*	*Almost none*	*Increased resistance to movement*	*Very firm and elastic*	*Triggers reported pain*	*Especially in middle region of thoracic spine*
▪ Lateral flexion, right	*Slightly hypo 2–3*	*< 5°*	*Slightly increased resistance to movement*	*Firm and elastic*	*None*	
▪ Lateral flexion, left	*Somewhat hypo 2–3*	*< 5°*	*Slightly increased resistance to movement*	*Firm and elastic*	*None*	

Continued ▶

Pain in thoracic spine					
▪ Rotation, right	*No findings*	*ca. 10°*	*No findings*	*Firm and elastic*	*None*	
▪ Rotation, left	*No findings*	*ca. 10°*	*No findings*	*Firm and elastic*	*None*	
▪ Combined movements	*Not tested today*					

Translatoric tests	Quantity	Quality	End-feel	Symptoms/pain	Comments
▪ Traction, intervertebral disk plane	*Hardly felt*	*Hardly felt*	*Hardly felt*	*No changes*	
▪ Compression, intervertebral disk plane	*No findings*	*No findings*	*Very firm*	*None*	
▪ Traction (and compression) of the zygapophyseal joints	*Generally hypo, esp. T7 (score: 2)*	*Increased resistance to movement*	*Very firm and elastic*	*Pressure applied to approx. T8 triggers the reported pain*	

Summary Formulation aid: ▪ Symptoms ▪ Direction ▪ Contraindications ▪ Site (joint) ▪ Restricted mobility, hypermobility, or physiological mobility ▪ Structure: muscle, joint, etc.	*Text:* ▪ *The patient has pain in the middle of the thoracic spine when attempting to sit upright.* ▪ *Movement in the direction of dorsiflexion triggers the reported pain.* ▪ *There are no contraindications today to further movement testing.* ▪ *The symptom-changing region is the mid thoracic spine, especially approx. T7,* ▪ *which is hypomobile* ▪ *due to capsuloligamentous shrinkage affecting the zygapophyseal joints.*
Trial treatment	▪ *5-minute pain-relieving intermittent grade I–II traction using the technique from the springing test, after which the patient reports less pain when trying to sit upright.* ▪ *This is followed by 3-minute long grade III mobilization of the approx. T7 segment with a mobilization wedge, which provides even stronger relief of pain when the patient is sitting.*
Physical therapy diagnosis	*See above*
Treatment plan with treatment goal and prognosis	▪ *After initial pain-relieving traction, continue grade III mobilization using a wedge, treating especially the pain-triggering segment approx. T7 as well as adjacent hypomobile segments.* ▪ *Treatment goal: pain-free physiological mobility.* **(Further information on examination and treatment techniques may be obtained by attending further education.)**
Treatment with periodic control tests	
Final examination	

15.6 | The Costal Joints

(Articulationes costales)

15.6.1 | Anatomy

▦ Costovertebral Joint

Joint type: plane joint (nearly flat gliding joint; arthrodial joint)

Joint surface: nearly flat; in manual therapy the head of the rib is considered slightly convex

> **!** The 1st, 10th, 11th, and 12th ribs each articulate with a single vertebral body. The remainder of the ribs is connected with two vertebral bodies and the intervertebral disk in between. The intra-articular ligament of the head of the rib divides each of these articulations into two compartments.

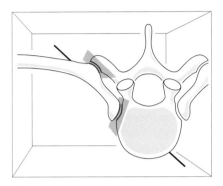

Fig. 15.75

▦ Costotransverse Joint

Joint type: plane joint (nearly flat gliding joint; arthrodial joint)

Joint surface: nearly flat; in manual therapy the articular surface of tubercle of rib is considered convex

> **!** This joint does not occur at the 11th or 12th rib.

▦ Sternocostal Joints

The costal cartilage forms the extension of the rib. It connects the 1st to 9th ribs—and in about one-third of people also the 10th rib—to the sternum. The 2nd to 5th ribs each form diarthroses (= true joints), while the 1st, 6th, and 7th are attached to the sternum by a synchondrosis. The 6th to 9th ribs are connected by their costal cartilages to each other by their interchondral joints and form the costal arch. The costal cartilages of the 11th and 12th ribs—and in two-thirds of people also the 10th rib—end at the abdominal wall and are called free ribs.

Resting position: the thorax is in the resting expiratory position, e.g., at the end of resting expiration

Close packed position: not described

Capsular pattern: not described

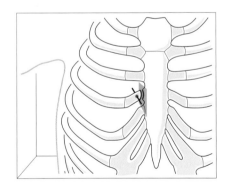

Fig. 15.76

Biomechanics

The mobility of the costal joints is the foundation for physiological respiratory mechanics. The level of mobility depends on the mobility of the costal joints and on the elasticity of the costal cartilage and of the ribs. The costal cartilages tend to ossify with increasing age with loss of elasticity.

All joints of a single rib move simultaneously—their movements are necessarily coupled. A movement axis passes through both costotransverse and costovertebral joints. Both joints are quite firm and primarily permit small gliding movements. Yet given its distance from the axis of rotation, there is considerable movement of the anterior end of the rib. In the upper region the axis is directed more toward the frontal plane and in the lower region more toward the sagittal plane. Inspiration thus tends to enlarge the sagittal diameter of the upper thorax and the transverse diameter of the lower thorax. This produces the visible raising of the sternum during inspiration forward and upward while the flanks move laterally.

The ribs curve in a semicircle from posterior to anterior and inferior. Because the posterior end of the rib is connected to the spine, and its anterior end to the sternum, a second, more sagittal movement axis may be placed through these two points. The anatomist Henry Gray compared this structure to that of a bucket handle (Gray 1901), the ribs being represented by the curved handle and the spinal column and sternum being where the handle attaches to the bucket. If one were to lift the handle, which may be compared to the movement of the rib that occurs during inspiration, the transverse diameter of the thorax would increase.

Because the two movement axes move slightly with motion, rather than staying in one place, simultaneous movement around two axes is possible.

In human beings, active movements of the ribs cause all ribs to move simultaneously. It is, however, possible to emphasize certain regions by altering the breathing: sternocostal breathing, infracostal breathing into the flank region, etc.

In general, the ribs can be moved passively further only in the direction of expiration, by compressing the thorax. This simultaneously tests the mobility of the costal joints and the elasticity of the costal cartilages and of the ribs.

The range of movement between two ribs may be palpated in the intercostal space while the patient inhales and exhales, or while the thoracic spine moves in lateral flexion. The intercostal space "opens" during inspiration or lateral flexion (on the convex side) and "closes" during expiration or lateral flexion (on the concave side). The range of movement is limited, however, especially in the upper thorax, and very difficult to sense. If the therapist is unable to feel much movement, this step should be skipped in the examination.

During the examination, the therapist should avoid asking the patient to *repeatedly* inhale and exhale deeply. Expelling large amounts of CO2 can cause hyperventilation due to respiratory alkalosis with low levels of carbon dioxide in the blood and dizziness, a tingling sensation affecting the hands and face, and muscle spasms, especially in the hands (= hyperventilation tetany with sharp flexion of the hands). To prevent hyperventilation, the therapist should ask the patient to exhale deeply. Inspiration occurs automatically at sufficient CO_2 levels in the blood. A short respiratory pause follows.

15.6.2 Rotational Tests

Testing Nerve Mobility

If there is suspicion of highly acute involvement of the nervous system, the therapist should test the thoracic spine as described in the section on the thoracic spine. The reader is referred to the appropriate section (p. 224).

■ Active Movements, Comparing Sides—Inspiration and Expiration

a) Observing respiratory movements:

The patient is first asked to take a few calm breaths and then to inhale and exhale once as deeply as possible. The therapist may stand back and observe the amount of movement, especially during resting respiration. Alternatively, the therapist may stand closer to the patient, especially in order to stimulate maximum inspiration and expiration and, if necessary, to illustrate the rib movement with his hands.

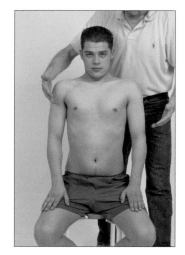

Fig. 15.77

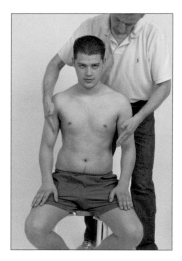

Fig. 15.78

In patients with hypomobility of the costal joints, one often observes the following:

- Inspiration:
  restricted elevation of the sternum and flanks, and increased protrusion of the abdomen
- Expiration:
  smaller decrease in the sagittal and transverse diameters of the thorax, stronger contraction of the abdomen

b) Palpation of respiratory movements:

- The therapist stands behind the seated patient and broadly palpates the rib cage during inspiration and expiration to get an idea of the general movements of the ribs. During expiration, the thorax may be compressed to test whether the movement continues passively. This provides information on the overall mobility of the joints and the elasticity of the ribs.
- Next, using a single finger, the therapist palpates the intercostal spaces, comparing sides, in the region in which the initial examination showed a potential problem. The therapist tests the difference in the distance between two ribs during respiration, comparing sides. To feel the greatest possible range of motion, in the caudal and middle regions the therapist primarily palpates laterally, and in the cranial region he palpates more ventrolaterally.

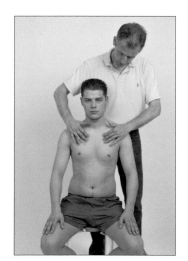

Fig. 15.79

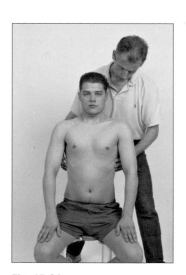

Fig. 15.80

- Up to this point, palpation has been during resting respiration. If a specific region has been identified with unusual movement, the therapist should ask the patient to inhale once as fully as possible. This increases the range of motion during inspiration and facilitates palpation. Immediately afterward, the patient should exhale as fully as possible and the therapist should palpate the range of motion during expiration.

Physiological end-feel during passive expiration: firm and elastic

■ Specific Movement Testing (Quantity and Quality)

Rib mobility during movement of the thoracic spine:

Because the active or passive movement of individual ribs is impossible, the therapist should palpate the movement of two ribs toward one another during movements of the thoracic spine. During lateral flexion, the ribs on the concave side of the thoracic spine move similarly to the movements during expiration, and on the convex side similarly to inspiratory movements.

The therapist should stand contralaterally to the seated patient who places each hand on the opposite shoulder. With his ventral hand, the therapist grasps the contralateral shoulder and supports the ipsilateral one with his body and ventral arm. With this grip

he leads the patient repeatedly into lateral flexion of the thoracic spine to the right and then to the left. The patient performs these movements actively. The palpating finger of the dorsal hand palpates the intercostal space on the lateral side of the thorax where the range of motion of the ribs is the greatest. In particular, the therapist should palpate the area in which the orienting examination has shown alterations in movement. At the uppermost ribs the movement may also be palpated during the primarily active flexion and extension of the thoracic spine. This palpation of movement is extremely difficult and may also be skipped.

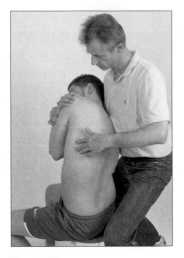

Fig. 15.81

> ❗ Students of manual therapy can easily practice palpation of this movement on themselves.

15.6.3 Translatoric Tests

Movements of the costovertebral joint in relation to the treatment plane are virtually impossible given the difficulty of the grip. The same is true for the joints connecting the ribs and sternum. Thus the following only discusses testing of the costotransverse joint, although this is associated with movements of the other two rib joints.

■ Traction on the Costotransverse Joint of the 1st to 10th Ribs

The patient is on a low seat with each hand placed on the opposite shoulder. The therapist stands contralaterally and with his ventral arm he grasps the shoulders of the patient to stabilize the starting position. Next he places the 2nd metacarpal head on the costal angle and pushes it ventrally and slightly laterally. Due to the orientation of the transverse costal facet, the force in the lower region is also directed slightly cranially and in the upper region slightly caudally.

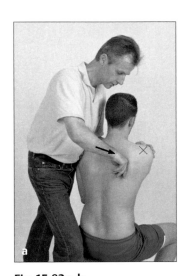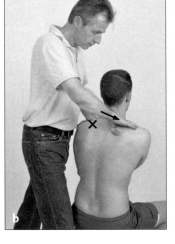

Fig. 15.82 a, b

To test the 1st rib in the resting position, the therapist holds the patient's sternum with his ventral hand. Pressure is applied by the 2nd metacarpal head ventrally, laterally, and slightly caudally. The force may be more caudally directed if necessary.

> ❗ The ventral hand is placed from above to prevent the thoracic spine from turning too far leftward. This may be enhanced by placing the patient in a position of right rotation beforehand.

Physiological end-feel:
firm and elastic

■ Compression of the Costotransverse Joint

Due to technical reasons, compression of the costotransverse joint is very difficult to perform. Theoretically the rib would have to be moved dorsally and slightly medially with a fixed thoracic spine – in the lower region it would in addition have to move slightly caudally and in the upper region cranially. This would be possible by applying force from ventral against the rib, although an uncertain amount of force would be absorbed by the elasticity of the ribs before reaching the costotransverse

joint. This technique is generally not performed.

In the springing test described in the section on the thoracic spine (p. 231), the patient is in the prone position and the ribs are held in place ventrally by the bench. The therapist presses a single thoracic vertebra ventrally. The transverse processes of a vertebra are pressed ventrally against the fixed rib, causing compression of the costotransverse joint. The reader is referred to the section on the springing test for further details.

If the springing test causes a change in symptoms, the possible involvement of the costotransverse joint should also be considered in addition to the thoracic spine. Additional specific movement tests of both regions should help find the difference.

■ Compression of the Costotransverse Joint of the 1st Rib

The above description also applies to compression of the joints of the 1st rib.

15.6.4 Treatment of Capsuloligamentous Hypomobility

■ Traction on the Costotransverse Joints of the 2nd to 10th Ribs in the Seated Patient

Pain-relieving treatment and grade III mobilization may be performed in the seated patient using the same technique as in the examination. The following alternative may be used to increase the intensity.

Alternative technique:

To reduce the accompanying rotation of the thoracic spine, the patient may be bent as far to the right as possible in the starting position with the grip as described above. This automatically rotates all thoracic vertebrae to the right (= coupled movement). Next, the therapist rotates the patient far enough to the left until there is a clear stop (= end of movement) of the thoracic spine (= uncoupled movement). The lateral flexion to the right must be maintained; this prevents the thoracic spine from rotating leftward—keeping it in the "locked position." The force is applied via the 2nd metacarpal head to the rib as described above.

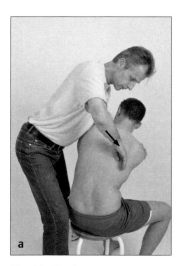 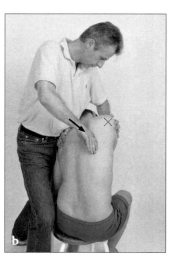

Fig. 15.83 a, b

! To develop a feeling for traction on the costotransverse joint and the uncoupled movements of the spine, it is advisable when practising to frequently alternate between both techniques, that is, with and without "locking" the thoracic spine. During the test, the therapist should note the movement quantity, quality, and end-feel, and any alteration in the patient's symptoms.

! In this position, with right lateral flexion of the thoracic spine and left rotation, the right rib is in the expiration position and the mobilization will improve expiration in particular. If the therapist moves the patient in left lateral flexion of the thoracic spine and right rotation, while holding his shoulder back, the right rib is in the inspiration position. This mobilization technique improves inspiration.

Physiological end-feel:
very firm and elastic (in the locked position)

■ Traction on the Costotransverse Joints of the 1st Rib in the Seated Patient

Pain-relieving treatment and grade III mobilization may begin in the resting position, as in the examination. For more intense grade III mobilizations, the patient is on a low seat with each hand resting on the opposite shoulder. The therapist stands contralaterally, grasps the patient's shoulders with his ventral arm and, emphasizing the upper region of the thoracic spine, bends the patient as far laterally to the right as possible. This causes automatic rotation all of the vertebrae to the right (= coupled movement). Next, the therapist rotates the patient leftward until there is a clear stop (= end of movement) of the thoracic spine. The lateral flexion to the right must be maintained. In this position the thoracic spine is prevented from rotating further leftward. Force is ap- plied via the 2nd metacarpal head to the 1st rib as described above. The cervical spine remains in the middle or resting position.

> **!** To develop a feel for traction on the costotransverse joint and uncoupled movements of the spine, it is advisable to alternate frequently during practice between both techniques, that is, with and without "locking" the thoracic spine. For both techniques the therapist pays attention to the movement quantity, quality, and end-feel, and any alteration in symptoms.

Physiological end-feel:
very firm and elastic (in the locked position)

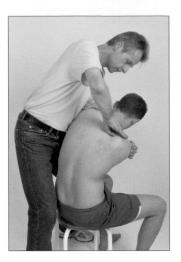

Fig. 15.84

Alternative technique:

If direct stabilization of the thoracic spine is not possible, and if the cervical spine is stable and pain-free, transmission of the movement to other segments may be limited by locking the cervical spine. The patient is again placed on a low seat. He or she should rotate the cervical spine to the side with the rib that is to be treated—in the example shown here, to the right. The therapist stabilizes the patient by placing his ventral forearm laterally against the patient's head. The soft part of his elbow stabilizes the lower cervical spine—especially C7—in rightward rotation. His fingertips rest lightly on the patient's head without applying pressure and bend it slightly (here to the left) in the cervical spine. In this position of rightward rotation and sidebending to the left, the lower cer- vical spine prevents the first thoracic vertebra from rotating further left; it is in the "locked position." Next, the therapist places the 2nd metacarpal head on the costal angle of the 1st rib and presses it ventrally, slightly laterally, and somewhat caudally.

> **!** This technique requires a stable cervical spine with no hypermobility. If that is not the case, we recommend the technique described above with "locking" of the thoracic spine in order to prevent transmission of movement to the first thoracic vertebra due to the uncoupled positioning of the thoracic spine.

Physiological end-feel:
very firm and elastic (if the cervical spine is stable)

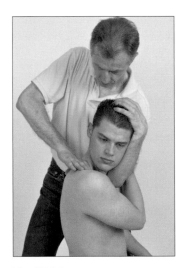

Fig. 15.85

■ Traction on the Costotransverse Joints of the 2nd to 10th Ribs in the Supine Patient

The patient is lying in the supine position. His or her hands are again resting on opposite shoulders. The arm on the side that is to be mobilized is crossed over the chest first, so that the scapula is in maximum abduction. The other arm is then crossed under the first one. The therapist stands laterally and rolls the patient toward him onto their side and places his tensed ("hardened") thenar eminence under the costal angle of the rib that is to be mobilized. Care should be taken that the thumb is placed lengthwise over a single rib rather than horizontally over several ribs. The tip of the thumb extends approximately to the spinous process line. The remaining fingers are loosely extended and the hand is held flat. With his cranial hand the

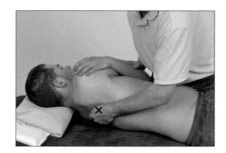

Fig. 15.86

therapist rolls the patient's torso onto his hand until his thenar eminence blocks the rib that is to be mobilized against the bench. If the upper body is then rolled further onto the fixating hand, there is further rotation of the thoracic spine—in the illustrated example, to the right—against the rib that is stabilized. During this, the transverse process moves away from the rib and there is traction on the

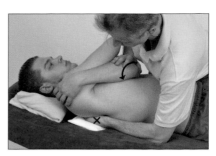

Fig. 15.87

costotransverse joint. To maintain this position for a longer time, the therapist may support himself on his contralateral elbow.

! The mobilization is more intense if the therapist places a sandbag or wedge under his hand which then gets closer to the rib.

■ Traction on the Costotransverse Joint of the 1st Rib in the Supine Patient

The patient is in the supine position. The hand on the mobilization side is placed on the contralateral shoulder. The therapist stands cranially and places the 2nd metacarpal head on the costal angle of the 1st rib and pushes it ventrally, slightly laterally, and rather caudally. The forearm of the mobilizing hand is lying on the edge of the bench, which it uses as a fulcrum for moving the hand forward and upward. The strength comes from the body which presses with the pelvis against the elbow. The other hand controls the patient's position or is used for support. The weight of the patient's own thorax is usually sufficient for fixation of the first thoracic vertebra. If necessary, simultaneously bending the thoracic spine laterally (to the right here) and rotating it in the opposite direction (to the left here) can prevent accompanying movement of the thoracic spine. Placement of a cushion under half of the thorax can help support this position of the thoracic spine.

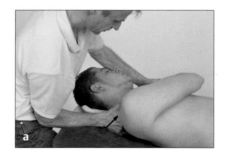

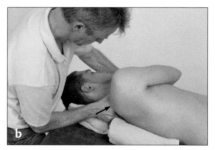

Fig. 15.88 a, b

Documentation Template: Practice Scheme

Costal joints	
Symptoms	
Symptom-altering direction	
Contraindications?	Nervous system: ▪ Mobility ▪ Impulse conduction Other:
Symptom-altering region	
General assessment of adjacent joints and the affected region	

Specific rotational tests	Active	Continues passively?	Passive	End-feel	Symptoms/ pain	Comments
▪ Inspiration						
▪ Expiration						
▪ Rib movements during inspiration with movement of the thoracic spine						
▪ Rib movements during expiration with movement of the thoracic spine						

Translatoric tests	Quantity	Quality	End-feel	Symptoms/pain	Comments
Traction, costotransverse joint					

Summary Formulation aid: ▪ Symptoms ▪ Direction ▪ Contraindications ▪ Site (joint) ▪ Restricted mobility, hypermobility, or physiological mobility ▪ Structure: muscle, joint, etc.	*Text:*
Trial treatment	
Physical therapy diagnosis	
Treatment plan with treatment goal and prognosis	
Treatment with periodic control tests	
Final examination	

Documentation: Practice Example

<table>
<tr><td colspan="7">Costal joints
(Pain on inspiration)</td></tr>
<tr><td>Symptoms</td><td colspan="6">Pain with inspiration in right mid thoracic region</td></tr>
<tr><td>Symptom-altering direction</td><td colspan="6">Elevation of the thorax during inspiration is less on the right side of the middle rib region than on the left. The pain occurs during inspiration even if the thoracic spine is held in slight flexion.</td></tr>
<tr><td>Contraindications?</td><td colspan="6">Nervous system: No findings
▪ Mobility
▪ Impulse conduction
Other: No findings</td></tr>
<tr><td>Symptom-altering region</td><td colspan="6">Middle ribs, right side</td></tr>
<tr><td>General assessment of adjacent joints and the affected region</td><td colspan="6">No findings</td></tr>
</table>

Specific rotational tests	Active	Continues passively?	Passive	End-feel	Symptoms/ pain	Comments
▪ Inspiration	*Right less than left, especially about the 4th rib*				*Provokes reported pain*	*Tested in the seated patient*
▪ Expiration	*No findings*	*Yes*	*No findings*	*Firm and elastic*		*None*
▪ Rib movements during inspiration with movement of the thoracic spine	*Limited on right between ca. 4th and 5th ribs*				*Provokes reported pain*	
▪ Rib movements during expiration with movement of the thoracic spine	*No findings*				*No findings*	

Translatoric tests	Quantity	Quality	End-feel	Symptoms/pain	Comments
Traction, costotransverse joint	*Hypo 2 at 4th rib*	*Increased resistance to movement*	*Very firm and elastic*	*Provokes reported pain*	

<table>
<tr><td>Summary
Formulation aid:
▪ Symptoms
▪ Direction
▪ Contraindications
▪ Site (joint)
▪ Restricted mobility, hypermobility, or physiological mobility
▪ Structure: muscle, joint, etc.</td><td>Text:
▪ Pain in right middle thoracic region
▪ during inspiration.
▪ There are no contraindications today to further movement testing.
▪ Symptom-altering joint is approx. 4th rib on the right side,
▪ which is hypomobile during inspiration

▪ due to capsuloligamentous restriction of the rib joint.</td></tr>
<tr><td>Trial treatment</td><td>▪ 5-minute pain-relieving traction on the costotransverse joint of the 4th rib in the seated patient, after which he reports less pain during inspiration.
▪ Next, 5-minute mobilizing traction on the costotransverse joint of the 4th rib in the supine patient, after which the patient reports a further decrease in pain during inspiration.</td></tr>
</table>

Continued ▶

Costal joints (Pain on inspiration)	
Physical therapy diagnosis	*See above*
Treatment plan with treatment goal and prognosis	▪ *After initial pain-relieving traction in the seated patient, continue mobilizing traction on the costotransverse joint of the approx. 4th rib in the supine patient.* ▪ *Treatment goal: pain-free physiological mobility (respiration).* **(Further information on examination and treatment techniques may be obtained by attending further education.)**
Treatment with periodic control tests	
Final examination	

15.7   Cervical Spine

(Columna cervicalis)

15.7.1   Anatomy

■ Lower Cervical Spine (C2–C7)

■ Intervertebral Disk Connection

Joint type: synchondrosis

Joint surface: the upper and lower vertebral end-plates move in the same direction as the vertebral body

■ Zygapophyseal Joint (Articulatio zygoapophysealis)

Joint type: plane joint (nearly flat gliding joint; arthrodial joint)

Joint surface: nearly flat; in manual therapy the inferior articular process is considered concave

> **!** The joint surfaces are tilted in relation to the upper vertebral plate by about 45° superiorly so that the inferior articular process "faces" ventrally and caudally.

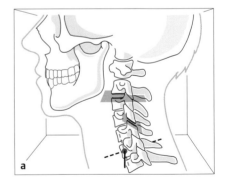

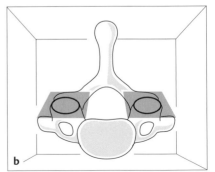

Fig. 15.89 a, b

Upper Cervical Spine (C0–C2)

Lateral Atlantoaxial Joints

Joint type: plane joint (not entirely flat gliding joint)

Joint surfaces: not entirely flat, but rather more ovoid: the superior articular facet of the axis is convex and the inferior articular facet of the atlas is also slightly convex. Both facets are cylindrical in cross-section and lie like wheels over each other.
The treatment plane is approximately parallel to a horizontal plane through the vertebra.

Median Atlantoaxial Joint

Joint type: pivot joint (articulatio trochoidea) consisting of a ventral compartment between the dens of the axis and anterior arch of the atlas (= diarthrosis) and a dorsal compartment between the dens of the axis and the fibrocartilaginous transverse ligament of the atlas (= bone–ligament joint with its own synovial capsule).

Joint surfaces: pass approximately in a frontal plane through the vertebral body. The dens is convex, while the corresponding surfaces on the anterior arch of the atlas and on the transverse ligament of the atlas are concave.

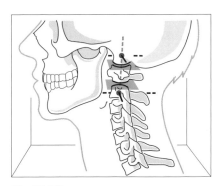

Fig. 15.90

> **!** Stability of this joint is crucial.

Atlanto-Occipital Joints

Joint type: ellipsoidal joint (Gray 1989)

Joint surfaces: the occipital condyles are convex while the superior articular facet of the atlas is concave.
The treatment plane is approximately parallel to a horizontal plane through the vertebra.

Resting position: physiological lordosis

Close packed position: end-range, uncoupled movement, i.e., for the lower cervical spine: lateral flexion with rotation in the opposite direction and for the upper cervical spine: lateral flexion with rotation in the same direction

Capsular pattern: not described

> **!** The lower and upper parts of the cervical spine act together in the orientation of the head in space. The C2–C3 segment is a key spinal segment. Dysfunction here influences both the lower and the upper cervical spine.

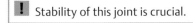

15.7.2 | Rotational Tests

Testing Nerve Mobility

The mobility of neural structures may be tested in the position in which the patient usually feels his or her symptoms most strongly. Because of gravity, symptoms are often stronger when upright than when lying down. Thus it is usually advisable to perform these tests in the standing or sitting patient, the latter being easier. We recommend allowing the patient to first perform active arm movements in order to lengthen the neural structures. The therapist should demonstrate these movements to the patient who may then be allowed to do them on their own. This simple test can already indicate the presence of larger lesions.

Active Movement for Maximum Elongation of Neural Structures of the Upper Extremities

The patient should be on a low seat with the cervical spine positioned just before where his or her symptoms begin. The therapist asks the patient to depress and retract their shoulders. Next, the patient performs the shoulder movements described in Figs. 15.94 to 15.96. The elbows should initially remain in a middle position between flexion and extension. The forearms, wrists, and fingers are moved into the end position. Finally, the elbows are also moved into end-range extension or flexion until symptoms occur or change.

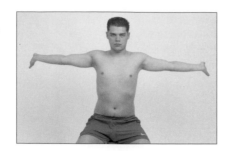

Fig. 15.91

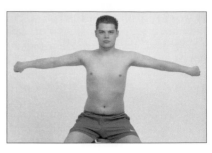

Fig. 15.92

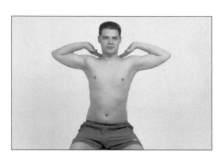

Fig. 15.93

> **!** A pulling or stretching feeling, often accompanied by a tingling sensation and warmth, is not uncommon in end-range movements of all joint components for a given nerve and often occurs before reaching the end position. This sensation is triggered by increased nerve tension with end-range movement and is physiological. Early onset of such sensations suggests that the neural structures are prematurely limiting the range of motion. Only if nerve mobility tests produce the reported symptoms or change them do they suggest that the neural structures may be related to the patient's symptoms. These should then be more closely examined and taken into consideration in further procedures.

> **Note**
> When one observes persons who wake up well-rested, they automatically stretch and reach out using typical arm movements. These roughly correspond to the joint positions in which the three major nerves of the upper extremity are elongated. The fact that the majority of people can clearly sense the tension on neural structures in the upper extremity—and in our "civilized" way of life are barely ever well-rested and thus do not stretch and move about in the morning—raises the intriguing question of a possible connection.

Median nerve:

The patient is seated on a stool. He or she holds the arm that is to be examined in the previously demonstrated position for elongation of the median nerve (see **Fig. 15.91**). The therapist stands laterally and behind the patient, supporting the patient's back with his own body. His medial elbow controls the depression and retraction of the patient's shoulder girdle. His forearm stabilizes the shoulder joint from ventral. His hand grasps the elbow and holds the abduction and external rotation in the shoulder joint. His lateral hand positions the movement components of the forearm (= supination), wrist (= dorsiflexion and ulnar abduction), and the three radial fingers (= extension). Next, the patient slowly extends their elbow and the therapist accompanies the movement. Then, for maximum effect the patient can bend and rotate the cervical spine to the contralateral side.

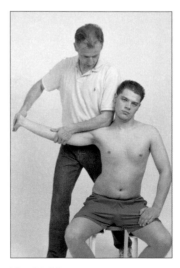

Fig. 15.94

Radial nerve:

The patient should be seated on a stool. He or she holds the arm that is to be examined in the previously demonstrated position for elongation of the radial nerve (see **Fig. 15.92**). The therapist stands laterally and behind the patient, supporting the patient's back with his own body. The elbow of the medial arm controls the depression and retraction of the shoulder girdle. His forearm stabilizes the shoulder joint from ventral.

His hand grasps the elbow and holds the shoulder joint in abduction and internal rotation. His lateral hand positions the movement components of the forearm (= pronation), wrist (= palmar flexion and ulnar abduction), and the three radial fingers (= flexion). Next, the patient slowly extends their elbow and the therapist accompanies the movement. Then, for maximum effect the patient can bend and rotate the cervical spine to the contralateral side.

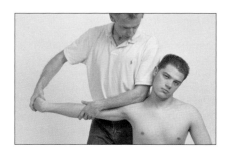

Fig. 15.95

Ulnar nerve:

The patient should be seated on a stool. He or she holds the arm that is to be examined in the previously demonstrated position for elongation the ulnar nerve (see **Fig. 15.93**). The therapist stands laterally and behind the patient, supporting the patient's back with his own body. The elbow of the medial arm controls the depression and retraction of the shoulder girdle. His forearm stabilizes the shoulder joint from ventral. His hand grasps the elbow and holds the shoulder joint in abduction and external rotation. His lateral hand positions the movement components of the forearm (= pronation), wrist (= dorsiflexion and radial abduction), and two ulnar fingers (= extension). Next, the patient slowly flexes their elbow and the therapist accompanies the movement. Then, for maximum effect the patient can bend and rotate the cervical spine to the contralateral side.

! Owing to the high sensitivity of the neural structures, these tests must be performed carefully and slowly. The patient should perform each of the movements on their own with the therapist guiding and supporting the movement. As soon as symptoms occur or change, movement in the symptom-altering direction should stop. However, one may try to alter joint positions further away from the site of symptoms in order to better differentiate between pain correlated to the musculoskeletal system or to the neural sytem. For instance, in patients with pain in the shoulder region, one could change the position of the wrist and cervical spine. If this changes the symptoms, they are probably related to the neural structures. Depending on the severity of symptoms, the therapist must decide whether to continue movement testing or whether it is contraindicated on that day and instead to perform a specific examination of the nervous system.

! After performing safety tests (see below), the foraminal compression test (see below) may be used to identify suspected spinal nerve compression in the cervical spine.

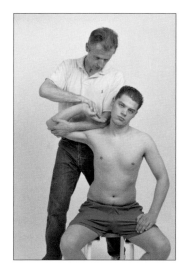

Fig. 15.96

■ Active Movements

The patient is typically seated (or possibly standing). The therapist should ask the patient to bend his or her head as far forward and backward as possible and to the right and left, and then to turn it in both directions. He should observe the head flexion/extension from the side as well as the lateral flexion from anterior and the rotation from above. The therapist may use his fingers to mark and compare the distance between the nose or chin and the acromion in the final position of rotation.

One often observes the following:

- Ventral flexion:
  more marked in the lower cervical spine and less so in the upper (often too little)
- Dorsiflexion:
  strong curve just above about C7 and then again stronger in the upper cervical spine (often too much)
- Lateral flexion:
  in the lower and upper cervical spine (physiological if there is a harmonious transition to the thoracic spine)
- Rotation:
  in the lower and upper cervical spine (physiological if there is a harmonious transition to the thoracic spine)

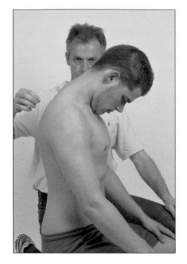

Fig. 15.97

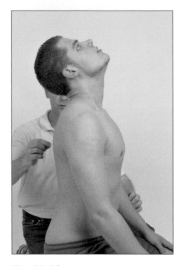

Fig. 15.98

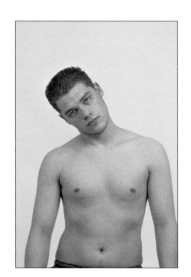

Fig. 15.99

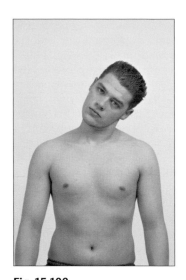

Fig. 15.100

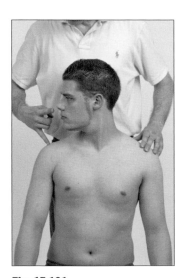

Fig. 15.101

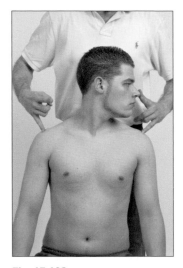

Fig. 15.102

■ Examples of Symptom Localization

If ventral flexion changes symptoms, simple active movement testing can help ascertain whether the lower or upper cervical spine is involved.

- First the patient is asked to draw their chin in toward the throat as far as possible while simultaneously drawing their head slightly backward. This produces flexion in the cervical spine, while the lower part remains still or tends to move in the opposite direction (= extension).
- Next the therapist asks the patient to push their chin far forward and then raise it slightly. This flexes the lower region of the cervical spine while the upper part is more extended.

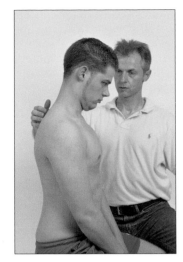

Fig. 15.103

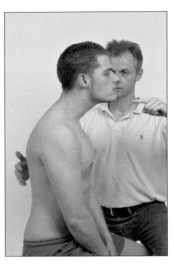

Fig. 15.104

If the first movement produces symptoms, but the second does not, then it is likely that the upper cervical spine is responsible. If the opposite is true, namely that the second movement triggers symptoms and the first does not, then it is likely that the lower region of the cervical spine is related to the patient's symptoms.

If forward bending of the cervical spine as a whole is painful, but not that of the upper or lower parts, then flexion of the middle cervical spine may correlate with the patient's symptoms. This portion bends only slightly during targeted ventral flexion of the upper or lower cervical spine.

If **dorsiflexion** causes symptoms, one may similarly test whether the lower or upper cervical spine is responsible.

- The patient should first be asked to push their chin far forward and then to slightly raise it. This produces extension in the upper part of the cervical spine with simultaneous flexion of the lower part.
- Next the therapist asks the patient to slightly shorten the distance between the chin and throat and to hold this position and then to draw the head backward. This causes extension in the lower cervical spine while the upper part remains neutral or flexed.

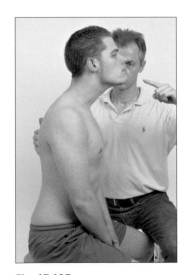

Fig. 15.105

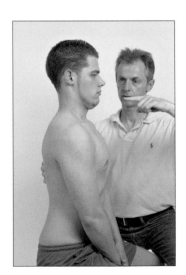

Fig. 15.106

Again, the upper cervical spine may correlate with the symptoms if the first movement produces them but the second does not. The lower cervical spine is probably related to the symptoms if the second movement provokes symptoms and the first does not.

If general dorsiflexion of the cervical spine is painful, while that targeting the upper and lower cervical spine is not, then, as in the previous example, one should consider the middle cervical spine.

These two examples are intended to illustrate how easily specific movements can be used to identify the symptom-provoking area that correlates with movement. Further tests for symptom localization may be obtained from appropriate further education courses.

Safety Tests

Before performing larger passive movements on the cervical spine, the therapist should look for any significant risks. These may arise due to lesions affecting vessels and/or instability of the cervical spine segments, especially in the upper cervical spine. Dreaded vascular complications include the release of a thrombus, which could travel to the brain and obstruct blood flow to the brain (Rivett et al. 2006). Instability can lead to spinal cord compression, and in the upper cervical spine to compression of the medulla oblongata, which contains life-sustaining centers for respiration and circulation.

All test movements should first be actively performed by the patient. Only if there are no symptoms or changes in symptoms may the therapist then carefully proceed with passive movements. This is the best way to avoid major damage if any lesions are indeed present.

! These safety tests can no more rule out the possibility of a coincidental injury than can a car's seatbelt prevent an accident completely. However, they can help therapists with prompt detection of significant problems.

The lowest-risk "safety test" is traction on C0–C1 and C1–C2 as described below (see p. 259). If the therapist senses an unusually high degree of movement, stability is possibly inadequate.

Test of the Vertebral Artery (and Internal Carotid Artery)

Prior to manipulation, it is advisable to test blood flow to the head. Decreased circulation and vascular lesions may occur due to manipulation or as a result of longer mobilizations or muscle stretching at the end of movement (Schomacher 2007). We therefore recommend testing circulation before performing any larger passive movements. This also applies to tests of craniocervical instability, which may be a cause of vascular lesions (Osmotherly and Rivett 2011).

It is important first to carefully question the patient about any minor blunt trauma such as a fall as well as manipulations, as these can damage the vertebral artery and other cervical arteries without causing any significant lesions of the cervical spine itself and corresponding sequelae (Inamasu and Guiot 2006). Dizziness is commonly considered to be a warning sign of vertebrobasilar insufficiency (Sweeney and Doody 2010). Yet one study reported that only 52% of patients examined had vertebrobasilar insufficiency; physiotherapists should therefore heed other subtle neurological symptoms and signs as well such as disorders of equilibrium, ptosis, and vision disturbances (Thomas et al 2011).

The usefulness of these tests is limited, however, because it is impossible to reliably evaluate the clinical risk of negative effects of treatment resulting from vascular complications (Moran and Mullany 2003; Kerry et al 2008). Pre-existing vascular risk factors and abnormalities found during the physical examination, including the "safety tests," can alert the therapist to potential risks (Rivett et al 2006; Kerry et al 2008). Rotation of the cervical spine significantly diminishes blood flow through the vertebral artery (Mitchell et al 2004), which is why it is recommended as a test movement. It is performed in the position of flexion/extension and/or lateral flexion in which the symptoms are most easily triggered with the least amount of risk. The easiest test movement, however, is the active movement with which patients can evoke the symptoms themselves.

It is difficult to distinguish circulatory disturbances from autonomic responses, which may occur with end-range movements of the cervical spine (Christe and Balthazard 2010) or the safety tests (Schomacher 2000). These symptoms—which are sometimes alarming, such as loss of consciousness—are harmless and pass without intervention.

A detailed consensus document on cervical examination of cervical artery dysfunction can be found at www.ifompt.org.

The patient should be seated on the end of the treatment bench. The therapist stands laterally and, as a precaution, holds his dorsal hand behind the patient's back. The patient is asked to actively slowly turn his or her head and to bend it backward and slightly laterally. This combination of movements should be performed to the right and to the left and held for a few seconds at the end. The therapist observes the patient's eyes and asks whether he or she experiences any discomfort such as dizziness, nausea, visual/hearing disturbances, or other such symptoms. Should symptoms like dizziness occur, the patient should stop the movement, remain in the position for a few seconds and then say whether the dizziness worsens (= crescendo dizziness) or improves (= decrescendo dizziness).

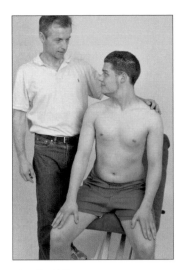

Fig. 15.107

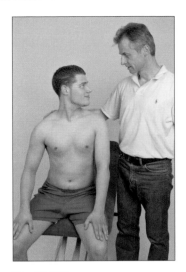

Fig. 15.108

! If the cause of dizziness is insufficient blood supply to the brain, the symptoms are progressive (= increasing)—just as in music when the volume increases during a crescendo. If, however, the afferent information triggered by the movement, for example, from the joints in the cervical spine, is causing the dizziness, then the symptoms will gradually subside once the movement stops—similar to a decrease in musical volume during a decrescendo.

This evaluation provides the therapist with essential information. If there are crescendo symptoms, any movement in the symptom-altering direction should be avoided and the treating physician should be informed. In decrescendo symptoms, the therapist should test using specific movements whether the disorder is caused by the cervical spine or other structures, like the inner ear (e.g., benign paroxysmal postural vertigo), which may be treated by the physical therapist (Wiemer 2011).

! The patient complaining of symptoms should be seated on the treatment bench so that in the event of dizziness or loss of consciousness he or she can easily lie down.

Test of the Alar Ligaments

Given its course from the posterolateral surface of the dens of the axis—passing obliquely ventrally, laterally, and cranially to the border of the foramen magnum in the occipital bone—bending the occiput laterally to the left places tension on the right alar ligament. This pulls on the dens of the axis rotating it to the left. Rotation to the left of the axis results and the spinous process of C2 moves to the right. If the alar ligament is insufficient, the movement of the spinous process of C2 is delayed during lateral flexion of the head. The therapist can feel this during the test movement.

Lateral movement of the spinous process of C2 may also be absent if lateral bending of the head does not occur in

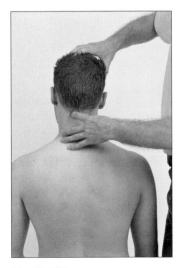

Fig. 15.109

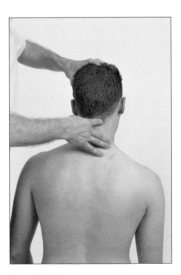

Fig. 15.110

the upper cervical spine, but rather in the lower portion. This is not a sign of insufficiency of the alar ligaments. The therapist must thus observe the patient's nose during the test, as this is approximately where the sagittal axis passes for lateral flexion of the upper cervical spine. If the patient's nose appears to remain in the same position during lateral flexion, then flexion is occurring in the upper cervical spine. If the patient's nose moves toward the bending side, then flexion is occurring more in the lower cervical spine.

The patient should be seated on a low seat while the therapist is standing laterally. His dorsal index finger palpates the spinous process of C2 on the contralateral side. His ventral hand guides the patient's head (using minimal force) in a small lateral bend toward the therapist. The test is performed to both sides.

> **!** As soon as the head bends to the side, the spinous process of C2 should move toward the opposite side while the patient's nose does not change its position in space.

Test of the Transverse Ligament of the Atlas

The transverse ligament of the atlas fixates the dens of the axis to the anterior arch of the atlas. This function is especially necessary for ventral flexion when the occiput first bends forward and then pulls the atlas with it. If the dens of the axis does not immediately follow the movement of the anterior arch of the atlas ventrally, the posterior arch of the atlas presses the medulla oblongata against the dens, which has remained in place. This results in CNS symptoms, which range from paravertebral tingling sensations (Lhermitte sign), paresthesia and/or weakness in both legs and/or arms (with compression of the ascending and descending pathways of the spinal cord) to nausea, respiratory or pulse rate changes, and other autonomous nervous system symptoms.

Instability of the transverse ligament of the atlas may occur, for instance, in inflammatory disorders such as primary chronic polyarthritis and Grisel syndrome, in children with Down syndrome, and after trauma such as sprains involving the cervical spine ("whiplash").

Manual testing to assess any hypermobility or instability between the atlas and axis are difficult and not entirely reliable scientifically (Cattrysse et al 1997). Thus we recommend a variation of the Sharp-Purser test, in which the therapist tries to sense mobility, but also should observe any change in the patient's symptoms.

The patient should be seated on a low stool or chair. He or she actively bends the head far enough forward that the symptoms just begin to be felt. In this tolerable and controllable position, the therapist, who is standing alongside, fixes the patient's head between his ventral hand and thorax or ventral shoulder. With the index finger and thumb of his dorsal hand, he carefully pushes the spinous process of C2 ventrally. The therapist should note whether he feels any movement and whether the patient's symptoms change.

> **!** Pressing the spinous process of C2 ventrally presses the dens of the axis forward toward the anterior arch of the atlas. If there is insufficiency of the transverse ligament of the atlas, this movement is possible. Symptoms which previously occurred due to compression of the medulla oblongata between the dens of the axis and the posterior arch of the atlas subside during this movement. Relief of symptoms is a sign of insufficiency of the transverse ligament of the atlas. If, in addition, the therapist senses the movement and even the hard impact of the dens of the axis against the anterior arch of the atlas, the suspicion of instability is strengthened.

With such findings, the patient should avoid ventral flexion and his or her physician should be informed.

If the test exacerbates the CNS symptoms, possible fracture of the dens of the axis or a similar problem should be considered. Again, the patient must avoid ventral flexion and his or her physician should be informed.

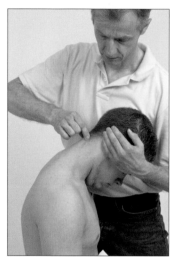

Fig. 15.111

Local tenderness without any CNS symptoms is not a sign of ligamentous instability, and the examination may proceed.

> **!** If the patient can perform maximum ventral flexion without symptoms, then the likelihood of highly acute instability symptoms is low. Nevertheless, momentary asymptomatic instability is still possible.

Symptoms may occur in the supine position as well, if C2 slides dorsally to C1. If this occurs, C2 should be pushed ventrally in this position. To do so, the therapist should place his index or middle finger (or guide the patient's finger) from dorsal on the spinous process of C2 and carefully push it ventrally. The test is done in the symptom-altering position.

▣ Foraminal Compression Test

If the patient's history of symptoms, protective posture, and tests of neural mobility are suggestive of nerve root compression at the intervertebral foramen, the size of the foramen may be further decreased in order to increase neural structure compression.

To perform this provocation test, the patient should be sitting on a low seat. He or she then bends the head backward, rotates it, and bends it to the same side until symptoms appear. The therapist stands contralaterally and with his dorsal hand fixes the thorax and thus the thoracic spine. His ventral hand is placed on the patient's head to perform additional axial compression of the cervical spine. His ventral forearm supports the patient's face from ventral and prevents the pressure from the hand from increasing the lateral flexion of the cervical spine. The test may be performed to both sides, taking care to observe the symptomatic side in particular.

The therapist's dorsal hand may also be placed on a vertebra and hold the

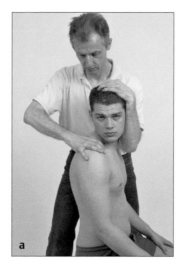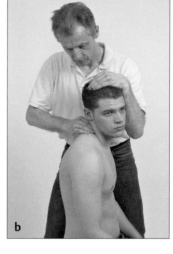

Fig. 15.112 a, b

cervical spine caudal to it in the resting position. His ventral hand again performs the movement, which now occurs cranial to the dorsal hand. The examination now focuses more on this region. One can test from cranial to caudal in this fashion until the symptom-altering region has been identified.

❗ The vertebral artery test, as well as the above-described stability tests, should have already been performed. In the vertebral artery test, the therapist should also look for the reported radiating pain, which must be radicular in order to be a sign of nerve root compression.

▣ Active and Passive Movement Testing (Quantity and Quality)

a) **Ventral flexion** from the zero position:

- The patient is sitting on a low seat, and the therapist is standing next to his or her shoulder. The therapist holds the patient's upper thoracic spine by placing the fingers of his dorsal hand contralaterally on the upper ribs and his thumb on the spinous process of about T1. The patient is asked to actively move their chin downward toward the sternum as far possible.
- Next the therapist takes the patient's head, which he grasps from the opposite side with his ventral hand, and slightly presses it against his ventral shoulder or thorax. With this grip he tests whether the movement continues passively.
- Without changing his grip, the therapist now moves the patient

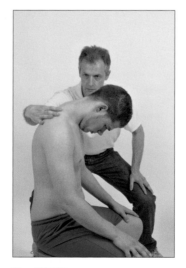

Fig. 15.113

back to the zero position. If indicated, he next moves from here again passively through the entire range of motion and tests the end-feel.

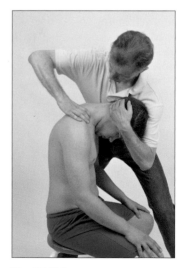

Fig. 15.114

Physiological end of movement or end-feel: firm and elastic

b) **Dorsiflexion** from the zero position:

- The starting position and fixation are the same. The patient is asked to bend their head <u>actively</u> back as far as possible.
- Next the therapist takes the patient's head with the grip described above and tests whether the movement <u>continues passively</u>.
- Without changing his grip, the therapist moves the patient back to the zero position. If indicated, he next moves from here again <u>passively</u> through the entire range of motion and tests the <u>end-feel</u>.

Physiological end of movement or end-feel: firm and elastic

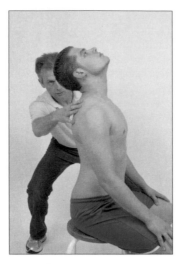

Fig. 15.115

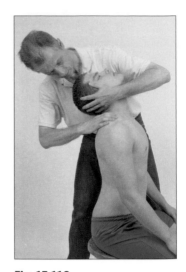

Fig. 15.116

c) **Lateral flexion** from the zero position:

- The therapist stands alongside the seated patient. The patient is asked to <u>actively</u> bend their head as far as possible to the side.
- Next the therapist takes the patient's head with the grip described above and tests whether the movement <u>continues passively</u>.
- Without changing his grip, the therapist moves the patient back to the zero position. If indicated, he moves from here again <u>passively</u> through the entire range of motion and tests the <u>end-feel</u>.

Lateral flexion should be performed to both sides.

Physiological end of movement or end-feel: firm and elastic

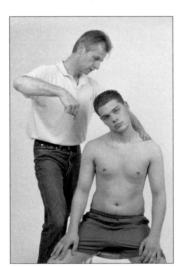

Fig. 15.117

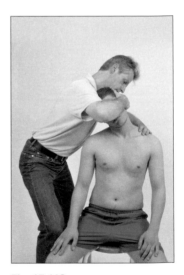

Fig. 15.118

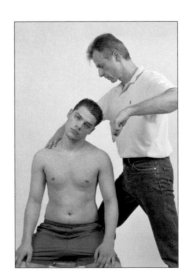

Fig. 15.119

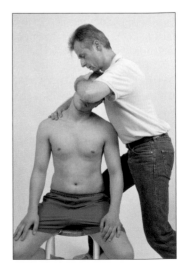

Fig. 15.120

d) **Rotation** from the zero position:

- The therapist stands laterally and behind the seated patient. The patient is asked to <u>actively</u> turn their head as far as possible to the side.
- Next the therapist takes the patient's head with the grip described above and tests whether the movement <u>continues passively</u>.
- Without changing his grip, the therapist moves the patient back to the zero position. If indicated, he moves from here again <u>passively</u> through the entire range of motion and tests the <u>end-feel</u>.

Rotation should be performed to both sides.

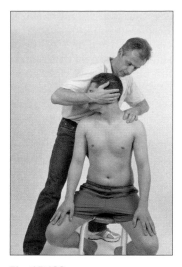

Fig. 15.121

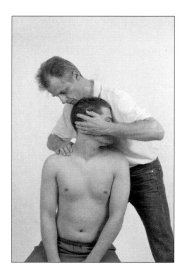

Fig. 15.122

> ! Increased care and attention is required when passively rotating beyond the active range of motion and beyond the first stop.

Physiological end of movement or end-feel: firm and elastic

> ! In the grip with the ventral hand around the patient's head, the therapist must take care not to crush the ear. He should cup his hand and place it around the ear in order to avoid placing any pressure directly on it.

In all movements it is important that the therapist himself also moves around the axes of the patient's cervical spine. The therapist should therefore start in a lunge, with bent knees, as this allows him to move as needed.

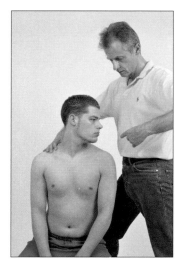

Fig. 15.123

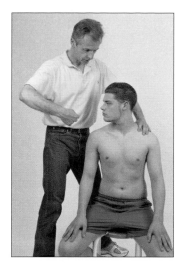

Fig. 15.124

> ! Moving both hands closer together the therapist can perform all these rotational tests with more specificity.

15.7.3 Translatoric Tests

■ Intervertebral Disk Connection

Traction:

The patient should be sitting on a low seat in the position in which he or she just begins to feel the symptoms. The therapist stands in a lunge behind the patient and places the balls of his thumbs on the patient's head under the ears. The patient's head thus rests in the "bowl" formed by the therapist's hands. The therapist's forearms lightly touch the patient's shoulders and help perform the technique in a steady and controlled manner. Next the therapist moves his elbows closer to the median plane which automatically lifts the patient's head at a right angle away from the treatment plane of the intervertebral disk, producing traction.

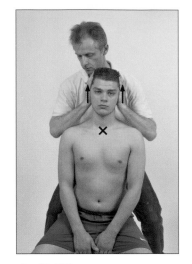

Fig. 15.125

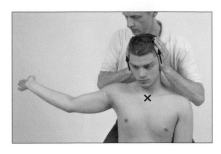

Fig. 15.126

The therapist should note any change in (neurological) symptoms in particular.

Physiological end-feel:
firm and elastic

Compression:

The patient should be seated and move until just before where the pain begins. The therapist stands behind him or her and places both hands on the patient's head. His forearms again lightly rest on the patient's shoulders to ensure proper control. Next the therapist presses the patient's head at a right angle toward the treatment plane of the intervertebral disk connection. This is also a simultaneous compression test between the occiput and atlas as well as between the atlas and axis.

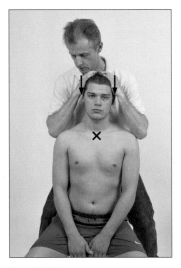

Fig. 15.127

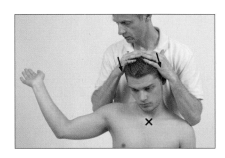

Fig. 15.128

The therapist should note any change in (neurological) symptoms in particular.

Physiological end-feel:
firm or hard and elastic

> **!** These general traction and compression tests don't give the therapist any information on the range of motion, but only whether the symptoms—especially neurological ones—change. If there is suspected neurological compression, traction and compression tests should be done in the position in which the patient feels his or her neurological symptoms. The therapist may then ask the patient to move the cervical spine correspondingly and to move their arm to the position that produces end-range movement of a nerve related to the symptoms.

■ Zygapophyseal Joints from C2 to C7

The joint surfaces are at an angle of 45° to the upper vertebral end-plate. Traction may be performed on the supine patient by moving the superior articular process of the caudal vertebra away from the inferior articular process of the cranial vertebra at a right angle to the treatment plane. This difficult technique is all the more challenging due to the surrounding soft tissues. Therefore, in everyday practice it is supplemented by other tests before drawing any conclusions on zygapophyseal joint mobility. The reader is referred to further education.

■ Traction on the Occiput/Atlas

The patient is on a low seat while the therapist stands laterally with slightly bent knees and in front of the shoulder. His ventral hand holds the patient's head against his ventral shoulder or thorax. His dorsal index finger palpates the space between the contralateral transverse process of the atlas and mastoid process. Next, he extends his knees, which pulls the patient's head away from the treatment plane at a right angle.

> ❗ The technique is performed once while palpating the right side and once palpating the left; the therapist stands on the contralateral side each time. During the test, he should evaluate the quantity, quality with end-feel, and any change in symptoms.

Physiological end-feel:

firm and elastic

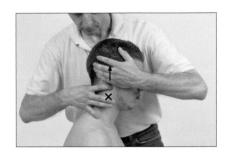

Fig. 15.129

■ Traction on the Atlas/Axis

The starting position is the same. The grip of the ventral hand is nearly identical to that used for traction on the occiput and atlas, but a little lower, and there is contact between the little finger and the neck at the level of the arch of the atlas. The index finger of the therapist's dorsal hand palpates at the level between the posterior arches of the atlas and axis. To get a rough sense of the vertebral arches, it helps to lean the patient's torso slightly back so that the head's center of gravity is behind the axes of flexion and extension in the upper cervical spine. This relaxes the suboccipital neck extensors, which makes palpation easier. Next, the therapist stretches his knees which pulls the occiput and atlas away at a right angle to the treatment plane between the atlas and axis. The contact between the little finger and the arch of the atlas emphasizes the movement between the atlas and axis. This phenomenon can probably not be explained in purely mechanical terms.

> ❗ The technique is performed with palpation once on the right and left with the therapist standing on the contralateral side each time. Quantity, quality with end-feel, and symptom-alteration should be evaluated.

> ❗ If there is a very large amount of traction movement of C0–C1 and C1–C2, one should consider potentially decreased stability in the upper cervical spine. This is a low-risk safety test of stability of the upper cervical spine.

> ❗ Both hands can move one vertebra caudally to perform traction on the lower cervical spine segments using the same grip (see **Fig. 15.130b**).

Physiological end-feel:
firm and elastic

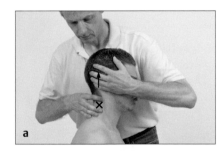

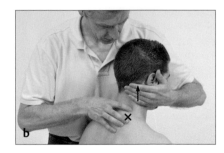

Fig. 15.130 a, b

15.7.4   Treatment of Capsuloligamentous Hypomobility

■ Traction in Relation to the Intervertebral Disk Plane: General Traction in the Supine Patient

The patient is in the supine position. The therapist stands cranially and grasps the occiput with both hands without lifting the patient's head off the underlying surface. Then he pulls the occiput at a right angle away from the treatment plane.

Variation with belt:
The starting position and the grip are identical. However, the therapist first loops a belt around the backs of both hands. The other end of the belt is around his pelvis. By leaning back with his pelvis, the tension is transmitted to his hands and thus to the cervical spine. The belt automatically tightens around his hands, and the grip on the occiput is more stable.

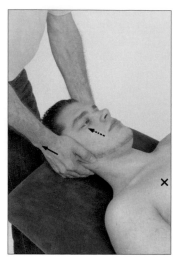

Fig. 15.131

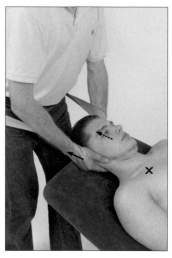

Fig. 15.132

■ Traction in Relation to the Intervertebral Disk Plane: Accentuated Segmental Technique in the Supine Patient

The patient should be in the supine position. The therapist stands cranially and places the radial borders of both index fingers on the posterior arch to the left and right of the spinous process of the vertebra, below which traction should begin. In general, the index fingers should be placed at a 45° angle to the plane of the treatment table. With this grip, the therapist firmly holds the vertebra and pulls it at a right angle away from the treatment plane.

Variation with belt:
The starting position and grip are identical to the previously described general technique. The therapist's index fingers grasp the posterior arch of the vertebra, below which traction should take place. By displacing his pelvis backward, the belt transmits the tension to this vertebra. Looping

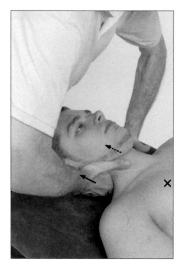

Fig. 15.133

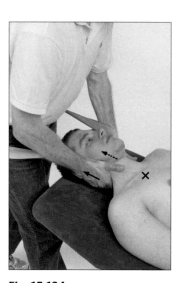

Fig. 15.134

the belt around the hands makes it easier to achieve a firm grasp on the vertebral arch.

Both traction techniques are used in grade I–II for their relieving effects, especially in the treatment of acute intervertebral disk protrusion/prolapse.

! To control the success of treatment, rather than merely asking the patient about any changes in symptoms, the therapist should also test nervous system functioning including neurodynamics.

Traction between Occiput and Atlas in the Seated Patient

The patient should be sitting on a low seat. The therapist stands alongside and in front of his shoulder and holds the patient's head with his ventral hand as before. His dorsal thumb and index finger grasp the posterior arch of the atlas and press it slightly caudally to fixate it. Next, the therapist extends his knees and lifts the patient's head away from the treatment plane.

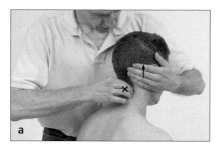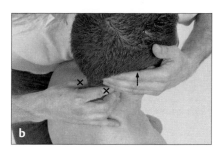

Fig. 15.135 a, b

Traction between the Atlas and Axis in the Seated Patient

The starting position and grip are nearly identical to the previous technique. The border of the little finger of the ventral hand moves slightly down, however, onto the level of the arch of the atlas. The thumb and index finger of the dorsal hand are also placed somewhat lower in order to be on the level of the arch of the axis which is pressed slightly caudally to fixate it. Extension of the knees produces traction.

Both of these techniques are suitable for patients with hypomobility and for joint-specific pain-relief in the upper cervical spine.

! Using this grip, the therapist may move both hands one vertebra down in caudal direction to perform traction on the lower cervical spine segments.

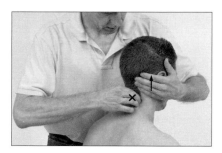

Fig. 15.136

Traction on C0–C1 and C1–C2 in the Supine Patient

The therapist grasps the posterior arch of the atlas or axis with his thumb and index finger for fixation and supports himself on his elbows. His other hand (or thumb and index finger) grasps the occiput and his ipsilateral shoulder is on the patient's forehead. His cranial hand and shoulder perform traction while his caudal hand is used for fixation. This technique can also be used in the segments of the lower cervical spine. The therapist fixates the caudal vertebra and moves the cranial one using the same grip.

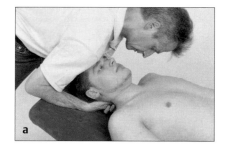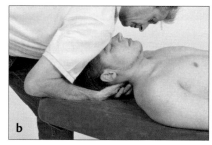

Fig. 15.137 a, b

Documentation Template: Practice Scheme

Cervical spine	
Symptoms	
Symptom-altering direction	
Contraindications?	Nervous system: ▪ Mobility ▪ Impulse conduction ▪ Safety tests Other:
Symptom-altering segmental region	
General assessment of adjacent joints and affected spinal region	

Rotational tests	Active	Continues passively?	Passive	End of movement and end-feel	Symptoms/ pain	Comments
▪ Ventral flexion						
▪ Dorsal flexion						
▪ Lateral flexion, right						
▪ Lateral flexion, left						
▪ Rotation, right						
▪ Rotation, left						
▪ Combined movements						

Translatoric tests	Quantity	Quality	End-feel	Symptoms/pain	Comments
▪ Traction					
▪ Compression					

Summary Formulation aid: ▪ Symptoms ▪ Direction ▪ Contraindications ▪ Site (joint) ▪ Restricted mobility, hypermobility, or physiological mobility ▪ Structure: muscle, joint, etc.	*Text:*
Trial treatment	
Physical therapy diagnosis	
Treatment plan with treatment goal and prognosis	
Treatment with periodic control tests	
Final examination	

Documentation: Practice Example 1

Cervical spine (Cervicobrachialgia)		
Symptoms	*Highly acute pain in the middle right neck region which is radiating into the lateral arm and down to the lateral three fingers*	
Symptom-altering direction	*Dorsiflexion, lateral bending to the right and right rotation. The patient is facing in the opposite direction, i. e., in a pain-relieving posture.*	
Contraindications?	Nervous system:	
	▪ Mobility	*Movement of the median nerve provokes the pain. The radial nerve is also contributing somewhat.*
	▪ Impulse conduction	*The sensation in the right thumb region is diminished (dermatome C6), the brachioradialis muscle is weakened and has a score of 4 (myotome C6). The brachioradialis reflex is also diminished.*
	▪ Safety tests	*No findings*
	Other:	*No findings*
Symptom-altering segmental region	*Not tested today.*	
General assessment of adjacent joints and affected spinal region		

Rotational tests	Active	Conti-nues passi-vely?	Passive	End of mo-vement and end-feel	Symptoms/pain	Comments
▪ Ventral flexion						
▪ Dorsal flexion						
▪ Lateral flexion, right						
▪ Lateral flexion, left			*Not tested today.*			
▪ Rotation, right						
▪ Rotation, left						
▪ Combined movements						

Translatoric tests	Quantity	Quality	End-feel	Symptoms/pain	Comments
▪ Traction intervertebral disk plane	*Barely palpable*	*Increased muscu-lar resistance*	*Soft and elastic or empty*	*Grade I–II relieves reported symp-toms, especially accentuated seg-mental traction caudal to C5*	*Tested in the actual resting position, accen-tuated segmental traction in the supine position*
▪ Compression intervertebral disk plane	*Barely palpable*	*Guarding tension*	*Empty*	*Early provoca-tion of reported symptoms*	*Tested in the actual resting position*

Continued ▶

Cervical spine (Cervicobrachialgia)	
Summary Formulation aid: ▪ Symptoms ▪ Direction ▪ Contraindications ▪ Site (joint) ▪ Restricted mobility, hypermobility, or physiological mobility ▪ Structure: muscle, joint, etc.	*Text:* ▪ *Highly acute pain in the middle right region of the neck radiating to the lateral arm and lateral three fingers.* ▪ *Pain worsens with dorsiflexion, lateral flexion to the right and rotation to the right of the cervical spine. Mobility tests of the median nerve, and to a lesser extent the radial nerve, provoke the reported pain. The impulse conduction of the C6 nerve root is diminished. Traction alleviates symptoms, especially traction caudally from C5; compression worsens them.* ▪ *There is a contraindication today to movement for both further examination and treatment. Therefore, the examination is stopped for today.* ▪ *The cause is presumably highly acute symptoms from the C6 nerve root which may be associated with mechanical compression.*
Trial treatment	*Static segmental grade I–II traction caudally from C5 after which there is mild improvement in symptoms.*
Physical therapy diagnosis	*See above*
Treatment plan with treatment goal and prognosis	▪ *Inform the treating physician. If physical therapy (PT) is prescribed to treat the symptoms, the following measures may be used:* ▪ *Traction:* *Static grade I–II traction in the actual resting position with the goal of relief and increasing space. In the intermittent form, traction serves to stimulate metabolism and inhibition of pain.* ▪ *Immobilization:* *Movement limitation with a neck brace to maintain the spine in the actual resting position may be helpful during this highly acute phase for 1–2 days (not much more).* ▪ *Protection:* *Rest is advised for a few days. If the patient needs to move about, he should wear a neck brace.* ▪ *Analgesia:* *Pain-relieving PT measures such as heat and massage may be used.* ▪ *Information/Instruction:* *The patient is informed about his condition and instructed in appropriate movements to protect the site such as how to get up from the supine position as well as self-help measures such as auto-traction.* ▪ *Treatment goal: relief of neural structure compression, pain relief.* *The mobility of the neural structures, the impulse conduction function of the nervous system, and active movement may be used as control tests along with status of pain symptoms.* *Only after the highly acute symptoms have subsided may the initial examination be continued.* **(Further information on examination and treatment techniques may be obtained by attending further education.)**
Treatment with periodic control tests	
Final examination	

Documentation tool: Practice Example 2

<table>
<tr><td colspan="7" align="center">Cervical spine
(Neck pain with headache)</td></tr>
<tr><td>Symptoms</td><td colspan="6">Right-sided pain in the suboccipital neck region which is associated with headache on the right side</td></tr>
<tr><td>Symptom-altering direction</td><td colspan="6">Ventral flexion</td></tr>
<tr><td>Contraindications?</td><td colspan="3">Nervous system:
▪ Mobility
▪ Impulse conduction
▪ Safety tests
Other:</td><td colspan="3">No findings</td></tr>
<tr><td>Symptom-altering segmental region</td><td colspan="6">Upper cervical spine, given that flexion of the upper cervical spine (double chin) provokes pain while flexion of the lower cervical spine (push chin forward) does not.</td></tr>
<tr><td>General assessment of adjacent joints and affected spinal segment</td><td colspan="6">Hyperkyphosis of the thoracic spine and marked ventral flexion position at cervicothoracic junction</td></tr>
</table>

Rotational tests	Active	Continues passively?	Passive	End of movement and end-feel	Symptoms/ pain	Comments
▪ Ventral flexion	*Diminished*	*< 5°*	*Increased resistance to movement*	*Soft to firm and elastic*	*Provokes reported pain*	*Flexion of lower cervical spine seems asymptomatic*
▪ Dorsiflexion	*More in the lower (around C6) and upper cervical spine*	*> 10°*	*Slight resistance to movement*	*Soft to firm and elastic*	*Local end-range pain in lower cervical spine*	*Extreme curve in lower cervical spine (C6)*
▪ Lateral flexion, right	*No findings*	*ca. 10°*	*No findings*	*Firm and elastic*	*None*	
▪ Lateral flexion, left	*No findings*	*ca. 10°*	*No findings*	*Firm and elastic*	*None*	
▪ Rotation, right	*Somewhat limited*	*ca. 5°*	*Slightly increased resistance to movement*	*Firm and elastic*	*None*	
▪ Rotation, left	*No findings*	*ca. 10°*	*No findings*	*Less firm and elastic*	*None*	
▪ Combined movements	*Not tested today.*					

Translatoric tests	Quantity	Quality	End-feel	Symptoms/pain	Comments
▪ Traction C0–C1	*Hypo 2 right*	*Increased resistance to movement*	*Very firm and elastic right > left*	*Grade III rather provokes reported pain*	
▪ Traction C1–C2	*No findings*	*No findings*	*No findings*	*No findings*	
▪ Compression	*No findings*	*No findings*	*Hard*	*None*	

Continued ▶

Documentation tool: Practice Example 2 *(Continued)*

<table>
<tr><td colspan="2" align="center">Cervical spine
(Neck pain with headache)</td></tr>
<tr>
<td>
Summary
Formulation aid:
<ul>
<li>Symptoms</li>
<li>Direction</li>
<li>Contraindications</li>
<li>Site (joint)</li>
<li>Restricted mobility, hypermobility, or physiological mobility</li>
<li>Structure: muscle, joint, etc.</li>
<li>Additional factors</li>
</ul>
</td>
<td>
Text:
<ul>
<li>Pain mainly on the right side of the suboccipital neck region, associated with headache on the right side.</li>
<li>The pain occurs especially with ventral flexion.</li>
<li>There are no contraindications today to further movement testing.</li>
<li>The symptoms are in correlation with the upper cervical spine, particularly the right atlanto-occipital joint,</li>
<li>which appears to be hypomobile</li>
<li>due to capsuloligamentous shrinkage.</li>
<li>The partly soft and elastic end-feel suggests additional tension in the suboccipital neck muscles.</li>
</ul>
</td>
</tr>
<tr>
<td>Trial treatment</td>
<td>
<ul>
<li>5-minute pain-relieving grade I–II intermittent traction on the right atlanto-occipital joint. Afterward the patient said he had less pain during ventral flexion.</li>
<li>This was followed by 5-minute static grade III traction on the right atlanto-occipital joint after which the patient reports a further reduction in pain. The next day he says his headache was less severe than usual the evening after the trial treatment.</li>
</ul>
</td>
</tr>
<tr>
<td>Physical therapy diagnosis</td>
<td>See above</td>
</tr>
<tr>
<td>Treatment plan
with treatment goal
and prognosis</td>
<td>
<ul>
<li>After initial pain-relieving traction on the right atlanto-occipital joint, continue treatment with static grade III traction.</li>
<li>Treatment goal: pain-free physiological mobility.</li>
</ul>
(Further information on examination and treatment techniques may be obtained by attending further education.)
</td>
</tr>
<tr>
<td>Treatment with periodic control tests</td>
<td></td>
</tr>
<tr>
<td>Final examination</td>
<td></td>
</tr>
</table>

15.8 | Temporomandibular Joint

(Articulatio temporomandibularis)

15.8.1 | Anatomy

Joint type:	condylar or ellipsoidal joint; together the right and left joints form a bicondylar joint (Gray 1989)
Joint surface:	the articular surface of the mandibular head is convex, while the mandibular fossa is concave with the ventrally situated convex articular tubercle
Articular disk:	a bi-concave disk, which in rare instances is perforated, divides the joint into two separate compartments
Resting position:	relaxed, hanging mandible with a slightly opened mouth, and the tongue resting against the palate
Close packed position:	closed mouth with full dental occlusion
Capsular pattern:	not described

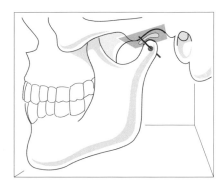

Fig. 15.138

■ Biomechanics

Rotation occurs in the lower compartments, between the mandibular head and the articular disk, around a transverse axis passing through both heads. This is known as "small mouth opening," the first phase of the movement cycle. Holding the tongue flat against the palate and opening the mouth limits the movement to the small mouth opening. In the upper compartments, gliding movements of the articular disk start in the mandibular fossa, moving forward to under the articular tubercle. In what is referred to as "large mouth opening," the mandibular head and articular disk glide ventrally as a unit under the articular tubercle. End-range mouth opening often causes major stress on the articular disk and stabilizing structures, especially retrodiskal structures. Clicking sounds are often the result of unphysiological movements of the articular disk.

> **!** Students of manual therapy can palpate the movements of the temporomandibular joint's articular surfaces on themselves and even hear any gliding disturbances. Simply place the index finger of each hand in the external acoustic meatus on either side and then actively move the jaw.

15.8.2 Rotational Tests

■ Active Movements

The patient should be seated in front of the therapist. He or she then moves the mandible to open and close their mouth as well as to perform protraction, retraction, and lateral deviation to the right and left. While doing so, patients should show their teeth so that the therapist can evaluate the amount of movement based on the teeth. A thin toothpick placed between the top and bottom middle incisors can help assess movement, which is measured with a ruler in millimeters or based on the width of the teeth. One should note especially any deviations from a straight line of movement.

If the right temporomandibular joint is more mobile than the left, for instance, one sees that

- opening the mouth causes deviation of the mandible to the left,
- lateral deviation is more pronounced to the left than right, and
- with protraction there is again deviation to the left.

! The therapist should then stand behind the patient and with his index fingers palpate the mandibular head movements in both temporomandibular joints while the patient actively moves the joints.

Painful hypermobility may suggest increased sensitivity of the retrodiskal tissue. Mouth closing is associated with compression, especially when one bites down strongly. Pain may be an indication of a lesion affecting the articular disk, degeneration of joint surfaces, or a fracture.

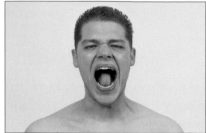

Fig. 15.139

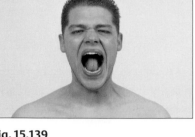

Fig. 15.140

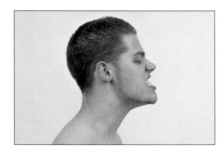

Fig. 15.141

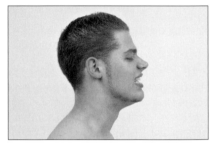

Fig. 15.142

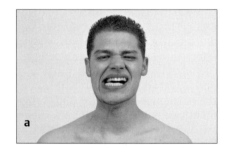

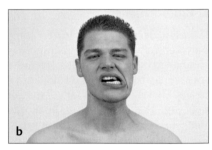

Fig. 15.143 a, b

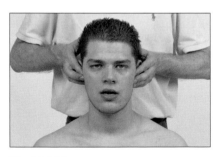

Fig. 15.144

◼ Specific Active and Passive Movement Testing (Quantity and Quality)

> **!** In all of the following tests, the starting position is the resting position (= zero position) with the tongue resting flat against the palate in order not to restrict pro-/retraction and lateral deviation by the contact of the teeth. The hand performing the movement feels the quantity and quality. The palpating finger in the joint space also gathers additional information. The tests must be performed twice so that the right and left sides may be palpated. The patient should be asked before active/passive movement testing whether he or she has a removable dental prosthesis and if so whether they would like to leave it in or remove it.

a) Mouth opening:

- The patient should be sitting on a low seat. The therapist stands laterally (in front of) the patient's shoulder and holds the head between his own dorsal hand and dorsal shoulder or chest. The index finger of his dorsal hand can palpate the movement in the contralateral joint space. Next the therapist asks the patient to actively open their mouth.
- Then the therapist takes the patient's mandible in the thumb and index finger of his ventral hand and places his bent middle finger against the mental protuberance (middle of the lower jaw). Using this grip, he tests whether the movement continues passively.
- Finally, he moves the joint from the zero position (= closed mouth) passively through the entire range of motion and tests the end-feel.

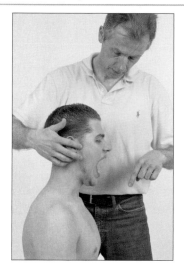

Fig. 15.145

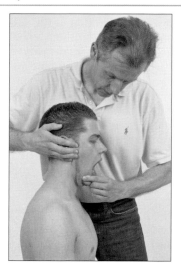

Fig. 15.146

Physiological end-feel:
firm and elastic

b) Mouth closing:

- The starting position, fixation of the head, and the position of the palpating finger are the same as before. The patient opens his or her mouth slightly and the therapist asks them to actively close it.
- Next the therapist takes the patient's mandible with the thumb and index finger of his ventral hand and places his bent middle finger under the ventral part of the mandible. Alternatively, he might place the palm of his hand under the mandible. With this grip, he tests whether the movement continues passively.

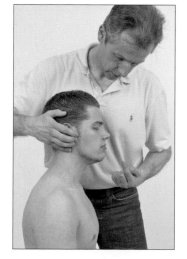

Fig. 15.147

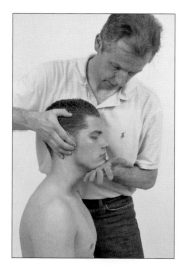

Fig. 15.148

- Finally, starting from a slightly opened position of the mouth, he moves the joint passively through the entire range of motion and tests the end-feel.

Physiological end-feel:
hard and not elastic

c) Protraction:

- The starting position, fixation of the head, and position of the palpating finger are the same as before. The therapist asks the patient to actively push the mandible forward.
- Next the therapist grasps the patient's mandible, placing the index finger of his ventral hand behind the ramus of the mandible while the remaining medial fingers grasp the mandible from below. Then he tests whether the movement continues passively.
- Finally, he moves the joint from the zero position (= closed mouth) passively through the entire range of motion and tests the end-feel.

Physiological end-feel:
firm and elastic

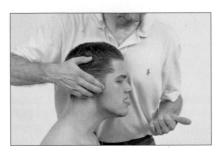

Fig. 15.149

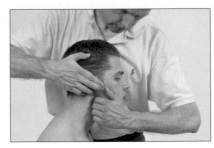

Fig. 15.150

> **!** Passive (continuing) protraction primarily occurs on one side. The right and left sides must therefore be tested separately.

d) Retraction:

- The starting position, fixation of the head, and placement of the palpating finger are the same as before. The therapist asks the patient to actively push his or her mandible dorsally.
- Next the therapist places the thumb and index finger of his ventral hand on the mandible from anterior and places his bent middle finger against the front of it. With this grip, he tests whether the movement continues passively.
- Finally, he moves the joint from the zero position passively through the entire range of motion and tests the end-feel.

Physiological end-feel:
firm and elastic

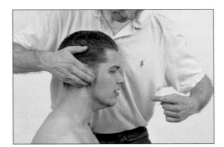

Fig. 15.151

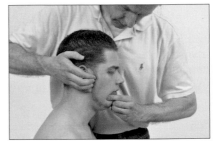

Fig. 15.152

> **!** Pain on retraction may be due to compression of the retrodiskal tissue.

e) **Lateral deviation:**

- The starting position, fixation of the head, and placement of the palpating finger are the same as before. The therapist asks the patient to <u>actively</u> shift the mandible to the right (or left).
- Then the therapist grasps the mandible by placing the ball of his thumb from lateral against the mandibular body while supporting the mandible from below with his fingers. With this grip, he tests whether the movement <u>continues passively</u>.
- Finally, he moves the joint from the zero position <u>passively</u> through the entire range of motion and tests the <u>end-feel</u>.

> **!** Lateral deviation should be tested to the right and left.

Physiological end-feel:
firm and elastic

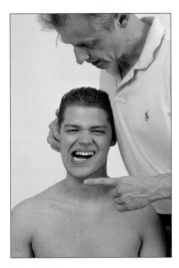

Fig. 15.153

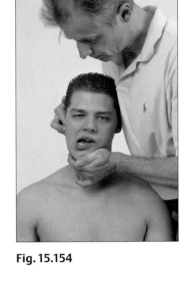

Fig. 15.154

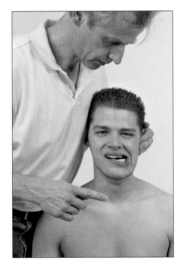

Fig. 15.155

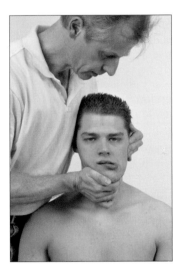

Fig. 15.156

15.8.3 Translatoric Tests

Traction:

The starting position, fixation of the head, and the placement of the palpating finger are the same as in the previous section. Wearing a disposable glove, the thumb of the therapist's ventral hand is placed on the patient's back molars. His index finger is placed laterally around the ramus of the mandible, and his remaining fingers are flexed and resting underneath the mandible. With this grip he moves the mandible <u>at a right angle</u> away from the treatment plane. The direction of traction may slightly vary: caudally/dorsally or caudally/ventrally.

Physiological end-feel:
firm and elastic

! This test is performed on the right and left.

Suitable gloves should be worn given that friction between a loose glove and palate could irritate it. Disposable gloves are often powdered and must therefore be washed before use. The patient should be given a paper tissue to wipe any saliva away during the test. As when visiting the dentist, the therapist and patient should agree on a sign, such as raising the hand, if the patient needs to say something or swallow, and then the therapist should remove his thumb from the patient's mouth.

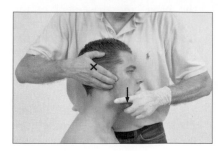

Fig. 15.157

Compression:

The starting position, fixation of the head, and the placement of the palpating finger are the same as before. The ulnar border of the therapist's ventral hand is placed from below against the ramus of the mandible and presses it <u>perpendicularly</u> toward the treatment plane.

! This test is performed on the left and right sides. The direction of compression may vary: cranially/ventrally or cranially/dorsally.

Physiological end-feel:
hard and elastic

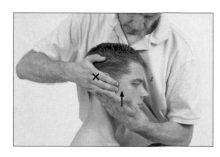

Fig. 15.158

15.8.4 Treatment of Capsuloligamentous Hypomobility

The starting position, fixation of the head, and the placement of the palpating finger are nearly the same. The fingers of the stabilizing hand no longer palpate the joint space, however, but instead rest on the temporal bone to better stabilize the head. As in the traction test, the gloved ventral hand grasps the mandible and moves it <u>at a right angle</u> away from the treatment plane.

! Traction may also be performed in the supine patient or with the patient in a partially reclined position with his upper body on the raised foot piece of the treatment bench.

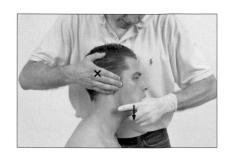

Fig. 15.159

Documentation Template: Practice Scheme

Temporomandibular joint	
Symptoms	
Symptom-altering direction	
Contraindications?	Fractures: Other:
Symptom-altering joint	
General assessment of adjacent joints	

Active movements, comparing sides (observation and palpation)	

Specific rotational tests	**Active**	**Continues passively?**	**Passive**	**End-feel**	**Symptoms/pain**	**Comments**
Mouth opening						
Mouth closing (from the resting position)						
Protraction, right						
Retraction, right						
Protraction, left						
Retraction, left						
Lateral deviation, right						
Lateral deviation, left						

Translatoric tests	**Quantity**	**Quality**	**End-feel**	**Symptoms/pain**	**Comments**
Traction, right					
Compression, right					
Traction, left					
Compression, left					

Summary Formulation aid: - Symptoms - Direction - Contraindications - Site (joint) - Restricted mobility, hypermobility, or physiological mobility - Structure: muscle, joint, etc.	*Text:*
Trial treatment	
Physical therapy diagnosis	
Treatment plan with treatment goal and prognosis	
Treatment with periodic control tests	
Final examination	

Documentation: Practice Example

<table>
<tr><td colspan="7">Temporomandibular joint
(Pain in right temporomandibular joint)</td></tr>
<tr><td>Symptoms</td><td colspan="6">Pain and "clicking noises" in the right temporomandibular joint</td></tr>
<tr><td>Symptom-altering direction</td><td colspan="6">Mouth opening</td></tr>
<tr><td>Contraindications?</td><td colspan="6">Fractures: No findings
Other: No findings</td></tr>
<tr><td>Symptom-altering joint</td><td colspan="6">Right temporomandibular joint</td></tr>
<tr><td>General assessment of adjacent joints</td><td colspan="6">No findings</td></tr>
<tr><td>Active movements, comparing sides

(observation and palpation)</td><td colspan="6">Active mouth opening and protraction occur with leftward deviation of the mandible; lateral deviation to the left is larger than to the right (inspection).

The right mandibular head moves more quickly and further ventrally during mouth opening and protraction than the left. During lateral deviation to the left, the right mandibular head also moves further ventrally than the left during lateral deviation to the right (palpation).</td></tr>
</table>

Specific rotational tests	Active	Continues passively?	Passive	End-feel	Symptoms/pain	Comments
Mouth opening	*ca. 3½ finger widths*	*ca. 1 finger width*	*Slight resistance to movement, jerky movement*	*Firm and elastic with a tendency toward a soft end-feel*	*Triggers end-range pain as reported by the patient as well as "clicking" on the right side*	
Mouth closing (from the resting position)	*No findings*	*No (= no findings)*	*No findings*	*Hard (= no findings)*		
Protraction, right	*Nearly 10 mm*	*ca. 2 mm*	*Slight resistance to movement*	*Firm to soft/elastic*	*Triggers end-range pain as reported by the patient*	
Retraction, right	*ca. 1 mm*	*< 1 mm*	*Somewhat further left*	*Firm and elastic and painful*	*Triggers some end-range pain as reported by the patient*	
Protraction, left	*ca. 7 mm*	*< 1 mm*	*Increased resistance to movement*	*Very firm and elastic*	*No findings*	
Retraction, left	*ca. 1 mm*	*< 1 mm*	*No findings*	*Firm and elastic*	*No findings*	
Lateral deviation, right	*Up to 1st Incisor*	*Hardly 1 tooth width*	*Increased resistance to movement*	*Very firm and elastic*		
Lateral deviation, left	*Nearly to the canine tooth*	*ca. 1½ tooth-widths*	*Slight resistance to movement*	*Firm to soft/elastic*	*Triggers end-range pain as reported by the patient*	

Continued ▶

Documentation: Practice Example *(Continued)*

<table>
<tr><td colspan="6">Temporomandibular joint
(Pain in right temporomandibular joint)</td></tr>
<tr><th>Translatoric tests</th><th>Quantity</th><th>Quality</th><th>End-feel</th><th>Symptoms/pain</th><th>Comments</th></tr>
<tr><td>Traction, right</td><td>Hyper 4</td><td>Slight resistance to movement</td><td>Firm or soft/elastic</td><td>Triggers end-range pain as reported by the patient</td><td></td></tr>
<tr><td>Compression, right</td><td>No findings</td><td>No findings</td><td>Hard</td><td>No findings</td><td></td></tr>
<tr><td>Traction, left</td><td>Hypo 2</td><td>No findings</td><td>Very firm and elastic</td><td>No findings</td><td></td></tr>
<tr><td>Compression, left</td><td>No findings</td><td>No findings</td><td>Hard</td><td>No findings</td><td></td></tr>
</table>

Summary Formulation aid: <ul><li>Symptoms</li><li>Direction</li><li>Contraindications</li><li>Site (joint)</li><li>Restricted mobility, hypermobility, or physiological mobility</li><li>Structure: muscle, joint, etc.</li><li>Additional causal and influencing factors</li></ul>	*Text:* <ul><li>*Pain in right mandible*</li><li>*during mouth opening.*</li><li>*There are no contraindications today to further movement tests.*</li><li>*The symptoms are in correlation with the right temporomandibular joint,*</li><li>*which is hypermobile with end-range pain*</li></ul> <ul><li>*due to a loose capsuloligamentous unit. Associated with this are jerky movement and "clicking noises" produced by the temporomandibular joint.*</li><li>*The hypomobility of the left temporomandibular joint is worsening the situation. During end-range mouth opening and protraction, it leads to deviation of the mandible to the left and limits the lateral deviation of the mandible to the right.*</li></ul>
Trial treatment	<ul><li>*5-minute grade I–II intermittent traction on the right temporomandibular joint for pain relief, after which there is somewhat less pain.*</li><li>*Afterward, 5-minute mobilizing grade III traction on the left temporomandibular joint, after which the pain on the right continues to decrease and the mobility on the left appears to increase.*</li></ul>
Physical therapy diagnosis	*See above*
Treatment plan with treatment goal and prognosis	<ul><li>*Continue initial pain-relieving traction on the right temporomandibular joint and advise patient to strictly avoid end-range movements (opening mouth widely, etc.).*</li><li>*Mobilizing grade III traction on the left to relieve movement stress on the right.*</li><li>*Treatment goal: pain-free physiological mobility.*</li></ul>***(Further information on examination and treatment techniques may be obtained by attending further education.)***
Treatment with periodic control tests	
Final examination	

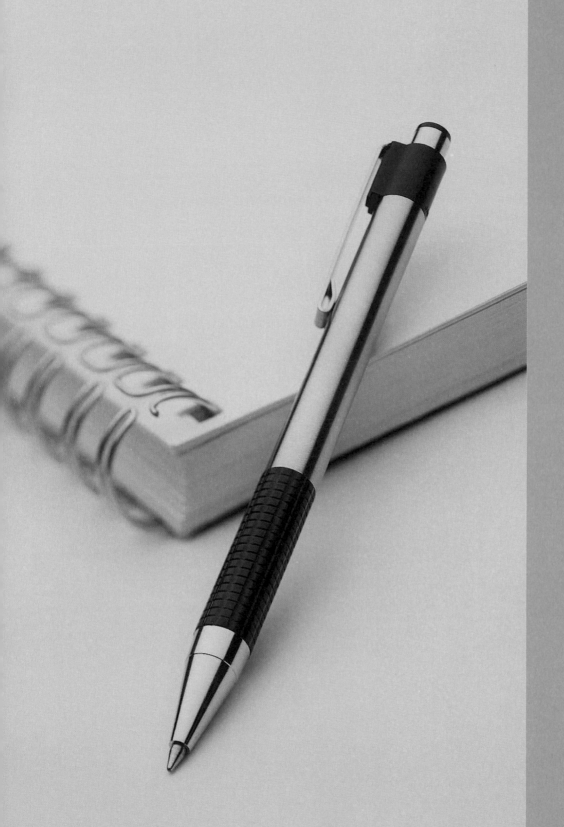

Appendix

16.1   Lower Extremity

(The degree values given here serve as a rough guide and are approximate only.)

Joint	Joint type	Distal joint surface	Resting position	Close packed position	Capsular pattern
Proximal interphalangeal joint (PIP) and distal interphalangeal joint (DIP) of the toes as well as the interphalangeal joint of the big toe.	Ginglymus, hinge joint, modified sellar	Distal phalanx is concave	Slight flexion	Max. extension	Limited in both directions, flexion affected the most
Metatarsophalangeal joint (MTP)	Condylar joint (Mac Conaill 1977), modified ovoid	Phalanx is concave	ca. 10° extension	MTP I max. ext., MTP II–V max. flexion	Limited in all directions, flexion affected the most
Distal intermetatarsal joint	Syndesmosis (deep transverse metatarsal ligament)	No true joint surfaces	Not described	Not described	Not described
Proximal intermetatarsal joint only between 2nd to 5th metatarsals	Amphiarthrosis, modified sellar	Metatarsal base is considered concave in manual therapy	Not described	Not described	Not described
Tarsometatarsal joints	Amphiarthrosis	Metatarsal base is considered concave in manual therapy	Not described	Not described	Equally in all directions
Subtalar joint and talocalcaneonavicular joint	Combined joint with 2 compartments that are coupled functionally. Subtalar joint: ginglymus, modified sellar Talocalcaneonavicular joint: spheroidal joint, unmodified ovoid	Subtalar joint: calcaneus is convex. Talocalcaneonavicular joint: calcaneus and navicular are concave	Middle position between max. eversion and max. inversion	Max. inversion	Not described
Ankle joint	Ginglymus, hinge joint, modified sellar	Talus is convex	10° plantar flexion	Max. dorsiflexion	Plantar flexion > dorsiflexion

Continued ▶

Joint	Joint type	Distal joint surface	Resting position	Close packed position	Capsular pattern
Tibiofibular syndesmosis (distal)	Syndesmosis, unmodified sellar	Variously described, in manual therapy for gliding anterior/posterior considered concave	10° plantar flexion in ankle joint	Max. dorsiflexion in ankle joint	Not described
Tibiofibular joint (proximal)	Amphiarthrosis, unmodified sellar	Fibular head: anatomic variants are common (Lazennec et al 1994)	10° plantar flexion in ankle joint	Max. dorsiflexion in ankle joint	Not described
Femorotibial joint	Pivotal hinge joint, modified ovoid	Tibial plateau glides during rotatory movements based on the principle of a concave surface	30° Flexion	Max. extension and external rotation	Flexion > extension
Femoropatellar joint	Gliding joint	Patella is concave (3 facets)	Extension of the knee joint	Knee in max. flexion	Not described
Hip joint	Enarthrodial joint, unmodified sellar	Femoral head is convex	30° flexion, 30° abduction and slight external rotation	Extension, inward rotation and abduction	Internal rotation > extension > abduction > external rotation

16.2   Upper Extremity

Joint	Joint type	Distal joint surface	Resting position	Close packed position	Capsular pattern
Proximal interphalangeal joint (PIP) and distal interphalangeal joint (DIP) of the fingers as well as the interphalangeal joint of the thumb.	Ginglymus, hinge joint, modified sellar	Concave	Slight flexion	Max. extension	Flexion > extension
Metacarpophalangeal joint (MCP)	Condylar joint, modified ovoid	Concave	Slight flexion MCP II–V additional slight ulnar abduction	MCP I: max. extension MCP II–V: max. flexion	Flexion is more limited than any other direction
Distal intermetacarpal syndesmosis	Syndesmosis (deep transverse metacarpal ligament)	No true joint surfaces	Not described	Not described	Not described
Proximal intermetacarpal joint	Amphiarthrosis	Base of metacarpal is irregularly shaped; in manual therapy considered concave	Not described	Not described	Not described

Continued ▶

Joint	Joint type	Distal joint surface	Resting position	Close packed position	Capsular pattern
Carpometacarpal joints II–V (CMC II–V)	Amphiarthrosis	Bases of metacarpals are considered concave in manual therapy	Not described	Not described	Equally in all directions
Carpometacarpal joint I (CMC I)	Saddle-shaped joint, unmodified sellar	Base of metacarpal joint I is concave for flexion/extension, convex for abduction/adduction	Midway between abduction/adduction and flexion/extension	Max. opposition	Abduction > extension
Radiocarpal joint	Ellipsoidal joint, ovoid joint, modified oval shape	Carpal bones are convex proximally	Zero position with slight ulnar abduction	Max. dorsiflexion	Equally in all directions
Midcarpal joint	Ellipsoidal joint, ovoid joint with S-shaped joint space, modified ovoid	Distal carpal bones are convex proximally except for trapezium and trapezoid, which are concave proximally	Similar to radiocarpal joint	Similar to radiocarpal joint	Similar to radiocarpal joint
Intercarpal joints	Amphiarthrosis	Irregularly shaped joint surfaces	Similar to radiocarpal joint	Similar to radiocarpal joint	Similar to radiocarpal joint
Distal radioulnar joint	Trochoidal joint, pivot joint	Radius is concave	10° supination	Maximum end-range joint position	Only with strong flexion/extension limitation in elbow are pronation and supination equally limited
Proximal radioulnar joint	Trochoidal joint, pivot joint	Radius is convex	70° flexion and 35° supination	Maximum end-range joint position	Similar to distal radioulnar joint
Humeroulnar joint	Saddle-shaped joint; sellar joint, unmodified sellar shape (Kaltenborn 2004), simplified description as a hinge joint (Platzer 2008)	Ulna for flexion/extension concave, for abduction/adduction convex	70° flexion and 10° supination	Max. extension and supination	Flexion > extension
Humeroradial joint	Spheroidal joint, ball-and-socket joint, unmodified ovoid	Radius is concave	Max. extension and supination	90° flexion and 5° supination	Similar to humeroulnar joint
Glenohumeral joint	Spheroidal joint, ball-and-socket joint, unmodified ovoid	Humerus is convex	55° abduction, 30° horizontal adduction and forearm in horizontal plane	Max. abduction and external rotation	External rotation > abduction > internal rotation

Continued ▶

Joint	Joint type	Distal joint surface	Resting position	Close packed position	Capsular pattern
Acromioclavicular joint	Plane joint, unmodified ovoid	Acromion is considered concave in manual therapy	Physiological position of the shoulder girdle	90° abduction of glenohumeral joint	Not described
Sternoclavicular joint	Saddle-shaped joint; sellar joint, unmodified sellar shape	Clavicles are convex for elevation/depression, concave for protraction/retraction	Physiological position of the shoulder girdle	Arm fully elevated	Not described
Scapulo-serrato-thoracic "gliding space"	"Muscular gliding joint"	Scapula is concave	Physiological position of the shoulder girdle	Not described	No joint capsule

16.3   Spinal Column

Joint	Joint type	Distal joint surface	Resting position	Close packed position	Capsular pattern
Sacroiliac joint	Amphiarthrosis	Sacrum considered convex in manual therapy (see p. 196)	Not described	Not described	Not described
Intervertebral joints	Synchondrosis	Cranial vertebra considered concave in manual therapy	Physiological position	Uncoupled movement at the end of range	Not described
Zygoapophyseal joints	Gliding joint	Joint surface of the inferior articular process is considered concave in manual therapy. Exception: occipital condyles are convex, atlas is slightly convex	Physiological position	Uncoupled movement at the end of range	Not described
Costovertebral joint	Gliding joint	Head of rib considered convex in manual therapy	Resting expiratory position	Not described	Not described
Costotransverse joint	Gliding joint	Articular surface of costal tubercles is convex	Resting expiratory position	Not described	Not described
Sternocostal joints	Synchondrosis	Not described	Resting expiratory position	Not described	Not described
Temporomandibular joint	Condylar joint	Head of mandible is convex, articular disk is bi-concave	Slightly opened mouth, lower jaw is relaxed and hanging, and tongue is resting flat against palate	Closed mouth with dental occlusion	Not described

17.1 Extremity Joints

Region	Rotatory tests of movement	Translatoric tests of movement	Translatoric mobilization
Toes: DIP, PIP, IP[a]	Flexion, extension, tibial and fibular stability	Traction and compression	Traction
Metatarsophalangeal (MTP) joint	Flexion, extension, abduction, adduction	Traction and compression	Traction
Intermetatarsal joints	Raising and flattening the arch of the foot, movement of individual metatarsal bones against each other (2nd metatarsal is most stable)	Compression, gliding plantarly and dorsally	Gliding plantarly and dorsally (mostly only in grade I–II)
Tarsometatarsal joints	Tested in intermetatarsal joint tests, specific flexion and extension	Traction and compression	Traction
Intertarsal joints	Similar to the ankle joint with the distal hand placed on the forefoot	Gliding	Gliding (mostly only in grade I–II)
Subtalar joint	Inversion and eversion	Traction and compression	Traction
Ankle joint	Plantar flexion and dorsiflexion, tibial and fibular stability	Traction and compression	Traction
Tibiofibular syndesmosis and joint	Like upper ankle joint: plantar flexion and dorsiflexion, tibial and fibular stability for the syndesmosis	Anterior and posterior gliding	Anterior and posterior gliding (mostly only in grade I–II)
Femorotibial joint	Flexion, extension, external and internal rotation, medial and lateral stability	Traction and compression	Traction
Femoropatellar joint	Tested with the femorotibial joint (flexion is especially important)	Traction global, compression and gliding distally and proximally, medially, and laterally	Distal gliding
Hip joint	Flexion, extension, abduction, adduction, external and internal rotation	Traction caudally and compression	Traction caudally
Fingers: DIP, PIP, IP	Flexion and extension, radial and ulnar stability	Traction and compression	Traction
Metacarpophalangeal joint (MCP)	Flexion, extension, abduction, and adduction	Traction and compression	Traction
Intermetacarpal joints proximal and distal	Hollowing the palm of the hand and flattening it, individual movements of the metacarpal bones against each other (3rd is the most stable)	Compression, gliding toward the palm and dorsally	Gliding toward the palm and dorsally (mostly only in grade I–II)

Continued ▶

Region	Rotatory tests of movement	Translatoric tests of movement	Translatoric mobilization
Carpometacarpal joints: CMC II–V	Tested with the intermetacarpal joints, specific flexion and extension	Traction and compression	Traction (mostly only in grade I–II)
Carpometacarpal joint of the thumb: CMC I	Flexion, extension, abduction, and adduction; several possibilities for opposition and reposition	Traction and compression	Traction
Wrist, global	Flexion, extension, radial and ulnar abduction	Traction and compression	Traction
Intercarpal joints	See wrist (global)	Gliding	Gliding
Radioulnar joint, distal and proximal	Supination and pronation	Gliding anteriorly and posteriorly	Gliding anteriorly and posteriorly (distal: mostly only in grade I–II)
Humeroradial joint	Flexion and extension (stability tested with humeroulnar joint)	Traction and compression	Traction
Humeroulnar joint	Flexion and extension, medial and lateral stability	Traction and compression	Traction
Glenohumeral joint	Flexion, extension, abduction, adduction, external and internal rotation; horizontal abduction and adduction possible	Traction and compression	Traction
Acromioclavicular joint (ACJ)	Shoulder girdle joints: elevation, depression, protraction, and retraction, internal and external rotation of the scapula	Traction and compression	Traction (mostly only in grade I–II)
Sternoclavicular joint (SCJ)	See ACJ	Traction and compression	Traction (mostly only in grade I–II)
Scapulothoracic joint	See ACJ	Lifting of the scapula, pressure of the scapula against the thorax	Lifting of the scapula

[a] For abbreviation expansion, see Appendix 16.

17.2   Spinal Column

Region	Rotatory tests of movement	Translatoric tests of movement	Translatoric mobilization
Pubic symphysis	Palpation during abduction and adduction of the hip joints in the supine position	None	None
Sacroiliac joint	Interaction between nonsupporting leg and supporting leg, forward bending test, standing hip flexion test, nutation and counternutation in prone position	See nutation and counternutation test	Nutation and counternutation (= rotational movements)
Sacrococcygeal joint	Passive ventral flexion	None	Pulling dorsally using static resistance of the gluteus maximus muscle
Lumbar spine	Ventral and dorsiflexion, lateral flexion and rotation on both sides; combined movements possible	Traction and compression in relation to the intervertebral disk plane and the zygapophyseal joint plane	Unspecific and specific traction in relation to the intervertebral disk plane; traction in relation to the zygapophyseal joint plane
Thoracic spine	Ventral and dorsiflexion, lateral flexion and rotation on both sides; combined movements possible	Traction and compression in relation to the intervertebral disk plane and to the zygapophyseal joint plane	Unspecific and specific traction in relation to the intervertebral disk plane; traction in relation to zygapophyseal joint plane
Rib joints 2–10 and 1st rib	Inspiration and expiration; ribs move with during lateral flexion of thoracic spine	Traction on costotransverse joint	Traction on costotransverse joint
Cervical spine	Ventral and dorsiflexion, lateral flexion and rotation on both sides; combined movements possible. ■ Safety tests: ■ Traction C0–C1 and C1–C2 ■ Vertebral artery ■ Transverse ligament ■ Alar ligaments ■ Foraminal compression test	Global traction and compression toward the intervertebral disk plane, traction occiput/atlas and atlas/axis	Global and accentuated traction to the intervertebral disk plane, traction occiput atlas and atlas/axis
Temporomandibular joint	Mouth opening and closing, lateral deviation of the mandible to the right or left, protraction and retraction of the mandible	Traction and compression	Traction

■ Important Tests of the Spinal Column

Safety tests:
■ Traction C0–C1 and C1–C2
■ Test of vertebral artery
■ Test of alar ligaments
■ Test of transverse ligament of atlas
■ Foraminal compression test

Nerve mobility tests:
■ Sciatic nerve
■ Femoral nerve
■ Median nerve
■ Radial nerve
■ Ulnar nerve

Theoretical questions	
Question	Answer (enlarge space before completing)
1. Define the terms manual therapy and orthopedic manual therapy.	
2. Name the two physical therapy concepts of manual therapy that form the basis of IFOMPT.	
3. What are the three areas included in orthopedic manual therapy?	
4. Describe the (*name*) joint along with the shape of its articular surfaces, the joint type, and the positions of its movement axes.	
5. Define the term "treatment plane" and describe it using an example.	
6. Name four important joint positions in manual therapy and describe them in an example.	
7. Define the term "osteokinematics."	
8. Define the term "rotation" and give examples of various rotational movements.	
9. Name at least four coupled and uncoupled movements.	
10. Define the term "translation" and give examples of different translatoric movements.	
11. Define the term "arthrokinematics."	
12. Explain what the term "roll-gliding" means and give two examples.	
13. Explain the term "joint play" and give two examples.	
14. Explain why a joint should be examined using rotatory movements.	
15. Explain why a joint should be examined using translatoric movements.	
16. Name the aspects of evaluating the quantity of movement.	
17. Name the aspects of evaluating the quality of movement.	
18. Define the term "end-feel" and name the possible types of end-feel.	
19. Explain the simplified procedure for symptom localization.	
20. Explain why a joint with capsuloligamentous restriction should be treated with translatoric measures.	
21. Name the parameters for the dosage of the amount of traction or gliding force.	
22. Name the parameters for the duration of the application of traction or gliding force.	

Continued ▶

Theoretical questions (Continued)	
Question	Answer (enlarge space before completing)
23. Explain why three-dimensional positioning of the joint is useful prior to performing traction or gliding movements.	
24. Name the indications for translatoric joint treatment.	
25. Name the contraindications to grade III translatoric joint treatment.	
Practical questions	
Question	

1. Show the positions of the treatment plane for the (*name*) joint.

2. Show the resting position of the (*name*) joint.

3. Show the rotatory examination of the (*name*) joint for the direction (*name*).

4. Show the translatoric examination of the (*name*) joint for the direction (*name*).

5. Show the treatment of capsuloligamentous pain affecting the (*name*) joint.

6. Show the treatment of capsuloligamentous restriction of the (*name*) joint in the direction (*name*).

19.1   General Documentation Template for the Extremity Joints: Basic Scheme

I Orienting examination	
Symptoms	
Symptom-altering direction	
Contraindications?	Nervous system: ▪ Mobility ▪ Impulse conduction Other:
Symptom-altering joint	
General assessment of adjacent joints	

II Specific examination of the joint correlating with symptoms						
Movement testing **a) Rotatory movements**						
Active movements, comparing sides						
Rotatory tests	**Active**	**Continues passively?**	**Passive**	**End-feel**	**Symptoms/ Pain**	**Comments**
▪ Flexion						
▪ Extension						
▪ Abduction						
▪ Adduction						
▪ Internal rotation						
▪ External rotation						
▪ Supination/inversion						
▪ Pronation/eversion						

Stability tests	Quantity	Quality	End-feel	Symptoms/Pain	Comments
Tibial or ulnar gaping					
Fibular or radial gaping					

Continued ▶

II Specific examination of the joint correlating with symptoms (Continued)					
b) Translatoric movement tests	**Quantity**	**Quality**	**End-feel**	**Symptoms/Pain**	**Comments**
▪ Traction					
▪ Compression					
▪ Gliding, anterior					
▪ Gliding, posterior					
Summary evaluation					
Interpretation of positive and negative findings: Symptoms ↓ Movement direction ↓ Contraindications ↓ Region (joint) ↓ Hypomobile/hypermobile/physiologically mobile ↓ Structure ↓ Causal and influencing factors					
Trial treatment					
Physical therapy diagnosis					
Treatment					
▪ **Treatment plan with treatment goal and prognosis** ▪ **Treatment progress with periodic control tests**					
Final examination					

19.2   General Documentation Template for the Spine: Basic Scheme

I Orienting examination	
Symptoms	
Symptom-altering direction	
Contraindications?	Nervous system: ■ Mobility ■ Impulse conduction For the cervical spine: safety tests ■ Traction C0–C1 ■ Traction C1–C2 ■ Vertebral artery ■ Alar ligaments ■ Transverse ligament of atlas ■ Possibly foraminal compression test Other:
Symptom-altering segment region	
General assessment of adjacent joints and affected spinal segment	

II Specific examination of the region that correlated with symptoms					

Active movement tests compared with adjacent regions

a) Rotatory tests	Active	Continues passively?	Passive	End-feel	Symptoms/Pain
■ Ventral flexion					
■ Dorsiflexion					
■ Lateral flexion, right					
■ Lateral flexion, left					
■ Rotation, right					
■ Rotation, left					
■ Combined movements					

b) Translatoric movement tests:	Quantity	Quality	End-feel	Symptoms/Pain	Comments
■ Traction					
■ Compression					

Continued ▶

II Specific examination of the region that correlates with symptoms (Continued)	
Summary evaluation	
Interpretation of positive and negative findings: Symptoms ↓ Movement direction ↓ Contraindications ↓ Region (joint) ↓ Hypomobile/hypermobile/ physiologically mobile ↓ Structure ↓ Causal and influencing factors	
Trial treatment	
Physical therapy diagnosis	
Treatment ▪ **Treatment plan with treatment goal and prognosis** ▪ **Treatment progress with periodic control tests**	
Final examination	

19.3   Complete Documentation Scheme (For Practice)

Patient: .... Age: .... Date of PT examination:..........................

Physician diagnosis:....................................... Physical therapist: ....

PT prescription: .... Address or room/tel. no. of patient: ....

I Orienting examination					
Symptoms ▪ Where? ▪ Since when? ▪ How? ▪ When now and what causes it? ▪ What is it related to?	Night pain: Yes ❐ No ❐ *Intensity:* 0 1 2 3 4 5 6 7 8 9 10				
Symptom-changing direction or posture					
Contraindications to larger movements?	*Starting position:*	*Positive*	*Negative*	*Joint position:*	*Comments:*
Nervous system mobility:					
▪ Sciatic nerve		❐	❐		
▪ Femoral nerve		❐	❐		
▪ Median nerve		❐	❐		
▪ Radial nerve		❐	❐		
▪ Ulnar nerve		❐	❐		
▪ Function of organs of the lesser pelvis		❐	❐		
▪ Other (pathological reflexes etc., possibly add separate page for complete neurological examination)		❐	❐		

Continued ▶

I Orienting examination (Continued)						
Impulse conduction, motor function and sensitivity	*Lumbar*	*Positive*	*Negative*	*Cervical*	*Positive*	*Negative*
	L4	❏	❏	C5	❏	❏
	L5	❏	❏	C6	❏	❏
	S1	❏	❏	C7	❏	❏
	Other:	❏	❏	C8	❏	❏
				Th1	❏	❏
				Other:	❏	❏

Superficial palpation	Negative ❏ Positive ❏	Comments:

Safety tests:	*Starting position*	*Positive*	*Negative*	*Comments*
▪ Traction C0–C1		❏	❏	
▪ Traction C1–C2		❏	❏	
▪ Vertebral artery		❏	❏	
▪ Alar ligaments		❏	❏	
▪ Transverse ligament of atlas		❏	❏	
▪ Other		❏	❏	

Acuteness	*Acute*	*Subacute*	*Chronic*	*Continuous*	*Intermittently daily*	*Episodic* ↙ rarely　↘ often	
	❏	❏	❏	❏	❏	❏	❏
	(6 weeks)	(6–12 weeks)	(3 months)				

Assessment of pain management	*Positive*	*Questionable*	*Negative*	*Realistic*	*Emotional/ affective*	*Other:*
	❏	❏	❏	❏	❏	

Joint/region in which movement correlates with symptoms	
General assessment of adjacent joints (use separate page if necessary)	
General assessment of patient (respiration, circulation, . . .)	
Expectations of the patient from PT	

II Specific examination of the joint or segment (or region) that correlates with symptoms

1 Patient history *(use separate page if necessary)*	

Continued ▶

II Specific examination of the joint or segment (or region) that correlates with symptoms (Continued)

2 Inspection *Including superficial palpation: muscle tone, tissue change, contour, etc.*	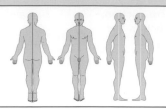

3 Movement testing Active	*Describe extremities, comparing sides:*

Draw position of end-range spinal movements and possibly add score from 0 to 6:

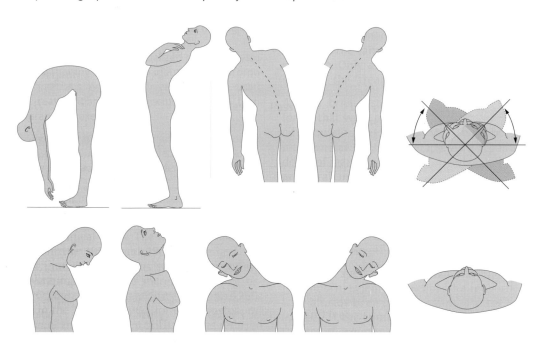

a) Rotatory tests	Active (angle or degree of movement 0–6)	Continues passively? (add degrees if possible)	Passive (resistance to movement)	End-feel	Symptoms/ pain (reported pain)	Comments
Flexion or ventral flexion						
Extension or dorsal flexion						
Abduction or lateral flexion, right						
Abduction or lateral flexion, left						
External rotation or rotation, right						

Continued ▶

II Specific examination of the joint or segment (or region) that correlates with symptoms (Continued)					
Internal rotation or rotation, left					
Pronation or eversion					
Supination or inversion					
Combined movements					
Stability tests of extremities		**Quality (resistance to movement)**	**End-feel or end of movement**	**Pain or symptoms (reported pain)**	**Comments**
Tibial/ulnar gaping:					
Fibular/radial gaping:					
b) Translatoric movement tests:	**Quantity (degree of movement 0–6)**	**Quality (resistance to movement)**	**End-feel or end of movement**	**Pain or symptoms (reported pain)**	**Comments**
Traction					
Compression					
Anterior gliding					
Posterior gliding					
4 Muscle tests	**Strength** *(score 0–5)*	**Symptoms** or pain with resistance test	**Length**	**Symptoms** or pain with length test	**Comments**
Coordination *(describe test and results)*					

Continued ▶

II Specific examination of the joint or segment (or region) that correlates with symptoms (Continued)	
Endurance *(describe test and results)*	
Other (speed, etc.)	
5 Palpation (structure-specific)	
6 Neurological and vascular tests	
❏ Neurology: segment-indicating muscles, sensitivity, reflexes, ANS function, mobility ❏ Vascular tests: pulse, blood, functional tests (Ratschow test. . .) etc.	
7 Physician examinations	
❏ Radiography, laboratory tests, punctures, excisions ❏ Electrodiagnostic tests (EEG, EMG, . . .) ❏ Organ examinations by the physician	

8 Summary evaluation			
Interpretation of positive and negative results: Symptoms ↓ Movement direction ↓ Contraindications/Acuteness/ Pain management ↓ Region (joint) ↓ Hypomobile/hypermobile/physiolo-gically mobile ↓ Structure ↓ Causal and influencing factors			
Assessment of the problem based on ICF (impaired health-related functional ability)	**Damage** *(bodily function or structure)* ❏	*Impaired* **activity** *(of the patient)* ❏	*Impaired* **participation** *(in areas of life with personal and environmental contextual factors)* ❏
Trial treatment			
Physical therapy diagnosis			

III Treatment				
Treatment plan with treatment goal and prognosis	**Treatment aspect**	**Treatment goal**	**Treatment measures and self-exercise**	**Prognosis**
	Symptoms:			
	Hypomobility: muscular articular neural			
	Maintenance of mobility:			
	Hypomobility: Passive stabilization Active stabilization Mobilization of hypo-mobile adjacent joints Avoid end-range move-ments including end-range postures			
	Tissue changes:			
	Information, Instruction:			

Treatment progress with periodic control tests (use separate page if necessary)	**Date:**	**Measure**	**Control test(s):**	**Result:**

Continued ▶

III Treatment (Continued)						
Final examination						
Date: .... (use separate page if necessary)	**Control test(s):**	**Measurement at initial examination**	**Measurement at final examination**	**Negative change**	**Unchanged**	**Positive change**
Patient satisfaction						
Other recommendations						

Date:.............................   *Signature of responsible physical therapist:* ....

19.3.1 Complementary Documentation Template: Temporomandibular Joint

Active movements, comparison of sides
(Observe and palpate)

Mouth closing

Lateral deviation to right

Lateral deviation to left

Mouth opening

Retrusion

Resting position

Protrusion

Specific rotatory tests	Active	Continues passively?	Passive	End-feel	Symptoms/pain	Active
Mouth opening						
Mouth closing (from resting position)						
Protrusion, right						
Protrusion, left						
Retrusion, right						
Retrusion, left						
Lateral deviation, right						
Lateral deviation, left						

Translatoric movement tests	Quantity	Quality	End-feel	Symptoms/pain	Comments
Traction, right					
Compression, right					
Traction, left					
Compression, left					

Muscle tests (primarily)	Strength (score 0–5)	Length	Coordination	Endurance	Symptoms/pain	Others
Mouth opening						
Mouth closing (from resting position)						
Protrusion						

Continued ▶

Complementary Documentation Template: Temporomandibular Joint (Continued)						
Retrusion, right						
Retrusion, left						
Lateral deviation, right						
Lateral deviation, left						

19.3.2 Complementary Documentation Template, Specific Examination of Sacroiliac Joint

Test		Results		Comments
Mobility test	Pubic symphysis			
	Shifting between supporting and free leg	Right	Left	
	Forward bending test	Right	Left	
	Standing hip flexion test	Right	Left	
	Nutation as mobility test	Right	Left	
	Counternutation as mobility test	Right	Left	
	Result:			
Symptom localization test	Nutation test			
	Counternutation test			
	Sacrum, caudal			
	Sacrum, cranial			
	Dorsal gaping			
	Ventral gaping			
	Active Straight Leg Raising (ASLR)			
	Result:			

19.4 Short Documentation for Everyday Use

Patient: .... Age: .... Date PT examination: ....

Physician diagnosis:...................................... Physical Therapist: ....

PT prescription: .... Address or room/tel. no. of patient: ....

I Orienting examination					
Symptoms • Where? • Since when? • How? • When now and what causes it? • What is it related to? Night pain: Yes ☐ No ☐ *Intensity:* 0 1 2 3 4 5 6 7 8 9 10					
Symptom-changing direction or posture					
Contraindications to larger movements?	*Starting position:*	*Positive*	*No findings*	*Joint position:*	*Comments:*
Nervous system mobility:					
• Sciatic nerve		☐	☐		
• Femoral nerve		☐	☐		
• Median nerve		☐	☐		
• Radial nerve		☐	☐		
• Ulnar nerve		☐	☐		
• Function of organs of the lesser pelvis		☐	☐		
• Other (pathological reflexes etc.)		☐	☐		
Superficial palpation	Negative ☐ Positive ☐	Comments:			
Safety tests:	*Starting position*	*Positive*	*No findings*	*Comments*	
Traction C0–C1		☐	☐		
Traction C1–C2		☐	☐		
Vertebral artery		☐	☐		

Continued ▶

I Orienting examination (Continued)					
Alar ligaments		☐	☐		
Transverse ligament of atlas		☐	☐		
Other		☐	☐		
Acuteness	Acute	Subacute	Chronic	Continuous	Intermittent daily	Episodic ↙ ↘ rarely often
	☐	☐	☐	☐	☐	☐ ☐
	(6 weeks)	(6–12 weeks)	(3 months)			
Assessment of pain management	Positive	Questionable	Negative	Realistic	Emotional/ affective	Other:
	☐	☐	☐	☐	☐	

Joint which correlates with symptoms	
General assessment of adjacent joints	
General assessment of the patient (respiration . . .)	
Expectations of the patient from PT	

Continued ▶

II Specific examination of the joint or segment (or region) that correlates with symptoms			
Mobility			
Structure			
Causal and influencing additional factors			
Summary			
Assessment of problem based on ICF	**Damage** *(bodily function and structure)*	*Impaired* **activity** *(of the patient)*	*Impaired* **participation** *(in areas of life with personal and environmental contextual factors)*
Trial treatment			
Physical therapy diagnosis			
Treatment			
Treatment plan with treatment goal and prognosis	**Treatment aspect**	**Treatment goal**	**Treatment measures** *Therapeutic and self-exercises*	**Prognosis**
	Symptoms:			
	Hypomobility: ■ muscular ■ articular ■ neural			
	Maintenance of mobility:			

Continued ▶

II Specific examination of the joint or segment (or region) that correlates with symptoms (Continued)				
	Hypermobility:			
	Tissue changes:			
	Information, instruction:			
Treatment progress with periodic control tests *(on a separate page if necessary)*	**Date:**	**Measure:**	**Control test(s):**	**Result:**

Final examination						
Date: *(on a separate page if necessary)*	**Control test(s):**	**Measurement of Orienting examination**	**Measurement of final assessment**	**Negative change**	**Un-changed**	**Positive change**
				☐	☐	☐
				☐	☐	☐
				☐	☐	☐
				☐	☐	☐
Patient satisfaction						
Further recommendations						

Date:.............................   Signature of responsible physical therapist: ....

Treatment progress with periodic control tests   Patient: . . . .

Date:	Measure:	Control test(s):	Result:

Date:. . . . .   Signature of responsible physical therapist: . . . .

References

Airaksinen O, Brox JI, Cedraschi C, et al. Chapter 4. European guidelines for the management of chronic non specific low back pain. Eur Spine J 2006; 15 (Suppl. 2): 193–300

Akeson, W. H., Amiel, D. Kwan, M., Abitbol, J.-J., Garfin, S. R.: Stress Dependence of Synovial Joints, in Hall BK (ed). Bone, Volume V: A Treatise. CRC Press, 1992, pp. 33–61

Allet L, Cieza A, Bürge E, et al. ICF-Interventionskategorien für die Physiotherapie bei muskuloskelettalen Gesundheitsstörungen. Physioscience 2007; 3(2): 54–62

Aquino RL, Caires PM, et al. Applying joint mobilization at different cervical vertebral levels does not influence immediate pain reduction in patients with chronic neck pain: a randomized clinical trial. J Manual Manip Ther 2009; 17(2): 95–100

Biedermann H. KISS und die Folgen: Leitsymptome manualtherapeutisch beeinflußbarer Beschwerdebilder bei Kindern und Jugendlichen. Manuelle Therapie 1997; 1(2): 10–15

Biedermann H. Vertebragene Faktoren bei Schreikindern – Diagnostische und therapeutische Konsequenzen. Manuelle Therapie 2000; 4(1): 27–31

Bogduk N. Klinische Anatomie von Lendenwirbelsäule und Sakrum. Berlin, Heidelberg: Springer; 2000

Brockhaus in fünf Bänden. Mannheim: Brockhaus; 1993

Bruggencate ten G. Sensomotorik: Funktionen des Rückenmarks und absteigender Bahnen. In: Klinke R, Silbernagl S, eds. Lehrbuch der Physiologie. Stuttgart, New York: Thieme; 1996: 631–649

Bucher-Dollenz G, Wiesner R, eds. Therapiekonzepte in der Physiotherapie: Maitland. Stuttgart, New York: Thieme; 2008

Bullough P, Goodfellow J, O'Conner J. The relationship between degenerative changes and load-bearing in the human hip. J Bone Joint Surg Br 1973; 55(4): 746–758

Bussey MD, Bell ML, Milosavljevic S. The influence of hip abduction and external rotation on sacroiliac motion. Man Ther 2009; 14(5): 520–525

Butler DP. Mobilisation des Nervensystems. Berlin, Heidelberg, New York: Springer; 1995

Calvillo O, Skaribas I, Turnipseed J. Anatomy and pathophysiology of the sacroiliac joint. Curr Rev Pain 2000; 4(5): 356–361

Cattrysse E, Swinkels R A H M, Oostendorp R A B, Duquet W. Upper cervical instability: are clinical tests reliable? Man Ther 1997; 2(2):91–97

Cervero F, Laird JMA. One pain or many pains? a new look at pain mechanisms. News Physiol Sci 1991; 6(December): 268–273

Christe G, Balthazard P. Episode of fainting and tetany after an evaluation technique of the upper cervical region: a case report. Man Ther 2011; 16(1): 94–96

Cibulka, M. T. and R. Koldehoff. Clinical usefulness of a cluster of sacroiliac joint tests in patients with and without low back pain. Journal of Orthopaedic & Sports Physical Therapy 1999; 29(2): 83–89

Cleland JA, Childs JD, McRae M, Palmer JA, Stowell T. Immediate effects of thoracic manipulation in patients with neck pain: a randomized clinical trial. Man Ther 2005; 10(2): 127–135

Cleland JA, Glynn P, Whitman JM, Eberhart SL, MacDonald C, Childs JD. Short-term effects of thrust versus nonthrust mobilization/manipulation directed at the thoracic spine in patients with neck pain: a randomized clinical trial. Phys Ther 2007; 87(4): 431–440

Coppieters MW, Butler DS. Do 'sliders' slide and 'tensioners' tension? An analysis of neurodynamic techniques and considerations regarding their application. Man Ther 2008; 13(3): 213–221

Cramer A, Doering J, Gutmann G. Geschichte der manuellen Medizin. Berlin: Springer; 1990

Cramer A. Gezielte manuelle Beeinflussung der oberen Atlasgelenke. Manuelle Medizin 1994; 32: 141–142

Cunnings GS, Tillman LJ. Remodeling of dense connective tissue in normal adult tissues. In: Currier DP, Nelson RM, eds. Dynamics of Human Biologic Tissues. Philadelphia: F.A. Davis Company; 1992: 45–73

Cutler P. Problem Solving in Clinical Medicine, From Data to Diagnosis. Philadelphia: Lippincott Williams & Wilkins; 1998

Cyriax J. Textbook of Orthopaedic Medicine, vol. 2. Treatment by Manipulation, Massage and Injection. London: Ballière Tindall; 1971

Cyriax J. Textbook of Orthopaedic Medicine, vol. 1. Diagnosis of Soft Tissue Lesions. 8th ed. London: Ballière Tindall; 1982

Dalichau S., Scheele K. Wirksamkeit eines Muskeltrainingsprogramms in der Therapie chronischer Rückenschmerzen bei Verwendung funktioneller Orthesen. Z Physiother 2004; 56(3): 414–427

Debrunner AM. Orthopädie, Orthopädische Chirurgie, Die Störungen des Bewegungsapparates in Klinik und Praxis. Bern: Verlag Hans Huber; 1995

de Morree JJ. Dynamik des menschlichen Bindegewebes, Funktion, Schädigung und Wiederherstellung. Munich, Jena: Urban & Fischer; 2001

Engel, G.L. The need for a new medical model: a challenge for biomedical science. Science 1977; 196: 129–136

Evjenth O, Hamberg J. Muscle Stretching in Manual Therapy, a Clinical Manual, vol. I: The Extremities. Alfta, Sweden: Alfta Rehab Förlag; 1984a

Evjenth O, Hamberg J. Muscle Stretching in Manual Therapy, a Clinical Manual, vol II: The Spinal column and the TM Joint. Alfta, Sweden: Alfta Rehab Förlag; 1984b

Evjenth O, Hamberg J. Autostretching. Alfta, Sweden: Alfta Rehab Förlag; 1990

Evjenth O, Schomacher J. Wie trainieren? Praktisches Vorgehen beim Erstellen eines Trainingsplans. Manuelle Therapie 1997; 1(1): 44–49

Falla D, Jull G, Hodges PW. Training the cervical muscles with prescribed motor tasks does not change muscle activation during a functional activity. Man Ther 2008; 13(6): 507–512

Friedell E. Kulturgeschichte der Neuzeit. Munich: C. H. Beck; 1927

Frisch H. Programmierte Untersuchung des Bewegungsapparates. 3rd ed. Berlin: Springer; 2001

Giamberardino MA. Von den Eingeweiden her übertragene Hyperalgesie. In: van den Berg F, ed. Angewandte Physiologie, 4. Schmerz verstehen und beeinflussen. Stuttgart, New York: Thieme; 2003: 86–89

Gibbons SGT, Comerford MJ. Kraft versus Stabilität. Teil 2: Grenzen und positive Auswirkungen. Manuelle Therapie 2002; 6: 13–20

Gifford L. Perspektiven zum biopsychosozialen Modell. Teil 1: Müssen einige Aspekte vielleicht doch akzeptiert werden? Manuelle Therapie 2002a; 6(3): 139–145

Gifford L. Perspektiven zum biopsychosozialen Modell. Teil 2: Einkaufskorb-Ansatz. Manuelle Therapie 2002b; 6(4): 197–206

Gray H. Anatomy, Descriptive and Surgical. 1901 edition edited by Pick TP, Howden R. Philadelphia: Running Press; 1974: 217–293

Gray H. Gray's Anatomy, edited by Williams PL, Warwick R, Dyson M, Bannister LH. 37th ed. Edinburgh: Churchill Livingstone; 1989: 493–495

Greenmann PE. Lehrbuch der Osteopathischen Medizin. Heidelberg: Hüthig Fachverlage; 1998

Grimsby O, Rivard J, eds. Science, Theory and Clinical Application in Orthopaedic Manual Physical Therapy, vol. 1, Applied Science and Theory. Taylorsville: The Academy of Graduate Physical Therapy; 2008

Grimsby O. STEP–Scientific-Therapeutic-Exercise-Progressions, Ein wissenschaftlich fundierter Zugang zu therapeutischen Übungen. Manuelle Therapie 2000; 4: 112–118

Gross AR, Hoving JL, Haines TA, et al; Cervical overview group. Manipulation and mobilisation for mechanical neck disorders. Cochrane Database Syst Rev 2004; (1, Issue 1) CD004249 10.1002/14651858. CD004249.pub2

Gross AR, Kay T, Hondras M, et al. Manual therapy for mechanical neck disorders: a systematic review. Man Ther 2002a; 7(3): 131–149

Gross AR, Kay TM, Kennedy C, et al. Clinical practice guideline on the use of manipulation or mobilization in the treatment of adults with mechanical neck disorders. Man Ther 2002b; 7(4): 193–205

Haas M, Groupp E, Panzer D, Partna L, Lumsden S, Aickin M. Efficacy of cervical endplay assessment as an indicator for spinal manipulation. Spine 2003; 28(11): 1091–1096, discussion 1096

Hall T, Zusman M, Elvey R. Adverse mechanical tension in the nervous system? Analysis of straight leg raise. Manual Therapy 1998; 3(3): 140–146

Hengeveld E. Gedanken zum Indikationsbereich der Manuellen Therapie, Teil 1. Manuelle Therapie 1998; 4(2): 176–181

Heymann WV. Neck and back pain. Manuelle Medizin 2002; 3: 188–192

Higgs J, Jones M. Clinical Reasoning: An Introduction. In: Higgs J, Jones M, eds. Clinical Reasoning in the Health Professions. Oxford: Butterworth-Heinemann; 2002

Huber EO, Cieza A. Umsetzung der ICF in den klinischen Alltag der Physiotherapie. Physioscience 2007; 3(2): 48–53

Huber H, Winter E. Checkliste Schmerztherapie. Stuttgart, New York: Thieme; 2006

Hüter-Becker A. Ein Altmeister der Physiotherapie feiert Geburtstag: Freddy Kaltenborn. Krankengymnastik 1998; 50(6): 965–966

IFOMPT. Educational standards in Orthopaedic Manipulative Physical Therapy, 2008 www.ifompt.org (downloaded 21.08.2012)

IFOMPT. Standards Document, downloaded 17 August 2012: http://www.ifompt.com/ About+IFOMPT/Standards+Document. html

Inamasu J, Guiot BH. Vertebral artery injury after blunt cervical trauma: an update. Surg Neurol 2006; 65(3): 238–245, discussion 245–246

Jacobsen F. Medical Exercise Therapy. Fysioterapeuten 1992; 7(May): 19–22

Jänig W. Einfluss von Schmerz auf das vegetative Nervensystem, Sympathisches Nervensystem und Schmerz. In: van den Berg F, ed. Angewandte Physiologie, 4. Schmerz verstehen und beeinflussen. Stuttgart, New York: Thieme; 2003: 63–75

Jones MA. Clinical Reasoning: Fundament der klinischen Praxis und Brücke zwischen den Ansätzen der Manuellen Therapie. Teil 1. Manuelle Therapie 1997; 1(4): 3–9

Jones MA, Rivett DA. Clinical reasoning for manual therapists. Edinburgh: Butterworth Heinemann, 2004

Jordan HM. Orthopedic Appliances. 2nd ed. Springfield: Charles C. Thomas; 1963

Jull G. Management of cervical headache. Manuelle Therapie 1997; 2(4): 182–190

Jull G, Amiri M, Bullock-Saxton J, Darnell R, Lander C. Cervical musculoskeletal impairment in frequent intermittent headache. Part 1: Subjects with single headaches. Cephalalgia 2007; 27(7): 793–802

Jull G. Übungsansatz bei HWS-Störungen: Wie fließen die Ergebnisse der Forschung in die Praxis ein? Manuelle Therapie 2009; 13(3): 110–116

Kaltenborn FM. Manuelle Mobilisation der Extremitätengelenke. 9th ed. Oslo: Olaf Norlis Bokhandel; 1992a

Kaltenborn FM. Wirbelsäule, Manuelle Untersuchung und Mobilisation. Oslo: Olaf Norlis Bokhandel; 1992b

Kaltenborn FM. The Spine. Basic Evaluation and Mobilization Technics. Oslo: Olaf Norlis Bokhandel 1993; 32–33, 88–89

Kaltenborn FM, Evjenth O. Manuelle Therapie nach Kaltenborn. Untersuchung und Behandlung. Teil I: Extremitäten. Oslo: Olaf Norlis Bokhandel; 1999

Kaltenborn FM. Von der Rotation zur Translation bei Mobilisation und Manipulation. Z Physiother 2002; 54(11): 1786–1794

Kaltenborn FM. Manual Mobilization of the Joints, vol. II, The Spine. Oslo: Norlis, 2003

Kaltenborn FM. Manuelle Therapie nach Kaltenborn. Untersuchung und Behandlung. Teil II: Wirbelsäule. 4th ed. Oslo: Norli; 2004

Kaltenborn FM. Manuelle Therapie nach Kaltenborn. Untersuchung und Behandlung. Teil I: Extremitäten. 12th ed. Oslo: Norli; 2005

Kaltenborn FM. Wissenschaftlicher Männerberuf mit Primärkontakt, Physiotherapie im 19. Jahrhundert. Z Physiother 2007; 59(10): 1025–1030

Kaltenborn FM. Manual Mobilization of the Joints, vol. III. Traction Manipulation of the Extremities and Spine. Oslo: Norli; 2008

Kaltenborn FM. Traction Manipulation of the Extremities and Spine. Basic Thrust Techniques. Oslo: Norli; 2008

Kaltenborn FM. Manual Mobilization of the Joints, vol. II. The Spine. Oslo, Norli; 2012

Kaltenborn FM. Manual Mobilization of the Joints, vol. I. The Extremities. Oslo, Norway, Norli 2011

Kaltenborn FM. Manual Mobilization of the Joints, vol. II. The Spine: Oslo: Norli; 2012

Kay TM, Gross A, Goldsmith C, Santaguida PL, Hoving J, Bronfort G; Cervical Overview Group. Exercises for mechanical neck disorders. Cochrane Database Syst Rev 2005; (3, Issue 3) CD004250 10.1002/14651858. CD004250.pub3

Kerry R, Taylor AJ, Mitchell J, McCarthy C. Cervical arterial dysfunction and manual therapy: a critical literature review to inform professional practice. Manuelle Therapie 2008; 13(4): 278–288

Kirschneck M, Gläßel A, Wilke S, Stucki G. Umsetzung der ICF und der ICF-Core-Sets für lumbale Rückenschmerzen in der Rehabilitation, Teil 1. Manuelle Therapie 2007a; 11(3): 101–110

Kirschneck M, Gläßel A, Wilke S, Stucki G. Umsetzung der ICF und der ICF-Core-Sets für lumbale Rückenschmerzen in der Rehabilitation, Teil 2. Manuelle Therapie 2007b; 11(4): 188–195

Klemme B, Geuter G, Willimczik K. Physiotherapie – über eine Akademisierung zur Profession. Physioscience 2007; 3(2): 80–87

Klemme B, Siegmann G. Clinical Reasoning, Therapeutische Denkprozesse lernen. Stuttgart, New York: Thieme; 2006

Konrad B, Thue L, Robinson H S, Koch R Günther K-P. Wirksamkeit der neuralen Mobilisation in der postoperativen Physiotherapie nach nicht instrumentierten Bandscheibenoperationen. Manuelle Therapie 2008; 12(4): 153–157

Kool J. Wie misst man Gesundheit und Lebensqualität? In: Hüter-Becker A, Dölken M, eds. Beruf, Recht, Wissenschaftliches Arbeiten. Stuttgart, New York: Thieme; 2004: 212–218

Kräutler P. Der wissenschaftliche Nachweis für Stretching/Flexibilität in der Verletzungsprävention. Manuelle Therapie 2003; 7(1): 4–12

Krauss J, Creighton D, Ely JD, Podlewska-Ely J. The immediate effects of upper thoracic translatoric spinal manipulation on cervical pain and range of motion: a randomized clinical trial. J Manual Manip Ther 2008; 16(2): 93–99

Kügelgen B. Das Zeichen nach Lasègue—ein nur scheinbar banales Untersuchungsverfahren. Manuelle Medizin 1991; 5: 84–85

Kumar K. Historical Perspective Spinal Deformity and Axial Traction. Spine 1996; 21(5): 643–655

Lamb DW. A review of manual therapy for spinal pain. In: Boyling JD, Palastanga N, eds. Grieve's Modern Manual Therapy, The Vertebral Column. Edinburgh: Churchill Livingstone; 1994: 629–650

Lamb DW, Kaltenborn FM, Paris SV. History of IFOMT. J Manual Manip Ther 2003; 11(2): 73–76

Laslett M. Evidenzbasierte Diagnose und Behandlung bei schmerzhaftem Gelenk. [Evidence-based diagnosis and treatment of the painful sacroiliac joint] Manuelle Therapie 2009; 13: 124–134

Laslett M, Aprill CN, McDonald B, Young SB. Diagnosis of sacroiliac joint pain: validity of individual provocation tests and composites of tests. Man Ther 2005a; 10(3): 207–218

Laslett M, McDonald B, Tropp H, Aprill CN, Öberg B. Agreement between diagnoses reached by clinical examination and available reference standards: a prospective study of 216 patients with lumbopelvic pain. BMC Musculoskelet Disord 2005b; 6: 28

Lazennec JY, Besnahard J, Cabanal J. L'articulation péronéo-tibiale supérieure: une anatomie et une physiologie mal connues. Annales de Kinéisthérapie. 1994; 1: 1–5

Llopis E, Cerezal L, Kassarjian A, Higueras V, Fernandez E. Direct MR arthrography of the hip with leg traction: feasibility for assessing articular cartilage. AJR Am J Roentgenol 2008; 190(4): 1124–1128

Logiudice J. Schmerz und das Immunsystem. In: van den Berg F, ed. Angewandte Physiologie, 4. Schmerz verstehen und beeinflussen. Stuttgart, New York: Thieme; 2003: 89–99

Mac Conaill MA. Mechanical anatomy of motion and posture. In: Licht S, ed. Therapeutic Exercise. 2nd ed. Baltimore: Waverly Press 1965

Main, C. J., Williams A. C. d. C. ABC of psychological medicine: Musculoskeletal pain. BMJ 2002; 325: 534–537

Melzack R, Wall PD. Pain mechanisms: a new theory. Science 1965; 150(3699): 971–979

Melzack R, Wall PD. The Challenge of Pain. Harmondsworth: Penguin Books, 1996

Menell JB. Physical Treatment by Movement. Manipulation and Massage. 5th ed. London: J. & A. Churchill; 1945

Menell JB. The Science and Art of Joint Manipulation. Vol. I. London: Churchill; 1949

Mitchell J, Keene D, Dyson C, Harvey L, Pruvey C, Phillips R. Is cervical spine rotation, as used in the standard vertebrobasilar insufficiency test, associated with a measureable change in intracranial vertebral artery blood flow? Man Ther 2004; 9(4): 220–227

Moran R, Mullany A. What is the clinical utility of the cervical extension rotation test as routinely applied in the premanipulative screening process? Osteopathik Med. 2003; 6(1): 24–29

Newble D, Norman G, van der Vleuten C. Assessing clinical reasoning. In: Higgs J, Jones M. Clinical Reasoning in the Health Professions. Oxford: Butterworth-Heinemann, 2002: 156–165

Niethard FU, Pfeil J. Orthopädie. Stuttgart: Thieme; 2003

Nijs J, Van Houdenhove B. From acute musculoskeletal pain to chronic widespread pain and fibromyalgia: application of pain neurophysiology in manual therapy practice. Man Ther 2009; 14(1): 3–12

Nijs J, Van Houdenhove B, Oostendorp RA. Recognition of central sensitization in patients with musculoskeletal pain: Application of pain neurophysiology in manual therapy practice. Man Ther 2010; 15(2): 135–141

Osmotherly PG, Rivett DA. Knowledge and use of craniovertebral instability testing by Australian physiotherapists. Man Ther 2011; 16(4): 357–363

O'Sullivan PB. Lumbar segmental 'instability': clinical presentation and specific stabilizing exercise management. Man Ther 2000; 5(1):2–12

Ottosson A. Als Orthopäden noch Physiotherapeuten waren, oder warum es Physiotherapeuten an Geschichtsbewusstsein mangelt—Verhältnis von Orthopädie und Physiotherapie in Schweden im 19. Jahrhundert, Teil 1. Manuelle Therapie 2010a; 14: 14–21

Ottosson A. Als Orthopäden noch Physiotherapeuten waren, oder warum es Physiotherapeuten an Geschichtsbewusstsein mangelt—Verhältnis von Orthopädie und Physiotherapie, Teil 2. Manuelle Therapie 2010b; 14: 76–84

Ottosson A. The manipulated history of manipulations of spines and joints? Rethinking Orthopaedic Medicine through the 19th century discourse of European mechanical medicine. Med. Studies 2011; 3(2): 83–116

Paatelma M, Kilpikoski S, Simonen R, Heinonen A, Alen M, Videman T. Orthopaedic manual therapy, McKenzie method or advice only for low back pain in working adults: a randomized controlled trial with one year follow-up. J Rehabil Med 2008; 40(10): 858–863

Panjabi MM. The stabilizing system of the spine. Part II. Neutral zone and instability hypothesis. J Spinal Disord 1992; 5(4): 390–396, discussion 397

Panjabi MM, White AA III. Biomechanics in the Musculoskeletal System. New York: Churchill Livingstone, 2001

Pescioli A, Kool J. Die Zuverlässigkeit klinischer Iliosakralgelenktests. Manuelle Therapie. 1997; 1: 3–10

Platzer W. Color Atlas of Human Anatomy. Vol. 1: Locomotor System, 6th ed. Stuttgart, New York: Thieme; 2008

Powers CM, Beneck GJ, Kulig K, Landel RF, Fredericson M. Effects of a single session of posterior-to-anterior spinal mobilization and press-up exercise on pain response and lumbar spine extension in people with nonspecific low back pain. Phys Ther 2008; 88(4): 485–493

Pschyrembel W. Klinisches Wörterbuch. 261st ed. Berlin: Walter de Gruyter Verlag; 2007

Rauber A, Kopsch F. Anatomie des Menschen. Vol 1. Stuttgart: Thieme; 1987

Richardson CA, Jull GA. Muscle control-pain control. What exercises would you prescribe? Man Ther 1995; 1(1): 2–10

Richardson C, Jull G, Hodges P, Hides J. Therapeutic Exercise for Spinal Segmental Stabilization in Low Back Pain, Scientific Basis and Clinical Approach. Edinburgh: Churchill Livingstone; 1999

Rivett DA, Shirley D, Magarey M, Refshauge KM. Clinical guidelines for assessing vertebrobasilar insufficiency in the management of cervical spine disorders. Camberwell: Australian Physiotherapy Association; 2006: 1–14

Rölli D. Nozeboeffekt—unerwünschter Therapiebegleiter. Manuelle Therapie 2004; 8(2): 47–54

Ruhe A, Bos T, Herbert A. Pain originating from the sacroiliac joint is a common non-traumatic musculoskeletal complaint in elite in-line-speedskaters—an observational study. Chiroprac Manual Ther 2012; 20(1): 5

Ryf C, Weymann A. AO Neutral-0-Methode, Messung und Dokumenation: Measurement and Documentation. Stuttgart: Thieme; 1999

Sackett DL, Rosenberg WMC. The need for evidence-based medicine. J R Soc Med 1995; 88(11): 620–624

Schmid A, Brunner F, Wright A, Bachmann LM. Paradigm shift in manual therapy? Evidence for a central nervous system component in the response to passive cervical joint mobilisation. Man Ther 2008; 13(5): 387–396

Schomacher J. ICIDH-2—Internationale Klassifikation der Schäden, Aktivitäten und Partizipation. Manuelle Therapie 1999; 3(2): 81–84

Schomacher J. Falsch positiver Stabilitätstest der Ligamenta alaria. Manuelle Therapie 2000; 4: 127–132

Schomacher J. Diagnostik und Therapie des Bewegungsapparates in der Physiotherapie. Stuttgart, New York: Thieme; 2001a

Schomacher J. Schmerz—Entstehung, Leitung, Verarbeitung und physiotherapeutische Beeinflussung, Teil 1. Manuelle Therapie 2001b; 5(2): 93–103

Schomacher J. Schmerz—Entstehung, Leitung, Verarbeitung und physiotherapeutische Beeinflussung, Teil 2. Manuelle Therapie 2001c; 5(3): 112–120

Schomacher J. Diagnostik und Therapie des Bewegungsapparates in der Physiotherapie, Stuttgart, New York: Thieme; 2001d

Schomacher J. SIG—Handeln trotz fehlender Evidenz? Manuelle Therapie 2003; 7(4): 197–208

Schomacher J. Wer denkt, stellt Diagnosen—Plädoyer für die physiotherapeutische Diagnose. Physiopraxis 2004a; 4: 34–38

Schomacher J. Kommentar zu: Klässbo M, Harms-Ringdahl K, Larsson G. Examination of Passive ROM and Capsular Patterns in the Hip. Physiotherapy Research International, 1, 2003: 1–12. Manuelle Therapie 2004b; 8(3): 132–133

Schomacher J. Physiologie der Entstehung von Gelenkkontrakturen. Manuelle Therapie 2005a; 9(2): 82–95

Schomacher J. Biomechanik der Körperstrukturen. In: Hüter-Becker A, Dölken M (eds). Biomechanik, Bewegungslehre, Leistungsphysiologie, Trainingslehre – Physiolehrbuch Basis. Stuttgart, New York: Thieme; 2005b: 67–124

Schomacher J. The spine, 7.–9. Oktober 2005 in Rom. Editorial Manuelle Therapie 2005c; 9(5): 199–201

Schomacher J. Mechanische Aspekte zum Training lumbaler Hypermobilitäten. Manuelle Therapie 2005d; 9(5): 218–229

Schomacher J. Symptomlokalisation am Beispiel Rückenschmerz. Den Schmerzen auf der Spur. Physiopraxis 2006; 4(1): 18–22

Schomacher J. Manipulation der HWS und evidenzbasierte Medizin, Literaturstudie zur Manipulation für Physiotherapeuten. Manuelle Therapie 2007; 11: 229–239

Schomacher J. Gütekriterien der visuellen Analogskala zur Schmerzbewertung. Physioscience 2008a; 4(3): 125–133

Schomacher J. Fähigkeit des spezifischen manuellen Bewegens in einzelnen Wirbelsäulensegmenten. Manuelle Therapie 2008b; 12(3): 113–124

Schomacher J. The convex–concave rule and the lever law. Man Ther 2009a; 14(5): 579–582

Schomacher J. The effect of an analgesic mobilization technique when applied at symptomatic or asymptomatic levels of the cervical spine in subjects with neck pain: a randomized controlled trial. J Manual Manip Ther 2009b; 17(2): 101–108

Schomacher J. Impingement Syndrom des oberen Sprunggelenks. Manuelle Therapie 2010; 14: 91–97

Schomacher J, Learman K. Symptom localization tests in the cervical spine: a descriptive study using imaging verification. J Manual Manip Ther 2010; 18(2): 97–101

Schomacher J, Petzke F, Falla D. Localised resistance selectively activates the semispinalis cervicis muscle in patients with neck pain. Man Ther 2012; 17(6): 544–548

Scott I. Teaching clinical reasoning: A case-based approach. In: Higgs J, Jones M. Clinical Reasoning in the Health Professions. Oxford: Butterworth-Heinemann, 2002: 291–297

Shacklock M, ed. Biomechanics of The Nervous System: Breig Revisited. Adelaide: Neurodynamic Solutions; 2007

Shacklock M, Studer V. Manuelle Behandlung von Kreuzschmerzen und Ischialgie nach dem Konzept der Klinischen Neurodynamik. Manuelle Therapie 2007; 11(1): 17–23

Slater H. Vegetatives Nervensystem. In: van den Berg F, ed. Angewandte Physiologie, 3. Therapie, Training, Tests. Stuttgart, New York: Thieme; 2001: 497–528

Spalteholz W, Spanner R. Handatlas der Anatomie des Menschen. Erster Teil: Bewegungsapparat. 3. unv. Nachdruck. Utrecht: Scheltema & Holkema; 1989: 75

Sweeney A, Doody C. The clinical reasoning of musculoskeletal physiotherapists in relation to the assessment of vertebrobasilar insufficiency: a qualitative study. Man Ther 2010; 15(4): 394–399

Thacker M, Gifford L. Sympathetically maintained pain: myth or reality? In: Gifford L, ed. Topical Issues in Pain 3, Sympathetic Nervous System and Pain, Pain Management, Clinical Effectiveness. Kestrel, Swanpool: CNS Press; 2002

Thomas LC, Rivett DA, Attia JR, Parsons M, Levi C. Risk factors and clinical features of craniocervical arterial dissection. Man Ther 2011; 16(4): 351–356

Trudel G, Uhthoff HK. Contractures secondary to immobility: is the restriction articular or muscular? An experimental longitudinal study in the rat knee. Arch Phys Med Rehabil 2000; 81(1): 6–13

Trudel G, Desaulniers N, Uhthoff HK, Laneuville O. Different levels of COX-1 and COX-2 enzymes in synoviocytes and chondrocytes during joint contracture formation. J Rheumatol 2001; 28(9): 2066–2074

Ushida T, Willis WD. Changes in dorsal horn neuronal responses in an experimental wrist contracture model. J Orthop Sci 2001; 6(1): 46–52

van den Berg F. Therapeutische Effekte der Kompressionsbehandlung synovialer Gelenke. In: van den Berg F, ed. Angewandte Physiologie, 3. Therapie, Training, Tests. Stuttgart, New York: Thieme; 2001: 31–44

van den Berg F. Angewandte Physiologie. Das Bindegewebe des Bewegungsapparates verstehen und beeinflüssen. Stuttgart, New York: Thieme; 2010

Vleeming, A., M. D. Schuenke, et al. The sacroiliac joint: an overview of its anatomy, function and potential clinical implications. Journal of Anatomy 2012; 221: 537–567

Vleeming A, Albert HB, Östgaard HC, Sturesson B, Stuge B. European guidelines for the diagnosis and treatment of pelvic girdle pain. European Spine Journal 2008; 17: 794–819

von Eisenhart-Rothe R, Eckstein F, Müller-Gerbl M, Landgraf J, Rock C, Putz R. Direct comparison of contact areas, contact stress and subchondral mineralization in human hip joint specimens. Anat Embryol (Berl) 1997; 195(3): 279–288

von Eisenhart-Rothe R, Witte H, Steinlechner M, Müller-Gerbl M, Putz R, Eckstein F. Quantitative Bestimmung der Druckverteilung im Hüftgelenk während des Gangzyklus. [Quantitative determination of pressure distribution in the hip joint during the gait cycle.] Unfallchirurg 1999; 102(8): 625–631

Vleeming A, Albert HB, Östgaard HC, Stuge B, Sturesson B. Evidenz für die Diagnose und Therapie von Beckengürtelschmerz – Europäische Leitlinien. Physioscience 2006; 2: 48–58

Waddell G. The Back Pain Revolution. Edinburgh: Churchill Livingstone; 1998

Weiss T, Schaible H-G. Physiologie des Schmerzes und der Nozizeption. In: van den Berg F (ed). Angewandte Physiologie, 4. Schmerz verstehen und beeinflussen. Stuttgart, New York: Thieme; 2003a: 1–61

Weiss T. Plazebo-Effekte. In: van den Berg F, ed. Angewandte Physiologie, 4. Schmerz verstehen und beeinflussen. Stuttgart, New York: Thieme; 2003b: 369–381

White AA, Panjabi MM. Clinical Biomechanics of the Spine. Philadelphia: J. B. Lippincott; 1990

Wiemer, M. Benigner paroxysmaler Lagerungsschwindel (BPLS) – Befundung und Behandlung. Manuelle Therapie 2011; 15: 172–177

Wilkinson A. Stretching the truth. A review of the literature on muscle stretching. Austr Physiother 1992; 38(4): 283–287

Williams PL, Warwick R, Dyson M, Bannister LH. Gray's Anatomy. Edinburgh: Churchill Livingstone, 1989: 476–485

Wolf U. Evidenz für Kryotherapie bei Verletzungen und Erkrankungen des Bewegungsapparates. Physioscience 2005; 1(3): 120–128

Zahnd F, Mühlemann D. Einführung in manuelle Techniken, Oberflächen- und Röntgenanatomie, Palpation und Weichteiltechniken. Stuttgart, New York: Thieme; 1998

Zahnd F. Stretching—Suche nach Erklärungen, Physiotherapie in Sport und Orthopädie (theoretische Grundlagen). Manuelle Therapie 2005; 9(4): 171–178

Zelle BA, Gruen GS, Brown S, George S. Sacroiliac joint dysfunction: evaluation and management. Clin J Pain 2005; 21(5): 446–455

Zusman M. Gewebespezifischer Schmerz. In: van den Berg F, ed. Angewandte Physiologie, 4. Schmerz verstehen und beeinflussen. Stuttgart, New York: Thieme; 2003: 149–157

Zusman M, Moog-Egan M. Neurologisch begründete Mechanismen der Schmerzlinderung durch Physiotherapie. In: Angewandte Physiologie, 4. Schmerz verstehen und beeinflüssen. Stuttgart, New York: Thieme; 2003: 269–291

Glossary

English	Latin
Interphalangeal Joints of the Toes	Articulationes interphalangeales pedis
Metatarsophalangeal Joints of the Foot	Articulationes metatarsophalangeales pedis
Intermetatarsal and Tarsometatarsal Joints	Articulationes intermetatarsales and tarsometatarsales
Subtalar (talocalcaneal) Joint	Articulatio subtalaris et articulatio talocalcaneonavicularis
Ankle Joint	Articulatio talocruralis
Lower Leg	Syndesmosis tibiofibularis distalis et articulatio tibiofibularis proximalis
Knee Joint	Articulatio genu: articulationes femoropatellaris et femorotibialis
Hip Joint	Articulatio coxae
Interphalangeal Joints of the Fingers	Articulationes interphalangeae manus proximales et distales
Metacarpophalangeal Joints	Articulationes metacarpophalangeales manus
Metacarpal Joints II–V	Articulationes intermetacarpales distalis (syndesmosis) et proximales et articulationes carpometacarpales II–V
Carpometacarpal Joint of the Thumb	Articulatio carpometacarpalis I
Wrist Joint	Articulatio manus, consisting of the articulatio mediocarpalis, articulatio radiocarpalis, and articulatio ossis pisiformis
Forearm Joints	Articulationes radioulnaris distalis et proximalis
Elbow Joint	Articulatio cubiti, consisting of the articulatio humeroradialis and articulatio humeroulnaris
Shoulder Joint	Articulatio humeri
Should Girdle Region	Articulatio acromioclavicularis, articulatio sternoclavicularis, articulatio subacromiales and scapulo-serrato-thoracic gliding space
Pubic Symphysis and Sacroiliac Joints	Symphysis pubica and articulationes sacroiliacae
Sacrococcygeal Joint	Articulatio sacrococcygea
Lumbar Spine	Columna lumbalis
Thoracic Spine	Columna dorsales
The Costal Joints	Articulationes costales
Cervical Spine	Columna cervicalis
Temporomandibular Joint	Articulatio temporomandibularis

Index